CANCER RISK ASSESSMENT

OCCUPATIONAL SAFETY AND HEALTH

A Series of Reference Books and Textbooks
on Occupational Hazards ● Safety● Health ●
Fire Protection ● Security ● and Industrial Hygiene

Series Editor
ALAN L. KLING
Loss Prevention Consultant
Jamesburg, New Jersey

1. Occupational Safety, Health, and Fire Index *David E. Miller*
2. Crime Prevention Through Physical Security *Walter M. Strobl*
3. Fire Loss Control *Robert G. Planer*
4. MORT Safety Assurance Systems *William G. Johnson*
5. Management of Hotel and Motel Security *Harvey Burstein*
6. The Loss Rate Concept in Safety Engineering *R.L. Browning*
7. Clinical Medicine for the Occupational Physician *edited by Michael H. Alderman and Marshall J. Hanley*
8. Development and Control of Dust Explosions *John Nagy and Harry C. Verakis*
9. Reducing the Carcinogenic Risks in Industry *edited by Paul F. Deisler, Jr.*
10. Computer Systems for Occupational Safety and Health Management *Charles W. Ross*
11. Practical Laser Safety *D.C. Winburn*
12. Inhalation Toxicology: Research Methods, Applications, and Evaluation *edited by Harry Salem*
13. Investigating Accidents with STEP *Kingsley Hendrick and Ludwig Benner, Jr.*
14. Occupational Hearing Loss *Robert Thayer Sataloff and Joseph Sataloff*
15. Practical Electrical Safety *D.C. Winburn*
16. Fire: Fundamentals and Control *Walter M. Haessler*
17. Biohazards Management Handbook *Daniel F. Liberman and Judith Gordon*
18. Practical Laser Safety, Second Edition, Revised and Expanded *D.C. Winburn*
19. Systematic Safety Training *Kingsley Hendrick*
20. Cancer Risk Assessment: A Quantitative Approach *Samuel C. Morris*
21. Man and Risks: Technological and Human Risk Prevention *Annick Carnino, Jean-Louis Nicolet, and Jean-Claude Wanner*

Additional Volumes in Preparation

Fire Loss Control: A Management Guide. Second Edition, Revised and Expanded *Peter M. Bochnak*

CANCER RISK ASSESSMENT
A Quantitative Approach

Samuel C. Morris

Department of Applied Science
Brookhaven National Laboratory
Associated Universities, Inc.
Upton, New York

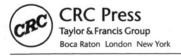

CRC Press
Taylor & Francis Group
Boca Raton London New York

CRC Press is an imprint of the
Taylor & Francis Group, an **informa** business

CRC Press
Taylor & Francis Group
6000 Broken Sound Parkway NW, Suite 300
Boca Raton, FL 33487-2742

First issued in paperback 2019

ISBN-13: 978-0-8247-8239-9 (hbk)
ISBN-13: 978-0-367-40318-8 (pbk)

Library of Congress Cataloging-in-Publication Data

Morris, Samuel C.
    Cancer risk assessment: a quantitative approach / Samuel C. Morris.
        p. cm. -- (Occupational safety and health; 20)
    Includes bibliographical references.
    Includes index.
    ISBN 0-8247-8239-9 (alk. paper)
    1. Cancer--Risk factors. 2. Health risk assessment. I. Title.
II. Series: Occupational Safety and Health (Marcel Dekker, Inc.);
20.
    [DNLM: 1. Carcinogens. 2. Neoplasms--etiology. 3. Risk. W1
OC597M v. 20 / QZ 202 M882c]
RC268.48.M67   1990
616.99'4071--dc20
DLC
for Library of Congress   90-3479
                                                            CIP

Visit the Taylor & Francis Web site at
http://www.taylorandfrancis.com

and the CRC Press Web site at
http://www.crcpress.com

Preface

Cancer risk assessment has a massive impact on the regulatory environment in the United States. It is widely used in government and industry, yet it remains a relatively new and evolving field. Risk assessment draws on many subareas of biology, chemistry, physics, engineering, and the social sciences. For an assessment to work well, the effort should be truly interdisciplinary—not multidisciplinary. Both approaches involve people from many disciplines, but in the latter they may work independently: the meteorologist and air chemist in their corner, the water modelers in theirs, the toxicologist and epidemiologist in their respective corners, perhaps an economist or a geographer thrown in, and the "risk analyst," off in another room or another state, pulling it together. That approach can work, but it is not a formula for success. *Interdisciplinary* means people from different disciplines working together, talking to each other, pulling together toward a common goal. To achieve this, each must know something about the others' fields and appreciate their contributions. Interdisciplinary knowledge comes partly from study and partly from doing. It is a slow and perhaps inefficient process, but effective.

This book is meant as a guide to interdisciplinary practice in risk assessment. It was written with five overall tenets: (1) it should be an introduction to the field but still be of value to the experienced practitioner, (2) it should be comprehensive, (3) it should examine critical problem areas, (4) it should be practical, and (5) it should maintain a consistent viewpoint. These points need some amplification.

That a book may aim to be both an introduction to a field and of interest to those experienced in that field may seem contradictory, but in risk assessment it is not. Risk assessment is not a well-established discipline, and it is still riddled with problem areas. The neophyte should learn about these right away. Moreover, one generally comes to risk assessment already well grounded in a contributing discipline and well able to understand that methodological problems remain to be solved. Indeed, it is common in interdisciplinary fields for a newcomer, given an understanding

iii

of the general approaches taken and the current problems faced by the field, to hit upon new approaches which make significant improvements. I urge the reader to approach the book with this in mind.

Emphasizing the interdisciplinary nature of risk assessment, the book shows how each discipline relates to the whole and interrelates with other contributing disciplines. To do this, it must be comprehensive. There are many books on cancer risk assessment that focus on toxicology, biostatistics, or exposure assessment. Here, the focus is holistic. Risk assessment requires that information from diverse sources be brought together. While not a handbook, the book includes much practical data needed in assessment and provides sources of much more.

Many books available on risk assessment originated as conference proceedings with each chapter by a different author. Such a format has the advantage that each chapter is written by a specialist in that particular area, but, despite the best editing, the topics covered are frequently too narrow, leaving many gaps. It is difficult for the reader to gain a holistic view of risk assessment. This book filters everything through the mind of a risk analyst; the topics covered are selected from that perspective, and every subject is covered with a consistent focus on how it relates to doing risk assessment.

I would like to express my thanks to many people. Nat Barr and Alan Moghissi provided me the opportunity to explore quantitative cancer risk assessment over a period of more than a decade through their programs at the Department of Energy and the Environmental Protection Agency. The entire field of risk assessment has benefited from their enlightened program management. I owe a special debt to my colleagues in the Biomedical and Environmental Assessment Division of Brookhaven National Laboratory. Constant interaction with them over the years has led to new and sharpened understanding. In particular, I must mention Leonard Hamilton, Paul Moskowitz, Michael Rowe, John Nagy, and Harris Fischer. Richie Tulipano did the artwork. Several editors at Marcel Dekker, Inc., have provided assistance and encouragement; special acknowledgment is due to Elizabeth Fox, who initiated the project, and Jon Tell, production editor of the final manuscript. Finally, I must acknowledge the support and understanding of my wife, Stephanie, and my children, Jennifer, Dan, and Laura, who suffered the absence of husband and father for many evenings and weekends during the preparation of this book.

The author's affiliation is given for information only. Opinions expressed in this book are those of the author alone and do not represent the views of Brookhaven National Laboratory or of any part of the U.S. Government.

Samuel C. Morris

Contents

Preface   *iii*

I. INTRODUCTION   1

1. Introduction   3
2. The Human Cancer Situation   17
3. Hazard Identification   54

II. EXPOSURE AND DOSE ASSESSMENT   71

4. Exposure Assessment: General Issues   73
5. Measurement of Exposure and Dose   83
6. Modeling Exposure   108
7. Pharmacokinetics   154

III. DOSE–RESPONSE ASSESSMENT   167

8. Toxicology   169
9. Mouse to Man: Extrapolation from Animals   200
10. Quick Methods: Structure–Activity Relationships and Short-
    Term Bioassay   225
11. Epidemiology   243
12. Combined Approaches to Dose–Response: Putting It All
    Together   290

IV. RISK CHARACTERIZATION AND IMPLICATIONS   303

13. Characterization of Uncertainty   305
14. Risk Characterization, Communication, and Perception   331
15. Quality Assurance, Validation, and Peer Review   348

16. Implications for Risk Management   359
17. Future Directions for Quantitative Health Risk Analysis   397
                                                                   397

Index   *403*

PART I

INTRODUCTION

1

Introduction

QCRA

In 1960 congress passed a law banning carcinogenic additives in food, cosmetics, and drugs. We were not going to have any exposure to carcinogens. But carcinogens were more ubiquitous than legislators thought and preventing exposure to carcinogens proved to be a more difficult task than just passing a law. The famous Delaney clause is still on the books, but subsequent legislation has more realistically attempted to regulate carcinogens rather than eliminate them. Regulating carcinogens has meant setting allowable exposure levels, and allowable levels are increasingly based on quantitative risk assessment. William Ruckelshaus, twice Administrator of the Environmental Protection Agency, noted a further change in the 1970s. "Risk," he says, "was hardly mentioned in the early years of EPA, and it does not have an important place in the Clean Air or Clean Water Acts passes in that period." Yet, the concept of risk, and especially a particular kind of risk, so captured regulatory thinking during the course of that decade, that Ruckelshaus (1985) wrote, "... environmental controversy is now largely focused on the carcinogenic risk to human health from toxic chemicals..." He goes on to say that concern with the removal of increasingly small increments of carcinogens in air and water shifted the regulatory base toward a dependence on science since, "... unlike the touchable, visible, and malodorous pollution that stimulated the initial environmental revolution [risks of toxic substances] are largely constructs or projections based on scientific findings."

One source of this science is toxicology. A number of bioassays are considered tools for assessing cancer risk. Indeed, quantitative risk assessment is sometimes defined as the use of experimental laboratory data to estimate the risk of cancer in exposed human populations. That is a narrow view, however; while dose–response data may most frequently

3

come from animal experiments, often, they are based on epidemiology. Beyond that, those who design and conduct the biomedical studies to determine the dose–response or carcinogenic potency of a chemical are not necessarily the same people who go on to use those results to estimate cancer risks in the human population. The new field of risk analysis has quickly taken over this niche. The term quantitative cancer risk assessment (QCRA) will be used here to reflect a process involving calculations as an extension of laboratory or field work. The two, however, are interdependent. Any toxicological or epidemiological study requires some degree of statistical analysis for its interpretation and use; likewise, calculations would be quite sterile without biological data. This is only the beginning. QCRA goes far beyond analysis of biological studies. It must consider the physical, chemical, and engineering aspects of where the carcinogenic agent comes from and how it is transported through the environment to expose people.

The stress on the word quantitative focuses attention on the aim of estimating how great the cancer risk is, not just whether a substance is or is not a carcinogen. QCRA involves more than determining the potentcy of a carcinogen. It runs the full gamut of estimating sources of environmental carcinogens; modeling their transport, transformation, and distribution in the environment; quantifying the population at risk; calculating exposure and dose; developing dose–response relationships; considering exposure and effect of confounding disease agents; and assessing expected increased cancer risk. Each step involves a body of knowledge that is a life work in itself. No one person can be an expert in all areas. QCRA thus must be an interdisciplinary team effort. Not all the contributors must work together. Some do their part independently, often not even aware of the rest of the process. Their results, published in the scientific literature, are drawn upon by others. Someone must have an understanding of all the needed disciplines to structure the assessment and to lead the team. All of the active members of the team need an understanding and appreciation of the other disciplines and of the way they fit together to make the team work effectively. Even narrowly focused scientists who conduct research with no thought as to its future application in a cancer risk assessment can improve the usefulness of their results by gaining a better understanding of how their contributions are used in integrated assessments.

Quantitative cancer risk assessment has become increasingly used as a part of government regulation, industrial process design and development, safety and hazard analyses for liability control and insurance coverage, and even financial analysis. More than 10 federal laws require QCRA (NAS, 1983). Issues addressed in cancer risk assessments are frequently of direct concern to the public, and public interest groups, news media, and individuals are increasingly interested in aspects of the assessments, in evaluating their validity, and in trying to use the results in their decision-making processes. As Flamm points out, in the past decade "we have gone from a situation where the majority of the scientific community opposed risk assessment on the grounds that it could not be done with adequate confidence that the public health is being protected to a situation where the debate is now focused, not on the question of whether it should be performed, but how and how the results should be applied" (Flamm, 1986). This is true not only in the United States; in Canada risk analysis is being used increasingly in regulation of chemical waste disposal (Somers, 1979). International organizations promote world-wide use of QCRA (e.g., WHO, 1982).

The traditional approach in epidemiology and public health was to identify excessive disease in a population, then seek out, identify, and control its cause. In contrast, risk assessment is anticipatory. It identifies and anticipates the problems or effects of proposed technologies or regulations. To do this, risk assessment brings together results of research from many fields which bear on a specific problem, organizes them in a logical framework from which estimates can be drawn, then puts these estimates in a context which will make them useful to decisionmakers. Its focus on management and integration of information is an important characteristic of risk analysis. Information available is sometimes scant, sometimes vast. Too often, it is complex and of poor quality. Risk assessment cannot improve on the state of the basic data available. If it is poor quality, it remains poor quality. Risk assessment is an organizing and focusing activity which can improve the understanding of existing data, help to set priorities for making improvements where they are most needed, and express uncertain results in ways that aid in decisionmaking.

Contributing fields include biology, chemistry, ecology, economics, engineering, epidemiology, law, medicine, psychology, statistics, and others. The risk analyst may have individual expertise in any of these areas, but must have an appreciation of the needs and methods of all disciplines involved, and often must draw on experts from other fields. Frequently, the scientific questions which must be answered go beyond the limits of current scientific knowledge or capabilities, yet any reasonable solution must be based on, or at least take into account, the best current understanding of the scientific issues involved. The issues treated usually involve technology as a source, scientific questions of environmental transport, and biological response. But these are not scientific and technical issues alone. They interact strongly with basic societal values, often raising unprecedented problems of legal issues or moral values.

Risk assessment is fast becoming a new scientific discipline, one that draws on, and integrates other disciplines. Cancer risk assessment has taken the lead in this development.

BACKGROUND

The first scientific evidence linking cancer to a chemical exposure is attributed to Potts (1775), who described an excessive incidence of cancer in London chimney sweeps. Since that time, many scientific studies have shown associations between environmental exposures and cancer. Today, a great deal of effort goes into testing substances for carcinogenicity. Products and byproducts of modern society such as nuclear power, toxic wastes, food additives, and air and water pollution have become major public issues largely because they represent potential risks to human health, particularly cancer. Government and industry have invested heavily in developing and validating tests to determine carcinogenicity. But identifying a substance as a carcinogen is not enough. It is also necessary to estimate how great the risk is to the general population. This need for quantification has not always had wide agreement; some believed it *could not* be done; others that it *should not* be done because quantifying risks leads to trade-offs between lives and economic factors. Nonetheless, quantitative cancer risk assessment is being done and its applications are increasing.

Since the 1950s, Higginson has reported that as much as 90% of cancer is of environmental origin. These estimates were made by comparing geographical variations around the world, examining cancer incidence in people who migrated from one environment to another, and considering etiological factors. Then, the smallest observed incidence of cancer for each organ was summed and the result assumed to be the achievable cancer rate. Until the 1950s, there had been very little regulation of exposure to chemical or physical agents on the basis of cancinogenic action (NAS, 1983, p. 54). Coupled with a markedly increasing cancer rate in the western world in the mid-20th century and increasing concern with environmental pollution, this *quantitative* estimate of the role of environment in cancer focused more attention on the issue. Part of the effect was based on a wide misunderstanding. By "environmental factors" Higginson meant everything which was not genetic: air and water pollution and food additives as well as natural environmental factors, social and cultural habits, and lifestyle factors. Higginson (1980) clarified the state of knowledge by pointing out that removing a single factor, cigarette smoking, would eliminate 80–90% of lung cancers and a significant proportion of cancers at several other sites. He noted, however, that while low frequencies of lesions found in Mormons and Seventh Day Adventists of most remaining tumors not related to tobacco or alcohol suggest that these tumors are related to "lifestyle" and are not inevitable, that their basic nature is ill-understood, and possibilities for their control have been exaggerated. Turning specifically to what are normally considered "environmental carcinogens," Higginson makes clear that, while it is desirable and necessary to control exposure of humans to these agents, regulatory action should not be expected to have much effect on these "lifestyle"-related tumors.

A later comprehensive study by Doll and Peto (1981) showed that only a few percent of this environmental effect is likely to be due to what we ordinarily think of as environmental pollution. Fifty percent is estimated to be related to diet and nutrition (Vuolo and Schuessier, 1985), not because of carcinogenic food additives but as a result of the principal constitutants of food and the changes they undergo during cooking. The full implications of this for putting carcinogenic risk in perspective and for determining where preventive action should be focused has not made much impact on public perceptions. Some argue there is misplaced emphasis on air and water pollution and occupational exposure as a source of cancer since Doll and Peto found that together these are responsible for only a few percent of the total cancer burden. Others counterargue that the exposure to chemical carcinogens has been increasing rapidly and, since cancers take decades to develop, the current cancer burden from these exposures is only the tip of the iceberg to come. The situation with asbestos is often cited as an example. The full answer to the argument is not yet available, and this is not the place to explore the argument further. New exposures are introduced daily, and current mores demand their introduction be accompanied by an assessment of their risks. Cancer is a dread disease in our society and public sentiment is great to reduce any environmental cancer threat. Government regulation of carcinogens on an ad hoc basis by different agencies with different approaches and in an atmosphere sometimes described as the "carcinogen of the month" does not result in rational public policy.

The first approaches to regulating carcinogens were not quantitative. The answer to carcinogens in food in the 1950s and 1960s was the Delaney Amendment to the Food and Drug Act which banned any food additive showing carcinogenic effects in humans or animals (21 USC 348). The ideal was seen to be zero exposure to carcinogens. Congress and the Food and Drug Administration maintained the policy that no risk can be tolerated in the nation's food supply. But in 1977, when saccharin, an artificial sweetener, was found to be carcinogenic in test animals, it was clear that much of the public was willing to make a trade-off. They were willing—and in fact demanded the right—to continue to sweeten food without the calories of sugar even if it meant a small possible cancer risk. Cancer is a thing to be avoided, but it is not the only concern people have. Congress passed specific legislation to permit continued marketing of saccharin (P.L. 95–203). Evidence soon became available ". . . that carcinogens and other toxic substances pervade the entire food supply . . . it is literally impossible to eliminate all carcinogens from our food. Moreover, many of the substances which pose a potential risk are part of long accepted components of food, and any attempt to prohibit their use would raise the most serious questions both of practicality in implementation and of individual free choice in the market place." (Hutt, 1979). Hutt proceeds to list 29 common substances in food which were found to be carcinogenic in test animals (e.g., benzo(a)pyrene in charcoal broiled steaks, caffeine and tannic acid in coffee, tea, and cocoa, chloroform in water, cyclochlorotine in rice). More recently, Ames (1983) describes the ". . . extraordinary variety of [natural] mutagens and possible carcinogens . . ." in ordinary food, concluding, ". . . no human diet can be entirely free of mutagens and carcinogens. . . ." No longer was regulation of carcinogens a matter of controlling a few substances.

WHY DO QCRA?

Food is a matter of individual choice, at least to some degree. The air we breath is something else. Yet the same carcinogens which affected the sweeps in London are generated in home oil burners and fireplaces today, and are emitted from our chimneys into the air (e.g., Alfheim and Ramdahl, 1984; Reali et al., 1984). Reducing this exposure to zero is simply not conceivable. The issue cannot be whether or not to eliminate the exposure, but must be how much to reduce it. Not everything is carcinogenic, but we live in a virtual sea of carcinogens. Increasingly sophisticated chemical analysis techniques allow us to identify them at smaller and smaller concentrations. We can commit great attention and resources into reducing a few, but massive reduction of all exposures to carcinogens may prove to be more than we, as a society, can handle. We sometimes forget that resources are limited and that eliminating small carcinogenic risks may not be the best use of them, even if the objective was solely to improve public health. Disruptions introduced into society by intensive regulatory focus on a few carcinogens can take its own toll in health costs. One state official recently noted that the demand for zero risk was leading his state into paralysis. Uneven and seemingly haphazard focus distorts allocation of funding to protect public health. Is it reasonable, for example, for a state to spend $800 million for hazardous waste site clean-up and nothing to reduce exposure to carcinogenic organic vapors in indoor air? There must be a way to at least set some priorities. There is. Biological research has demonstrated that all carcinogens are not equal. Some are much more potent than others. Further, exposure to a carcinogen does not automatically mean one will develop cancer. It depends not only on individual susceptibilities (which current research efforts may soon provide the ability to predict and measure (see Samuels and Adamson, 1985) but on dose. Carcinogens may or may not have thresholds of effect like common toxic substances, but the greater the dose, the greater the likelihood of developing cancer. The doses people are exposed to by different carcinogens vary greatly. In the face of this, it makes no sense to treat them all alike.

We need to be careful, however, about rushing ahead too fast. While "strong" and "weak" carcinogens may be identified in experiments, our ability to distinguish quantitatively among carcinogens at the generally low dose level of exposure in the environment is limited. Indeed, understanding the range of uncertainty in the results is generally more important than risk estimates themselves. If there has been one major failure in the development of QCRA, it has been the lack of adequate attention to this issue.

Quantitative risk assessment forms the basis of rational decisionmaking. Risk assessment is not a new concept; over the past two decades, however, it has grown substantially as a formally recognized effort. There are several reasons for this:

• Problems have become increasingly subtle and complex. Cancer is a much more difficult problem than smallpox was, for example. The sources of new risks are themselves usually complex and have complex interactions with the economy and the environment. For example, in 1906, at the time of the passage of the Food and Drug Act, FDA faced problems that dealt almost exclusively with acute hazards in the food supply. Decisions on food safety have become more difficult over the years. Acute food hazards have been brought under effective control, while remaining problems involve chronic, long-term health effects such as cancer (Novitch, 1981).
• Society is outgrowing the stage where we thought we could have everything. We are recognizing we must make choices.
• Society is demanding more accountability for how those choices are made. They are less likely to trust to the judgment of government officials. Formal risk assessments can provide a rational, documented basis for decisions.
• In making choices, we are faced with the need to trade-off costs and

benefits. Risk assessment can provide the basis of putting health effects in these terms.
* Society has become more sophisticated about risk. People are beginning to realize that zero risk is not a possible, or even a desirable goal.
* At the same time, society is not comfortable with new and unfamiliar risks, and demands that they be fully investigated and proved safe.

These forces acting in society, and the resulting demands of the public on government and industry, have led to increased use of quantitative risk assessment.

In seeking to manage cancer risks, Congress and regulatory agencies have invented many phrases to express their philosophy and approach: "zero release," "virtual safe dose," "no effect levels," "no measurable effect levels," "as low as practicable," "as low as reasonably achievable." In the end, quantitative decisions are made on what levels of exposure will be permitted. While, hopefully, no one will ever make important regulatory decisions solely on the basis of a mathematical equation, it is only reasonable if we are going to set quantitative exposure limits to do the best job we can at quantitatively estimating what the risks are. Lave states the case for QCRA in this context succinctly: "The object of risk assessment is not to eliminate judgment but to inform it. . . . A careful review of scientific evidence and a quantitative risk assessment should be the basis of regulatory decisions. Regulation without these elements is uninformed, arbitrary, and unlikely to withstand litigation, induce co-operation from those being regulated, or produce the results desired. . . . Despite its limitations, quantitative risk assessment has no logical alternative . . . risk assessment is the only systematic tool for analyzing various regulatory approaches to health and safety (Lave, 1983)

MAKE THE ANALYSIS FIT THE OBJECTIVE

The philosophy of public health has always been to err on the side of safety. The consequences of not controlling something which later proved to be an important health hazard were seen to be much worse than the consequences of controlling something which later proved to be innocuous. Thus, estimates of hazards or risks always had "conservative" assumptions built into them, that is, they overestimated the risk. This philosophy has continued into cancer risk assessment. Scientists in regulatory agencies understand the large degree of uncertainty in estimating cancer risks and seek to protect the public by using highly conservative estimates. Upper bounds of 95% are commonly used in cancer dose–response coefficients, for example. Too often, successive conservative assumptions built into each step of the analysis lead to absurd overestimates, or different levels of conservatism are unknowingly built into risk estimates of alternatives. The likelihood of such problems is increased by the complex nature of a cancer risk assessment, and the compartmentalization of the steps involved in different disciplinary teams which do not adquately understand the basis of results they receive from others or how their results will be used by those following. While clearly described as upper bounds, these highly conservative estimates lose this description as they move from the scientists to the enforcement people, to lawmakers, and to the public. Getting better estimates of the nature and distribution of uncertainty is a tough scientific problem. Dealing with this uncertainty in the rough and tumble of political decisions is a much tougher problem that extends far beyond science. The inability to deal with uncertainty in risk management and, worse, the lack of general recognition of the uncertainty behind the upper bound estimates can distort important decisions.

Interacting with the conservatism built into the risk estimates is the notion of acceptable risk now commonly used in risk management. Different people are willing to accept different levels of risk in different situations. Setting an acceptable level of risk for society as a whole is a practical approach, but one seemingly fraught with political difficulties. Although being careful not to formally establish an acceptable risk level, federal agencies are more and more often using an annual risk of 10^{-6} (a 1 in a million chance of cancer) as an insignificant or de minimus level. At least one state has adopted this into law. Explanations of the basis of this as an acceptable risk level usually fail to take into account that it is applied with an upper bound estimate of predicted risk rather than a well-defined "best" estimate. Different levels of "conservatism" may be appropriate in different situations. Most standards have been imposed on industry, requiring their environmental emissions or their products to meet certain standards to protect the public, but the justification for the same approach may seem diminished in other situations. You may demand that the local factory spend money to limit the risk the smoke from its chimney poses to the neighborhood to 10^{-6} or less. Will you spend the same proportional amount yourself to protect yourself and your family from carcinogenic agents in the air in your home due to radon gas, benzene vapors from your car in the attached garage, and other household sources of organic vapors? Will it make a difference that other health risks in the home such as fire, electric shock, or falls are far greater? Should the government mandate that radon levels be the safest aspect of a home?

A hazard in introducing quantitative risk assessment is that one group of risks may be regulated stringently according to "conservative" estimates, while other coexisting greater risks are ignored. Quantification of risk is clearly not enough by itself. QCRA should not become a tool for further ad hoc assessments made with the "blinders on," disregarding everything but one chemical and one effect. QCRA offers the opportunity to develop a more holistic approach to cancer risk management, but to do this it must be carried out in the context of costs, benefits, and other other risks.

WHO DOES QUANTITATIVE CANCER RISK ASSESSMENT?

Quantitative risk assessment has been used to various degrees by the Coast Guard (which regulates hazardous waste transportation), the Consumer Product Safety Commission, the Environmental Protection Agency, the Food and Drug Administration, the Nuclear Regulatory Commission, and the Occupational Safety and Health Administration in establishing regulations for human exposure to potentially carcinogenic agents. More than ten federal laws require some use of risk analysis (NAS, 1983).

Regulatory action, however, is not the only basis for risk assessment. The Department of Energy has used health risk assessment to provide guidance in energy technology development and for defining the focus for biomedical research. Private industry and insurance companies conduct health risk assessments to assure adequate protection of workers and the public, to help them estimate their potential liabilities, and to guide development of new products. The International Atomic Energy Agency and the United Nations Environment Programme operate risk analysis programs on an international scale to provide individual countries with an information base to make better decisions, and to provide an international perspective on risk which might not be considered in any national level analysis.

A risk assessment program in a government agency may be mandated by law or may result from the agency's interpretation of the law. Even when the law forbids agency decisions from taking risk into account, risk assessments may still be carried out under an executive order requiring a Regulatory Impact Analysis of all major decisions (Executive Order 12291, 17 Feb. 81). The purpose of this order was to make clear to the Office of Management and Budget, the Congress, and the public, the expected economic cost to society of a proposed regulation. A cost–benefit analysis is included. The legal mandate under which risk analysis is performed can shape the character and emphasis of the analysis.

The Environmental Protection Agency has perhaps been the most vigorous agency in applying QCRA. Cancer dose–response assessment is the responsibility of the Carcinogen Assessment Group (CAG). Complete QCRAs are conducted by CAG's parent organization, the Office of Health and Environmental Assessment, but are also done in the "program offices" of EPA, particularly the Water Office and the Office of Toxic Substances, using CAG's dose–response coefficients. EPA's regulations are based on several laws which treat risk assessment differently. EPA's interpretation of the Clean Air Act (CAA) is that primary air quality standards must preclude adverse health effects in the most susceptible subgroup of the population with an adequate margin of safety. Similarly, emission standards for new facilities require the "best available control technology." Costs must not be considered. These standards are for "criteria" pollutants such as sulfur dioxide which are not generally considered carcinogens. Their principal health impacts are respiratory or other diseases. The Clean Water Act also requires best available technology for control, and so formal risk analyses are not required. Some of the most extensive use of risk analysis, and some searching reports on the scientific basis, methods, and philosophy of risk analysis has been done by the National Research Council under the EPA Water Office's sponsorship. These have been published in the continuing series, Drinking Water and Health, of which eight volumes have been issued in the past 10 years.

Regulatory Impact Analyses, including some degree of risk analysis, is required when new regulations are issued under these acts. For "hazardous" pollutants, which include carcinogens, the Clean Air Act provides for quantitative consideration of risk, and thus requires QCRA. QCRA is also required for regulations of mobile source emissions under the Clean Air Act. Similarly, the Toxic Substances Control Act, the Safe Drinking Water Act, and the Insecticide, Fungicide, and Rodenticide Act, all administered by EPA, require QCRA.

Although the Delaney clause requires FDA to prohibit use of food additives that are carcinogenic without regard to the quantitative level of risk, FDA has still been a leader in QCRA. Under the Food, Drug, and Cosmetic Act, "food additive" was narrowly defined, and the agency has made liberal interpretations of the Act. For color additives, FDA has developed a "constituent policy" for cases in which a constituent of an additive is carcinogenic. The level of the carcinogenic constituent must be sufficiently low that the upper limit of cancer risk provides reasonable certainty of no harm and the complete additive must not be carcinogenic. This policy has caused great controversy.

Natural contaminants of food are treated differently than those added for specific reasons. Here, some balancing of the cancer risk with the food's nutritional value and the extent to which the contamination can be controlled, are allowed. Exemptions are also allowed for drugs or food additives administered to animals raised for food production if no residue can be found in the meat. This, of course, depends on their sensitivity to the methods used. FDA has proposed that the sensitivity needed be established by quantitative risk assessment and not be based on the constantly advancing state of the art of chemistry (HHS, 1986). Thus, QCRA is used extensively for foods to avoid banning many foods outright and to take into account some of the real trade-offs. In many cases these are not "lives for dollars" but "lives for lives," e.g., balancing cancer risk against nutrition.

THE PURPOSE AND APPROACH OF THE BOOK

Risk assessment is still a new field. Complex as they may sometimes seem, current methods of cancer risk assessment are simplistic. They do not take into account much of what has been learned about cancer in the last 20 years. They often require detailed exposure information which goes way beyond the state of the art of environmental transport modeling. They do not take into account factors which have been shown to affect risk and the way people perceive risk. These include voluntariness of exposure, knowledge of exposure and risk, individual ability to control the risk, familiarity of the risk, the degree of dread associated with the effect, the signal value of the effect as a warning for greater future effects, and finally, the benefits which may be bundled with the risk. Part of the role of this volume is to to show the way to improvements.

In fact, the purpose of this text is twofold: First it serves as an introduction to quantitative cancer risk assessment, to show how it is done, what considerations are and should be taken into account, what basic background understanding of the broad contributing disciplines is important to cancer risk analysis. This single volume does not give the reader all a risk assessor needs to know about these subjects; it highlights only particular aspects important in QCRA. Some of these basic background needs are developed in appropriate chapters to make the book self-contained, but one does not become a risk assessor by reading one book. The "well-rounded" risk assessor will need to explore several disciplines in greater depth than can be included here. Moreover, a full appreciation of these disciplines can be had only from texts written for that discipline. For those who have studied widely in other fields, this book serves to pull it together in a way that focuses on risk assessment; for those who have not studied widely, it will hopefully serve as an inspiration to do so.

The second purpose, as suggested earlier, is to critically review the field and point out problem areas. This is aimed in part at the experienced practitioner. The level of treatment required in an introductory text and in a critical review is usually so different as to make the two purposes incompatible. I believe the opposite is true in risk assessment. It is not a well established discipline and is still riddled with problem areas. The neophyte should be made aware of these at the start. Moreover, the entry level for risk assessment requires some intellectual maturity. I expect many readers to be well-grounded in at least one of the contributing disciplines. As is common in interdisciplinary fields, the newcomer from another disciplinary background, given an understanding of the general approaches taken and the current problems faced by the field may well hit upon new approaches which make significant improvements. I urge the reader to continue the book with this in mind.

The generally accepted approach to quantitative risk assessment was described by a National Academy of Sciences committee (NAS, 1983). It distinguished the generally scientific task of risk assessment as apart from the more political, administrative, and value-laden task of risk management, although clearly there must be interaction between the two processes. Four steps were identified in risk assessment: hazard identification, exposure assessment, dose–response assessment, and risk characterization. This general approach forms the basic structure of the book. It is organized into four parts: Part I is an introductory section, which includes hazard assessment; Part II covers Exposure assessment; Part III deals with dose–response assessment; and Part IV discusses risk characterization. Although a full discussion of the subject is beyond the scope of this book, a chapter on risk management is included in Part IV to discuss some of the direct implications of QCRA for risk management. If the purpose of QCRA is to provide the scientific basis for risk management decisions, the better the risk analyst understands what is needed for those decisions the more useful the information provided will be. While to some degree the scientific and political aspects of cancer risk can be separated, it should be kept in mind that, just as it would be inappropriate for public decisions on risk to be delegated to scientists, it is equally inappropriate for scientists to stop at the scientific estimation of risk and simply turn the ball over to others with different backgrounds who may either use or abuse the results (Bailar and Thomas, 1985).

REFERENCES

Alfheim, I. and T. Ramdahl. 1984. Contribution of wood combustion to indoor air pollution as measured by mutagenicity in Salmonella and polycyclic aromatic hydrocarbon concentration. *Environ. Mutagen.* 6:121–130.
Ames, B.N. 1983. Dietary carcinogens and anticarcinogens. *Science* 221:1256–1264.

Bailar, J.C. III and S.R. Thomas. 1985. What are we doing when we think we are doing risk analysis? In A.D. Woodhead, C.J. Shellabarger, and V. Pond (eds.), *Assessment of Risk from Low-Level Exposure to Radiation and Chemicals*. Plenum Press, New York, pp. 65–76.

Doll, R. and R. Peto. 1981. The causes of cancer: quantitative estimates of avoidable risks of cancer in the United States today. J. *Natl Cancer Inst. 66*: 1191–1308

Flamm, W.G. 1986. Risk assessment policy in the United States, in P. Oftendal and A. Brogger (eds.), *Risk and Reason*, Alan R. Liss, Inc., New York, pp. 141–149.

HHS. 1986. *Determining Risks to Health, Federal Policy and Practice.* U.S. Department of Health and Human Services, Task Force on Health Risk Assessment. Auburn House Publishing Company, Dover, MA.

Higginson, J. 1979. Interview by T. Maugh II, Cancer and environment: Higginson speaks out. *Science 205*:1363.

Higginson, J. 1980. Multiplicity of factors involved in cancer patterns and trends. In H.B. Demopoulos and M.A. Mehlman (eds.), *Cancer and the Environment*. Pathotox Publishers, Inc., Park Forest South, IL.

Hutt, P.B. 1979. Individual freedom and government control of food safety: saccharin and food additives. *Ann. NY Acad. Sci. 329*:221–241.

Lave, L.B. 1983 *Quantitative Risk Assessment in Regulation*. The Brookings Institution, Washington, D.C.

NAS Committee on the Institutional Means for Assessment of Risks to Public Health. 1983. *Risk Assessment in the Federal Government: Managing the Process*. National Academy Press, Washington, D.C.

Novitch, M. 1981. *The Nation's Health*. November, p. 5.

Pott, P. 1775. Cancer scroti, in Chirurgical Observations, Hawes, Clarke and Collins, London, as cited in J.K. Wagoner, *Annals of the New York Academy of Sciences 271*: 1–3, 1976.

Reali, D., H. Schlitt, C. Lohse, R. Barale, and N. Loprieno. 1984. Mutagenicity and chemical analysis of airborne particles from a rural area in Italy. *Environ. Mutagen. 6*:813–823.

Ruckelshaus, W.W. 1985. Risk, science, and democracy, Issues in Science and Techology, Spring, pp: 19–38.

Samuels, S.W. and R.H. Adamson. 1985. Quantitative risk assessment: report of the subcommittee on environmental carcinogenesis, National Cancer Advisory Board. *J. Natl. Cancer Inst. 74*:945–951.

Somers, E. 1979. Environmental chemicals—how do we assess the risk? In N.E. Gentner and P. Unraw (eds.), Proceedings, First International Conference on Health Effects of Energy Production (AECL 6958). Chalk River Laboratories, Ontario, Canada.

WHO. 1982. Rapid assessment of sources of air, water, and land pollution. World Health Organization, Offset publ. no. 62, Geneva, Switzerland.

2

The Human Cancer Situation

This chapter introduces cancer: what it is, how it begins, how it develops, how many people get it, why they get it, and how much of it is due to environmental carcinogens. Some of these things are only partly understood, and current theories may later prove to be wrong. Moreover, only the bare bones of what is currently known of cancer biology can be presented here. In the last two decades, cancer research has greatly outpaced its application in assessing cancer risk. Risk assessment focuses on quantifying the relationship between exposure and cancer incidence. If assessments were based on an overall theory of the process underlying that relationship, then new information from research could be fit into place as it became available, clarifying, improving, and expanding the theory and the assessment model. Unfortunately, the actual situation is far from that ideal. Two to three decades ago, when the bases of current cancer risk assessment methods were laid, overall understanding of the carcinogenic process was vague; no overall unifying theory existed. Mechanistic models focused on only parts of the process and there were insufficient data to lend substance to any unifying concepts. Models applicable only to parts of the process were used to span the gap left by empirical data on exposure and effect.

Meanwhile, cancer research followed the path of basic research, rather than applied research. The general aim was to find the cause of cancer. The ultimate applications most researchers had in mind were medically oriented: curing cancers or preventing them through a vaccine. Reducing the cancer risk through intervening in environmental exposures was a second-order consideration, and supporting risk assessment methods to organize and set priorities for such intervention was seldom in the minds of biomedical researchers at all. The task facing researchers also proved much more difficult than expected. Repeated expectations of finding a "cure" for cancer went unfulfilled.

17

Perhaps this emphasis was correct, but the result was that the type of research carried out, although much of it was or will be ultimately of value, did not produce results that could be fit into risk assessments. Further, since the researchers did not have risk assessment in mind, even results that might have been useful for risk assessment were reported in a form that risk analysts could not use and often did not even recognize as being applicable. Nonetheless, the body of basic research information grew. The nature of science is that as bits of information accumulate, the opportunities for constructing a unifying theory increase. The abundance of new knowledge produced over two or three decades appears to be ripe for the introduction of such a theory.

As the role of risk assessment became more institutionalized, its data needs, its shortcomings in underlying theory, and the regulatory chaos and social impact which can result from these shortcomings became more apparent to the scientific community. Constructing anything even approaching a unifying theory of cancer, or even reducing the body of biomedical knowledge to a form more easily used in quantitative assessments, is a task beyond the scope of this book. Hopefully, providing statisticians, environmental scientists, and other participants in the risk assessment process who are outside the biomedical community with some insight into the biological aspects of cancer development will help smooth the way for the movement toward a more substantial biological basis in quantitative cancer risk assessment.

WHAT IS CANCER?*

Cancer is a disease characterized by cells which proliferate without control, invading neighboring tissue and metastasizing, or spreading groups of cancerous cells through the circulatory or lymph systems to establish new "invasions" in remote tissues throughout the body. The general term for an uncontrolled proliferation of cells is neoplasia. Cancer is a neoplastic process, and a tumor is called a neoplasm. Tumors are described as either benign or malignant. Malignant tumors are distinguished from benign tumors by histopathological characteristics of cellular morphology, invasiveness, growth, and differentiation (Barrett and Wiseman, 1987). The key difference is that malignant tumors have the ability to metastasize; benign tumors remain confined in their original tissues. It is the malignancies which are the greater health threat, although "benign" tumors

---

*Much of the information presented in this and the following sections is drawn from OTA (1981), Guidelines (1986), Thomas (1986), Bishop (1987), and Weinberg (1988).

can be life-threatening in themselves. Some benign tumors remain so. In other cases, tumors go through a progression in which benign or apparently benign tumors become malignant and develop the ability to metastasize.

Malignant neoplasms fall into three classifications: (1) carcinomas are solid tumors which afflict epithelial tissues, including the skin and the surfaces and linings of internal glands; (2) sarcomas are solid tumors of the supportive tissues such as bone, muscle, and cartilage; and (3) leukemias and lymphomas are cancers of circulating cells. Carcinomas are the most common form of human cancer and, technically, the only form to which the term "cancer" actually applies. We will follow the more common definition and use the term "cancer" to refer to all malignant neoplasms. Cancers are generally labeled by their site of occurrence, e.g., lung cancer, bladder cancer. This classification sometimes extends to the specific class of cells within a given organ, e.g., oat-cell carcinoma of the lung. Although cancers have a common nature, each different class is treated as a separate disease. This is because among cancers of different organs and of different cell types within an organ, there are great differences in causative agents, symptoms produced, treatment methods, and curability. There are hundreds of clinically identifiable cancers. The International Classification of Diseases (WHO, 1977) lists over 70 major categories of cancer by site (Appendix I); each major category is further broken down into multiple subcategories. The subcategories can be further classified by morphology or histology. Nearly 50 major histological categories are listed in Appendix II; most of these are further broken down into multiple subcategories, some into over 50 subcategories (WHO, 1977).

HOW DOES CANCER BEGIN?

The most broadly held theory is that most, if not all, cancers begin with genetic damage in a single cell. A short digression on genetics is, thus, appropriate before proceeding with carcinogenesis. In the mid-19th century, Mendel, the Father of Genetics, hypothesized the existence of genes and experimentally demonstrated how genetically controlled traits are passed from generation to generation. Not for almost 100 years was the molecular basis of Mendel's discovery shown to be in the nucleic acids, and particularly deoxyribonucleic acid (DNA). The advance of biological science since then has brought us to the brink of a complete mapping of the human genome. The nucleic acids control cell processes and, by reproducing themselves, provide the chemical link between one generation and the next; they thus determine the nature of a cell and insure that the progeny of that cell maintain the same characteristics as the parent. The genetic code which stipulates this information is found in the arrangement of the nucleotides (the basic subunits of nucleic acids) along the long-chain DNA molecule. A change in the sequence of nucleotides in DNA results in a change in the genetic message. This is a mutation. Mutations occur spontaneously during cell division in viruses, bacteria, plants, and animals. These "spontaneous" mutations may be simply accidents or may have an underlying cause such as a shortage of a particular chemical base. Mutations can also be induced by outside mutagenic agents. Mutations in germ cells, the reproductive cells of an organism, lead to effects in offspring rather than in the organism itself. Mutations in somatic cells, if those cells replicate and multiply, lead to effects in the target organism itself.

In the course of millions of years of evolution, many possible alternatives have been tried before and found wanting. It should not be surprising, therefore, that most mutations are harmful. In population genetics, a mutant offspring represents a varient to the species. In the rare circumstance that the mutation gives an advantage to the offspring, a new species may develop. More frequently, the mutation is either fatal to the offspring or poses some disadvantage to the offspring and, although it may propagate through some future generations, is sooner or later eliminated through evolutionary pressure in the population. The single change in a nucleic-acid base responsible for the disease sickle-cell anemia, for example, in addition to causing a debilitating disease, apparently also conferred a resistance to malaria. The latter may have been the predominant effect when the genetic trait was confined to Africa, but its desirability is now outweighed by the sickle-cell disease.

The effects of a genetically induced disease depend not only on the original mutation, but on the interaction among the resulting offspring, the other members of the population, and the environment at large. The same will be seen to be true in the case of somatic mutations.

Factors which support the theory that cancers begin with genetic damage in a somatic cell include: (1) observed hereditary predisposition to cancer; (2) detection of damaged chromosomes in cancer cells; (3) an apparent connection between susceptibility to cancer and impaired ability of cells to repair damaged DNA; (4) evidence relating mutagenic potential of substances (determined in tests with bacteria) to their carcinogenicity in animal tests; (5) evidence that some carcinogenic substances bind with DNA in the cell, forming DNA adducts; (6) discovery of cellular genes (proto-oncogenes) that in another form (oncogenes) can cause neoplastic growth (Bishop, 1987). Although the precise molecular nature of the damage is unknown, it appears that certain genes are activated; these are known as oncogenes and a number of them have been identified. At least three different mechanisms may be involved in the activation of these otherwise normal genes (Land et al., 1983).

It is well established that various *ras* genes may be activated by single point mutations to oncogenes. The presence of mutated *ras* genes in benign polyps of the colon indicate that their activation is an early, and perhaps the initiating, event in the process of carcinogenesis. But this is not the only role these genes have; the same transformation, occuring at a later time, may initiate the transition of a benign polyp to a carcinoma (Bos, 1988). While the mystery of cancer is beginning to unravel, all is not yet clear. Evidence of activated oncogenes is currently only found in 20% of human tumor DNA (Weinberg, 1988). This may be due to inadequate detection methods; to existence of other, as yet unknown, oncogenes; or to the presence of other, alternative, cancer initiation methods.

The theory of somatic mutation orgin of cancer is the basis of the "1-hit" model of radiation and chemical carcinogenesis; this assumes that a single "hit" or damage to the genetic material of a cell leads inexorably to development of a cancer. The 1-hit philosophy was the guiding influence in the regulation and management of radiation and chemical cancer risks for two decades. It is generally believed now, however, that, although cancer may begin with a single mutation, this event does not lead inexorable to a cancer. Far from it; a complex and relatively improbable series of steps appears to be necessary for a cancer to result from a single mutation. Indeed, single DNA-damaging events apparently happen all the time; even without exposure to a mutagen or a carcinogen, cells experience spontaneous mutations at low frequency. But, either the cell dies, the damage is repaired, or the damage is insufficient for the task of creating a cancer. This is apparently why we survive continual exposure to the "sea of carcinogens" in our air, water, and food, and perhaps is the explanation of the 2-pack per day smoker who lives to be 100.

In one set of experiments (Weinberg, 1988), when a *ras* oncogene was introduced into normal cells, no tumorigenic cell clones appeared, indicating that the oncogene might not be sufficient in itself to initiate the process. When another kind of oncogene (*myc* oncogene) was added, the two acted together to produce tumorigenic cells. Each appeared to contribute in its distinct way to the transformation process, demonstrating that oncogenes are not uniform, but are a heterogeneous group of genes which, at least sometimes, must act together to initiate a cancer.

Repair of genetic damage in a cell and suppression of its results are natural processes. Some people have defective or reduced repair mechanisms, making them more susceptible to the effect of spontaneous mutations and to environmental carcinogens. A frequently cited example of this is xeroderma pigmentosum, an inherited inability to repair DNA damage caused by the UVB band in sunlight. This makes its victims highly susceptible to skin cancer. Since repair processes are inherited, there is bound to be a range of sensitivity to mutagens within the population. This variety in sensitivity is similar in some ways to the distribution in sensitivity to acute toxic agents, and provides the basis of applying a class of models (e.g., the probit model) to cancer assessment which were originally used to predict effects of toxic chemicals and which assume an underlying distribution of susceptability in the population.

The immune system provides continual surveillance of foreign agents into the body, and appears to recognize the uncontrolled cell proliferation of cancer as a foreign invasion. Evidence for this is seen in increased cancer incidence in patients on immunosuppressive therapy and in those with acquired immunodeficiency syndrome. The existance of a viligent repair mechanism provides a different way for a carcinogen to act. Rather than directly damage DNA, the carcinogen may act indirectly to inhibit DNA repair, allowing spontaneous mutations (or those induced by other agents) to develop into cancer when their development might otherwise be cut short by a repair mechanism.

In addition to the oncogenes which can cause neoplastic growth, there are tumor suppressor genes which prevent the growth and modulator genes which influence secondary properties of malignancy such as invasiveness, metastatic propensity, or the ability to generate an immune response (Klein, 1987).

It has been speculated that a critical lesion in the tumor cell DNA may cause the loss of a gene normally responsible for regulating cell growth. Retinoblastoma, an inherited cancer, apparently is activated through the loss of such a regulating, or tumor suppressing, gene. Inactivation of tumor suppressing genes has also been implicated as a contributing cause in lung and colon cancer. It appears there is a large class of tissue-specific tumor-suppressing genes which have an important role in the carcinogenic process (Weinberg, 1988).

Finally, some carcinogens appear to directly affect neither DNA nor specific repair nor supression mechanisms; they act on the cellular level environment to facilitate initiation or development of an initiated cell. Diethylstilbestrol (DES), for example, is not mutagenic, but apparently produces cancer by causing either hormonal imbalances or altered hormone response. Another example is asbestos fibers, which are not mutagenic, but may allow entry of carcinogenic organics into target cells (Thomas, 1986).

Another indirect carcinogenic mechanism may be to increase cell proliferation, thus increasing the frequency of spontaneous mutations and speeding promotion. An agent inducing a toxic response may do both; a relationship has been shown between acute toxicity and carcinogenicity. This is of special concern in interpreting animal bioassays. The high doses given in these studies may produce cancer through such a toxic effect which does not exist at lower doses to which the dose–response function is extrapolated. This may also relate in some way to the action of the immune system in tumor supression and repair. The cellular components of the immune system are derived from bone marrow stem cells, which, because they are among the most rapidly proliferating cells in the body, are themselves especially susceptable to mutations induced by toxic agents (Thomas, 1986).

As continuing research provides more insight into these variations in the way different agents initiate cancer, it may be possible to improve risk assessment. Different mechanisms are not mutually exclusive, however; a single carcinogen may act through more than one channel. In many cases, seemingly different channels may lead to the same initiating event by different routes. The initiating event may even prove not to be the most important part of the carcinogenic process.

HOW DOES CANCER DEVELOP?

Cancer develops through a series of stages, generally classed as initiation, promotion, and progression. These terms simply describe what is observed in experimental studies; the underlying mechanisms are not well defined or understood. There are undoubtedly many substeps and perhaps many different competing and synergistic processes involved in each stage. Moreover, each stage may be influenced by factors such as age, sex, diet, metabolic activity, immunosurveillance status, and the kind and dose level of various environmental exposures. In reviewing these stages, it is important to realize that, although other sources of information are used, much of the experimental evidence on which knowledge of the multistage process of carcinogenesis is based was developed with mouse skin and rat and mouse liver exposures.

Initiation

Initiators are the agents which cause the initial DNA damage. In general they are mutagens. They are likely to test positive in mutagenic bioassays. In many cases, there is a dose–response relationship between the dose of the initiator and the probability of a tumor developing or the number of tumors produced. Studies of oncogene activation provide strong evidence that mutations are the source of the activation and thus initiate the critical changes in initiation (Barrett and Wiseman, 1987). Formation of an initiated cell involves at least two steps: initiating damage to the DNA forming a promutagenic lesion, followed by cell replication to establish the altered cell line in the tissue (Anderson, 1987). The latter is an important difference between tests of mutagenic activity in cell cultures and what happens in a whole animal where cell replication may be controlled by factors outside the altered cell itself. Mechanisms of initiation may vary in different tissues or with different agents in the same tissue (Barrett and Wiseman, 1987). Because initiation begins with DNA damage, it is a process involving a single cell; this single initiated cell then establishes its altered state in all its progency. Once established, initiation appears to be long lasting; tumors have been produced by applying a promoting agent more than a year following initiation. Indeed, initiation is commonly considered to be an irreversible phenomenon.

While initiators are generally thought of as agents which directly produce DNA damage, other agents can act indirectly to induce a physiological state that results in DNA damage. Since DNA damage occurs "spontaneously," an agent producing a change that increases the rate of spontaneous DNA damage can produce the same end result as one which which damages DNA directly.

Although many models assume the initial initiating event is a single "hit" or a single action damaging DNA, there is evidence that at least two protooncogenes must be activated for a tumor cell to arise and that these may be initiated by different mechanisms (Barrett and Wiseman, 1987).

For decades, mouse skin has been used as the test bed for distinguishing iniation from promotion. Understanding of the differences between the two roles was gained and chemicals were identified as initiators or promotors, or as having some properties of both. The information was more qualitative than quantitative, however. Only recently, has an experimental procedure been developed that can quantitatively examine initiation independently from the later stages of the carcinogenic process (Pitot and Campbell, 1987). In this test system, initiators produce lesions called enzyme-altered foci in the rat liver. Each enzyme-altered focus is the clonal progeny of a single initiated cell in the same way that colonies on a cultured bacterial plate each develop from a single bacteria. The number of initiated cells induced is the number of foci found in the test animal minus the number found in a control animal (to account for spontaneously initiated cells). An initiation index can then be calculated as the number of cells initiated per unit dose.

Promotion

Promoters are agents which generally do not produce tumors on their own, but, when applied following an initiator, result in tumor development. Promotion is the process in which an initiated cell clonally expands into a visible tumor (Barrett and Wiseman, 1987). Initiated cells respond differently to promoting agents than normal cells. A promoter is not simply a nongenotoxic carcinogen. Promotion is further characterized by reversible expansion of the initiated cell population and reversable alteration of genetic expression (Pitot and Campbell, 1987). Reversablity is a key property of promotion which distinguishes it from initiation and progression. Multiple or continual doses of promoters are often necessary for them to be effective; if application of the promoting agent is stopped, the rate of tumor production decreases or stops. For this reason, many feel that cigarette smoke acts primarily as a promoter since the lung cancer incidence in those who quit smoking tends to decrease and to eventually approach that of nonsmokers. Promoters are generally not mutagenic and do not test positive on mutagenic bioassays. Agents, however, can be both initiators and promoters; these are called *complete carcinogens*. Cigarette smoke, for example, contains several chemicals known to have mutagenic capacity, so, while it may act primarily as a promoter, it is, at least weakly, a complete carcinogen.

The immune system can play a critical role in preventing the formation of a tumor or otherwise influencing its development. In one experimental tumor model, not all tumor cells must be killed to prevent tumor development and maintain a disease-free state (Vitetta et al., 1987). Tumor suppressor genes and modulator genes may act during this stage to block further cell proliferation or to inactivate oncogenes.

The rat liver test system described for initiators can also independently and quantitatively assess the effectiveness of promoters. The effectiveness of promotion is based on the increase in the number of cells in the enzyme-altered foci; this is assumed to be proportional to the volume occupied by those foci. The occupied volumes are determined by three-dimensional quantitative stereology. A promotion index is derived from the ratio of the total volume occupied by all the enzyme-altered foci in the livers of treated animals to that in the control animals, which were initiated, but not treated with a promoter, divided by the dose of promoter.

Time and dose-level considerations are of greater importance in evaluating promotion than for initiation. The end product of promotion is a benign lesion or a preneoplastic foci of cells. These cells must undergo one or more additional heritable changes to progress to a malignant neoplasm (Barrett and Wiseman, 1987).

Progression

Progression has been described as the gradual emancipation of a clone of somatic cells from the complex controls that regulate its growth (Klein, 1987). In other words, "the process whereby tumors go from bad to worse" (Rous and Beard, 1939). It is a dynamic process, since tumors may become increasingly malignant at different rates, and may even evidence remission. The process seems to involve changes within the cancer and interaction between the cancer and other body processes. Continued promotion may be a part of progression, but is not sufficient in itself. The role of carcinogens is not clear, but initiation-promotion experiments on mouse skin indicate distinct differences among chemicals in their ability to promote the appearance of benign papillomas and the ability to produce cancers. Some strong promoters, which produce multiple papillomas, are not effective in the continuing progression of these to cancers (Barrett and Wiseman, 1987).

Unlike promotion, progression is irreversible. It has been suggested that arsenic is a progresser (Barrett and Wiseman, 1987). Arsenic is recognized as a human carcinogen, but is not mutagenic in bacterial tests, does not generally test positive in animal bioassay, and is inactive as an initiator or promoter in mouse skin experiments. Moreover, occupationally induced lung cancer attributable to arsenic exposure appears to be irreversable as it does not show declining rates after exposures cease as lung cancer attributed to cigarette smoking does.

Progression does not require the intermediate stage of promotion. There are examples of carcinogenic processes which have no demonstrable reversible phase; initiation is apparently followed directly by progression (Pitot and Campbell, 1987).

Further direct DNA damage may also enter at this stage. There is some evidence that transformation of a benign tumor to a malignant tumor could be caused by a second-hit phenomenon in a benign tumor cell (Anderson, 1987). Mutagenic activation of *ras* oncogenes have been shown to occur late in the carcinogenic process, initiating the transition of a polyp to a malignant carcinoma or to convert a primary melanoma into a metastic tumor (Bos, 1988). DNA damage and other important forces of change may also be produced by the tumor's own growth. During the progression stage, the tumor becomes much more complex. In the early, high cell-proliferation stage, proliferating cells are usually located within a few cell layers of blood vessels. Quiescent and necrotic cells are further away from blood vessels (Sutherland, 1988). As the tumor grows, its microenvironment becomes more heterogeneous. Sharp gradients in availability of oxygen, glucose, lactate, H^+ ions, and other nutrients, hormones, and growth factors develop. These microenvironmental changes exert selective pressure and new and diverse cell phenotypes emerge. Differentiated quiescent cells also emerge under the influence of this altered cellular environment. At the same time, natural biological response modifiers are present which can induce either cell proliferation or quiescence. These may cause cells to become quiescent and, at a later stage, reactivate them to cause a resurgence of growth in the tumor.

A Continuous Process

The multistage theory of cancer has been demonstrated in animal experiments and is consistent with epidemiological evidence. The stages of initiation, promotion, and progression have been examined separately in experiments. It must be remembered that experiments are specifically designed to separate these stages as an aid to understanding the mechanisms underlying them. More detailed understanding of what happens in each stage will provide a basis for better risk assessment. The stages are not so separate and distinct, however, in the human population. People are continuously exposed to initiators, promoters, and progressers; there may be synergisms or antagonisms among them. A new exposure does not impact on a "clean slate" of uninitiated cells as might be the case in a laboratory experiment. It adds to an ongoing process. Different cells in a given organ may be at different stages. An agent's interaction in that complex, ongoing process may be quite different than its action alone under laboratory conditions.

HOW BIG IS THE CANCER PROBLEM?

To understand the problem requires a more specific statement of the question. One must ask how many new cancers are diagnosed annually, how many people die of cancer annually, how these numbers are apportioned among the different kinds of cancers and among different people (e.g, by age), how the annual rates compare with those of other diseases, if there are trends over time, and how these trends vary among different cancers and different population groups. While a problem can exist independent of a solution, to a large degree the size of the cancer "problem" in the public mind depends on the extent it is felt that something can or should be done about it. The "problem" takes on greater proportions if it seems to be growing. If cancer is increasing rapidly because of increasing exposure to industrial chemicals in the environment over the last several decades, and continuing increases in such exposures suggest that cancer rates will continue to climb, then we have a problem of considerable importance. Many feel this is, or may be, the case; others do not (e.g., Davis, 1988; Epstein et al., 1988; Ames and Gold, 1988a, 1988b).

This section describes the extent and distribution of cancer in the population, generally without regard to cause. Much of this information can be helpful in seeking causes of cancer or relationships between environmental factors and cancer. Trends in cancer rates and differences in rates in different population groups may indicate the working of environmental factors. This is taken up in the following section on Cancer and Environmental Factors.

How Many People Get Cancer?

Cancer is a common disease. Over six million new cancer cases are diagnosed annually worldwide, of which nearly 900,000 are in North America (Parkin et al., 1988). In the United States, cancer is the second leading cause of death, exceeded only by heart disease. About 20% of all deaths in the United States are from cancer, a total of 466,000 in 1986 (NCHS, 1987). Many cancers are killer diseases; their death rate is indicative of the incidence rate. This is not true of all cancers, however, a fact reflected in the overall cancer incidence rate being roughly twice the cancer mortality rate; many cancer victims do not die of the disease.

The period 1978-1981 is useful for rate comparisons because it spans the 1980 census for which the best population estimates are available. During those years, in the ten areas participating in the National Cancer Institute's Surveillance, Epidemiology, and End Results (SEER) program,* there were a total of 296,025 new cancer cases diagnosed for a standardized annual rate of 338 per 100,000 people (excludes nonmelanoma skin cancers). During the same period, there were 144,400 cancer deaths for a standardized annual rate of 164 per 100,000 in the SEER participating areas (Horm et al., 1985). Differences by sex and race are shown in Table 2-1. Blacks have higher rates than whites and men higher rates then women. As a comparison, the 1978-1981 cancer mortality rate for the total U.S. population was 167 per 100,000. In a detailed comparison of incidence and mortality rates, one would have to consider that a period of years usually exists between diagnosis and death, so the cancer death rate should be related to an earlier incidence rate.

---

*Connecticut, Iowa, New Mexico, Utah, Hawaii, Puerto Rico, Metropolitan Detroit, Metropolitan Atlanta, Seattle–Puget Sound, and San Francisco–Oakland SMSA.

TABLE 2-1 Cancer Incidence and Mortality Rates (per 100,000, Age-Adjusted to 1970 U.S. Sandard) in SEER Regions, 1978–1981 (Excludes Nonmelanoma Skin Cancers)

	All Races			Whites			Blacks		
	Total	Male	Female	Total	Male	Female	Total	Male	Female
Incidence	338	397	302	335	391	303	372	488	290
Mortality	164	209	134	163	206	134	209	289	152

Source: Horm et al., 1985.

Incidence rates are limited to SEER participants because, although cancer mortality is well known nationwide, cancer incidence is not. There is no national reporting system for cancer diagnoses. Individual hospitals maintain tumor registeries, and many states have cancer registeries, but the coverage is far from national. The National Cancer Institute (NCI) has conducted three National Cancer Surveys to measure cancer incidence, but they were far from national. Moreover, the coverage changed with each survey. The first was in 1937-1939, the second in 1947-1948, and the third in 1969-1971. Incidence trends from these surveys are examined in Devesa and Silverman (1978, 1980) and Pollack and Horm (1980). These were recently updated drawing on data from SEER and local cancer registries (Devesa et al., 1987).

Our knowledge of cancer in the human population is almost entirely based on either deaths or diagnoses of cancer. This is quite a different situation from animal experiments in which cancer rates are derived from data gained by killing and autopsying all animals at the end of the experiment. The information that 20% of all deaths are from cancer can be turned around to state that 20% of the population would die from cancer, assumming the situation remained constant over time. But perhaps more like 35% of the population would have experienced cancer during their lifetime. Statistics on deaths assign a single underlying cause to each death; the total number of people who have cancer recorded on their death certificate is about 14% higher than the number who are specified as dying of cancer (NCHS, 1984). Since some people with undiagnosed cancers die from other causes, it is impossible to know the human population equivalent of the cancer rate found in animal experiments.

Another way of looking at the number of cancer deaths in the population is to ask, "what would happen if cancer were eliminated?" Everyone does die eventually anyway. Doll and Peto (1981) estimated that if half the cancer deaths in the United States were magically prevented and nothing else changed, those people would live an average of 10 to 15 additional years. Even then, many would eventually die of a second cancer. Rice and Hodgson (1981) estimated that between 10 and 24 person-years were lost for each cancer death, depending on the site (see Table 2-8).

Distribution of Cancers by Site

Examining total cancer morbidity and mortality helps to provide an appreciation of the public health impact of cancer, but it paints the picture with a broad brush. It is similar to looking at the impact of infectious diseases; a real understanding requires that measles, tuberculosis, and the common cold be examined separately. Cancers at different sites in the body are highly heterogeneous in causative factors, incidence rate, rate of development, and survival rate. Cancer rates are highly dependent on age; age-specific or age-standarized rates are the only valid bases of comparison among cancer rates. Available data, however, are insufficient to age-standardize cancer rates on a worldwide basis. Total estimated

TABLE 2-2 Cancer Incidence by Site: Estimated Number of New Cases (Thousands) in 1980 Worldwide by Developed and Developing Countries

Site	Developed countries	Developing countries
Stomach	333	336
Lung	455	206
Breast	348	224
Colon-rectum	389	183
Cervix	961	370
Mouth-pharynx	106	272
Esophagus	59.6	254
Liver	59.6	192
Lymphoma	116	122
Prostate	177	58.6
Bladder	148	71.2
Leukemia	82.7	106
Corpus uteri	104	45.3
Ovary	70.4	67.2
Pancreas	90.0	47.4
Larynx	52.9	67.1

Source: Data from Parkin et al., 1988.

number of annual new cancers in 1980 are summarized in Table 2-2, which compares the developed and developing countries of the world. The most common cancers worldwide are lung, stomach, colon–rectum, and breast. The latter ranks among the top four in total numbers despite the fact that its impact falls almost entirely on on only half the population (women). The total number of cancers is about evenly divided between the developed and the developing world, although the latter, with three times the population, has a considerably lower cancer incidence rate. This in part reflects the much younger population in the developing world. The top four cancers worldwide are also topranked in the developed world. While they are important in the developing world, too, cancer of the cervix ranks first there, and cancers of the mouth, pharynx, esophagus, and liver are also important (Table 2-2). There is, of course, a wide gradation of level of development in the world. Greater contrast among cancer sites can be seen between the most developed and the least developed countries. Lung cancer seems to be be associated with develop-

TABLE 2-3 Average Annual Age-Adjusted (1970 Standard) Incidence Rates (per 100,000) Among Whites in 5 U.S. Geographical Regions (Atlanta, Connecticut, Detroit, Iowa, and San Francisco–Oakland) for 1979–1980

	Rates	
Site	Male	Female
Lung	86.7	28.9
Colon-rectum	62.6	46.4
Breast	0.8	87.4
Prostate	72.1	—
Corpus uteri	—	25.4
Bladder	31.3	7.5
Lymphoma	16.0	11.7
Mouth-pharynx	17.5	7.1
Leukemia	13.8	7.8
Stomach	12.8	5.4
Pancreas	11.4	7.3
Ovary	—	13.8
Larynx	9.4	1.5
Cervix	—	9.1
Esophagus	5.3	1.7

Source: Data from Devesa et al., 1987.

ment, while stomach cancer is associated with the less developed, econom-
ically poorer countries. Colorectal cancer may be a disease of countries
in transition toward urbanization and industrialization. While stomach
cancer is the only overlap among the top four cancers in the developed
and the developing world, in both instances the top four cancers represent
roughly 50% of the total number of cases.

Cancer incidence in the United States is best estimated from the
SEER results mentioned above. Table 2-3 provides rates for key sites.

Distribution of Cancer Among Population Subgroups

Age

Cancer is a disease of middle age and the elderly. Its incidence rate goes
up sharply with age (Fig. 2-1). This is why changes in age structure of
the population can sharply affect crude cancer rates with no underlying
change in age-specific cancer risk.

Urban/Rural

A common observation is that cancer rates for several sites are higher
among urban residents than among rural residents (Goldsmith, 1980).
Possible factors in an urban-rural gradient are differences in smoking,

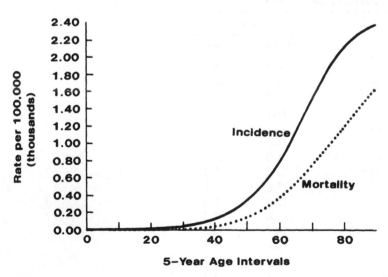

FIGURE 2-1 Cancer incidence and mortality rates by age, SEER areas 1978–81
(from Horm et al., 1985).

occupational exposures, and medical diagnosis. Goldsmith (1980) found similar ratios with educational level among U.S. counties that were neither completely urban nor completely rural. In another study, income and education by census tract were shown to inversely affect lung cancer incidence rates in males but not in females (Devesa and Diamond, 1983). Urban air pollution has been suggested as a possible cause of the urban/rural gradient. Robertson (1980) suggests motor vehicle exhaust is an important factor, pointing out that the number of motor vehicles per square mile tends to level off in densely populated cities similar to the way cancer rates do when correlated with population density. While this is a possibility, Goldsmith (1980) points out several drawbacks to an air pollution hypothesis:

> ... the urban gradient should be larger in those states or countries where there is the heaviest urban pollution. It is not.
> ... the rate should be higher in lifetime urban residents than in migrants to urban areas. They are not.
> ... A positive correlation has been shown with population density, but, when size of cities is controlled, not with levels of pollution.
> ... If the urban factor were community air pollution it should affect women at least as much as men. It doesn't apparently.

The underlying basis of an urban/rural ratio remains unclear; a leading hypothesis is that people begin to smoke at younger ages in cities (Doll and Peto, 1981).

International

Valid comparisons of cancer rates among communities throughout the world are difficult to obtain, but where efforts have been made to make such comparisons, the ratio of the highest to lowest standardized rates for the 35–65 age group is three for total cancers and six or greater for cancer at individual sites (Doll and Peto, 1981). Examples of the ratio of highest to lowest cancer rates (all in males) include: lung cancer, 35 (England/Nigeria); esophageal cancer, 300 (northeast Iran/Nigeria); liver cancer, 100 (Mozambique/England). One area may be high in one cancer and low in another. These differences are greater than expected from random variation of independent rates, indicating there is some etiological basis to the differences. Given that data are not available for many places, the actual variation is probably greater. The differences among international communities may be related to characteristics of the place, ethnic origin, religion, or economic factors.

CHAPTER 2

Ethnic and Religious Factors

Ethnic differences may be based on genetic, dietary, cultural, religious or economic factors. Numerous studies have been made of religious groups which prohibit the use of alcohol, tobacco, coffee, and tea. These groups have significantly lower cancer rates than comparison populations. Highly significant differences were found between Mormons and non-Mormons in Utah, for example, for all cancers combined and cancers of the mouth, esophagus, larynx, lung, bladder, colon, breast, and cervix. Much of the difference can be accounted for by known relationships between cancer and alcohol and tobacco use, but some residual effect remains (Lyon et al., 1980). An extensive discussion of this issue is found in Cairns et al. (1980).

Latent Period and Survival Rates

Cancer is characterized by a typically long latent period between initiation and manifestation of the disease. Despite multiple stages in the development of cancer, the often decades-long process is difficult to explain. It is related in some way to the aging process; tumors develop, not in calendar time, but in biological time. Thus, the full expression of cancers from a chemical or radiation exposure takes place in the 2-year lifetime of a mouse or the 70-year lifetime of a human.

In people, the actual time of initiation is almost never known. The first knowledge of the presence of the disease is the time of clinical diagnosis, which generally occurs 10-40 years later. The third, and final, mark on the time scale of cancer is death.

Estimates of latent period are based on studies of cancer following exposures well-defined in time such as radiation exposure in utero, childhood radiation exposure, and radiation exposure from the atomic bombs in Hiroshima and Nagasaki. Occupational exposures are often used for this purpose also, counting from the date first exposed. Initiation of a cancer might have occurred at anytime during an occupational exposure, however, leaving considerable uncertainty on one side of the range. Additional uncertainty is added because some of the cancers seen have been spontaneous and unrelated to the particular exposure. It has not been possible to definatively establish a cause and effect link for specific tumors. Smokers, for example, have a greatly increased lung cancer incidence, but nonsmokers also get lung cancer. While one can estimate the probability that a lung cancer in a smoker was related to tobacco, there is, so far, no way to precisely determine if a specific person's cancer was caused by smoking.

Limited work on cancers induced by radiation and occupational exposure to chemicals indicate latent periods to be lognormally distributed, with a geometric mean and standard deviation for each type of cancer (Armenian and Lilienfeld, 1974). These authors also conclude that, although animal data show that increasing dose levels of a carcinogen leads to a decreasing latent period, much larger doses of a carcinogen are needed to change the latent period in humans than the are required to change the cancer incidence.

A great deal of attention has been placed on cancer survival rates. Survival is the length of time between diagnosis and death and has been used primarily as a measure of effectiveness of treatment. All else being equal, introduction of a better treatment method should increase survival. The "war against cancer" has largely been directed to finding cures. As an operational definition, a person was considered cured if he survived 5 years. In the 1930s, the cure rate was 20%; in the 1940s, 25%; 1950-1970, 33%; 1976-1982, 50% (Hutter, 1988). The trend is encouraging, although overall survival rates are only a crude indicator. There are large differences in survival among different cancers; a shift in the incidence of the different cancers can affect the survival trend without changing the underlying phenomena.

There are additional, more subtle, factors which affect survival rates. The point at which a cancer is diagnosed is not fixed. It depends on the state of the art of diagnosis (which changes over time), and on factors such as the emphasis of public health agencies on screening and other means of early identification. If the cancer is diagnosed earlier, "survival" is lengthened even if no medical intervention is taken. The two are not independent, however. In most cases, early detection increases the effectiveness of treatment resulting in a real increase in survival; this is still confounded with the artifactual increase in measurements of survival. Paradoxically, early diagnosis may not influence measured survival rates in some cases. The following rationale is provided by Enstrom and Austin (1977): Because invasion of other tissues is the conclusive key to diagnosis of cancer, tumors which are not invasive (cancers in situ) may be confused with benign tumors. To avoid introducing this confusion into the survival calculation, only diagnoses of invasive cancers are counted. Early diagnosis may lead to detecting more cancers in the in situ stage for which the effectiveness of treatment is high, leading to a subtantial real increase in survival, but not affecting measured survival rates since these diagnoses are not counted when calculating survival rates.

Another phenomenon pointed out by Enstrom and Austin (1977) which may artificially decrease survival rates is the loss to follow-up. In order to know if a person has survived 5 years following diagnosis, one must keep track of the person over that time, or at least be able to find

TABLE 2-4 Percentage 5-Year Survival for Malignant Cancers Relative to Expected Survival Rate[a] Primary Site, Age, Sex, and Race

Primary site	Age (yr)	White		Black	
		Male	Female	Male	Female
Stomach	All	12	14	13[b]	16[b]
	<45	13[b]	15[b]	21[b]	22[b]
	45–54	16[b]	18[b]	7[b]	17[b]
	55–64	11[b]	17[b]	14[b]	13[b]
	65–74	13	14[b]	17[b]	19[b]
	75+	9[b]	12[b]	4[b1]	1[b]
Colon	All	47	49	41	46
	<45	47	58	42[b]	53[b]
	45–54	48	50	46[b]	50[b]
	55–64	48	50	45	45
	65–74	48	48	38[b]	50
	75+	44	46	32[b]	37[b]
Rectum	All	44	47	28[b]	41
	<45	48	52	20[b]	61[b]
	45–54	43	56	34[b]	39[b]
	55–64	47	50	29[b]	39[b]
	65–74	46	49	24[b]	49[b]
	75+	36	38	27[b]	25[b]
Pancreas	All	3[b]	2[b]	3[b]	6[b]
	<45	16[b]	8[b]	—	38[b]
	45–54	3[b]	4[b]	—	8[b]
	55–64	2[b]	2[b]	2[b]	7[b]
	65–74	1[b]	2[b]	3[b]	2[b]
	75+	2[b]	2[b]	3[b]	—
Lung and bronchus	All	10	14	8	11[b]
	<45	15	23	14[b]	16[b]
	45–54	12	16	11[b]	10[b]
	55–64	11	15	8[b]	14[b]
	65–74	9	12	6[b]	9[b]
	75+	6	9[b]	4[b]	8[b]
Melanoma	All	71	80	—	—
	<35	76	86	—	—
	35–44	73	85	—	—
	45–54	71	83	—	—
	55–64	71	83	—	—
	65–74	66	69	—	—
	75+	52[b]	62	−0	—
Breast	All	—	72	—	60
	<35	—	67	—	54
	35–44	—	74	62	

TABLE 2-4 *Continued.*

Primary site	Age (yr)	White		Black	
		Male	Female	Male	Female
	45–54	—	75	—	57
	55–64	—	70	—	60
	65–74	—	71	—	64
	75+	—	69	—	68
Cervix uteri	All	—	66	—	61
	<35	—	86	—	81
	35–44	—	78	—	70
	45–54	—	66	—	57
	55–64	—	58	—	54
	65–74	—	55	—	47[b]
	75+	—	38	—	50[b]
Corpus uteri	All	—	87	—	54
	<45	—	91	—	72[b]
	45–54	—	94	—	80
	55–64	—	91	—	56
	65–74	—	80	—	38[b]
	75+	—	65	—	47[b]
Ovary	All	—	34	—	35
	<45	—	61	—	66
	45–54	—	44	—	28[b]
	55–64	—	29	—	27[b]
	65–74	—	21	—	20[b]
	75+	—	19	—	23[b]
Prostate	All	64–54	—	45[b]	17[b]
	45–54	68	—	51[b]	—
	55–64	69	—	56	—
	65–74	67	—	56	—
	75+	56	—	47	—
Bladder	All	72	69	49	34[b]
	<45	93	91	57[b]	66[b]
	45–54	84	86	65[b]	—
	55–64	76	77	56[b]	38[b]
	65–74	68	65	43[b]	37[b]
	75+	59	56	37[b]	26[b]
Kidney	All	49	48	44	57
	<45	65	64	43[b]	68
	45–54	51	54	44[b]	64[b]
	55–64	48	47	44[b]	55[b]
	65–74	43	44	45[b]	42[b]
	75+	43	36	39[b]	—

TABLE 2-4 *Continued.*

Primary site	Age (yr)	White Male	White Female	Black Male	Black Female
Brain and nervous system	All	19	22	12[b]	32[b]
	<15	49	52	38[b]	53[b]
	15–24	47	58	20[b]	41[b]
	25–34	34[b]	45[b]	—	—
	35–44	24[b]	39[b]	—	51[b]
	45–54	14[b]	15[b]	4[b]	21[b]
	55–64	6[b]	5[b]	4[b]	—
	65–74	3[b]	4[b]	—	
	75+	—	4[b]	—	—
Non-Hodgkin's lymphoma	All	42	43	38[b]	49[b]
	<45	50	61	36[b]	68[b]
	45–54	54	56	38[b]	56[b]
	55–64	42	48	43[b]	50[b]
	65–74	37	37	48[b]	36[b]
	75+	21[b]	23[b]	—	22[b]

[a]Expected survival based on general population rates specific for age, sex, race, and calendar year of observation.
[b]Standard error >10% of rate.
— indicates not applicable or number of cases too small to yield a reliable rate.
Source: SEER data from Ries et al., 1983.

some record of him. Because of the completeness of death records, it is easier to discover a missing person if he is dead than if he remains alive; those lost to follow-up thus may be more likely to be alive. If they are ignored, or assumed to be dead or alive in the same proportion as those for which follow-up data are available, there is a bias toward artifically lowering the estimated survival rate. The U.S. population is especially mobile and follow-up can be difficult; still, the percentage lost to follow-up is not large. In the largest cancer survival study (Ries et al., 1983), out of 437,646 cases diagnosed, only 20,159 (less then 5%) had no follow-up information.

Risk analyses have generally focused on predicting numbers of cancers rather than the effect on population survival. A more sophisticated approach to cancer risk assessment would include years of life lost, or take differences in fatality rate of cancers at different sites into account in some other way. Table 2-4 provides survival rates for this purpose;

more detailed data are available (Ries et al., 1983). While these are imperfect and the factors discussed above must be considered, they allow survival rate to be included in a risk assessment. The relative survival rate given is the ratio of the observed survival rate to that expected in the general population, specific for age, sex, race, and calendar year. It thus corrects for other causes of death which might be expected even in someone who was not diagnosed with cancer and so estimates the chance of survival given that cancer diagnosis relative to expected survival without that cancer. Among the factors included in Table 2-4, differences in survival rate among primary site are the most striking, ranging from nil to nearly 90%. Females generally have a higher survival rate than males. The overall difference between men and women is about 15%, but most of this comes from the large difference in lung cancer incidence. Even after correcting for expected deaths from other causes, survival generally decreases with age. Finally, there is considerable variation by race in both size and direction of the differences in survival rate for different sites.

Is There a Cancer Epidemic?

There is sometimes talk of a cancer epidemic, often tied to rapidly increasing environmental exposure of the population to chemicals. An epidemic is a large but temporary increase in the number of cases of a disease in a population. An epidemic of food poisoning might last a couple of days; an epidemic of cholera, months. Chronic diseases are not usually discussed in terms of epidemics; because of its long latent period, a cancer "epidemic" might last many decades. The key is a rapid increase in disease incidence over time. Claims of a cancer epidemic are generally based on one of two possible foundations: (1) there is a current rapid increase in one or more cancers, or (2) there are current environmental exposures to known carcinogens which can be extrapolated to future rapid increases in cancer rates. The latter can only be discussed intelligently after the methods of extrapolation have been presented. The former, however, involves an investigation of current trends in cancer rates which is an appropriate task here. Because consideration of increasing trends of cancer is linked closely with the possibility of causative agents in the environment, the two will be discussed together in the next section.

Cancer and Environmental Factors

The purpose of this book is to outline the methods of quantative cancer risk assessment, not to prove or refute relationships between environmental factors and cancer. Analysis of these relationships is, of course, the bread and butter of QCRA, so it is appropriate to introduce the issues involved. Moreover, it is useful to gain some perspective on the existing cancer problem, as it can be observed in incidence and mortality data, before getting too deep into the methods of analysis which involve extrapolation from other sources.

Many agents found in the environment are known to be carcinogenic from toxicological and epidemiological studies. Moreover, wide differences in the rates of different cancers around the world suggest that a substantial fraction of cancers are attributable to environmental, as opposed to inheritable, causes. While some specific relationships are reasonably well-defined, such as radiation, tobacco use, and some occupational exposures to chemicals, the specific environmental factors associated with much of what appears to be avoidable cancers remain elusive. Although nearly a decade old, Doll and Peto (1981) remains the definitive work examining a broad range of potential environmental links with cancer. The following discussion draws on that work for the approach to the question, but on the most recent information on age-specific trends in cancer incidence (Devesa et al., 1987). Links can be discussed either in terms of potential environmental causes or in terms of the disease. Because this discussion draws primarily on incidence trends, the latter course will be followed. The discussion is not comprehensive; it includes the major cancer sites and some other sites that have increased in incidence or have been especially associated with environmental factors.

Trends in Cancer Rates and Environmental Linkages

Changes in age- and site-specific cancer rates over time provide strong evidence of involvement of environmental factors. Incidence is, in principle, a better measure of trend then mortality because it is not confounded by changes in survival rate over time. The time of diagnosis is also closer to the time of initiation, shortening the delay between cause and effect. There is no perfect measure, however; incidence trends may be affected by factors such as changes in diagnostic procedures and practices. Equally as important, incidence data are more limited in scope and time than mortality data. They may not be available for areas with the best exposure data. The data used are further limited because they include only whites. Although incidence data cover only about 10% of the U.S. population, they appear to track well with national cancer mortality rates. There are no general rules for interpretation of incidence trends. Each type of cancer must be examined separately to assess potential artifacts in the trend as well as potential environmental influences. Moreover, in examining trends, it is important to look at trends within age, sex, race and ethnic origin groups separately, as diagnostic practice, access to medical care, and other factors which may affect diagnosis and which may vary over time may vary within these groupings. Doll and Peto (1981) point out that diagnostic practice has changed especially among people over 65 making trends in those age groups particularly suspect. For that reason, their analysis was restricted to trends within those 35–64 years old. Particularly risky is analysis of trends in the last age-group (e.g., 85 +); since its upper range is open-ended, it is more subject than other age groups to changes over time in the age distribution within the group. Environmental exposures also may vary among these population subgroups.

Lung cancer has the highest rate in the United States where it has shown marked increases over the past three decades. It is also increasing throughout the world. In recent years, the U.S. rate of increase slowed and, in some age groups, appears to have peaked. Peaks in incidence appeared in 1970 for males 35–44, in 1977–1978 for males 45–54, and in 1981–1982 for males 55–74. Between 1970 and 1984, the rate of increase among older females rose, whereas it decreased in younger females. Because the survival rate for lung cancer is relatively low, mortality rates closely follow incidence. Cigarette smoking has been demonstrated to be the major cause of lung cancer; Doll and Peto (1981) attribute 90% of U.S. lung cancers to tobacco use; Schneiderman estimated 74% among men and 62% among women (Schneiderman, 1980). The pattern in the trends largely follow expectations from changes in smoking habits. Since incidence or mortality data themselves do not identify smokers and non-smokers separately, estimation of the proportion of, and trends in, lung cancer not related to smoking involves extrapolation from other studies. Estimates of changes in a small and uncertain fraction are always subject to greater uncertainty than estimates involving the whole. Schneiderman (1980) calculated the increase between 1970 and 1976 in lung cancer not related to smoking was at a rate 3 to 6 times higher than that of all lung cancer. Data on lung cancer among nonsmokers appear to support the finding of an increasing rate of lung cancer not related to smoking (Enstrom, 1979; Garfinkel, 1980) (Fig. 2-2). Occupational exposure and air pollution are prime suspects for the nontobacco related lung cancer, but whether there is an increasing trend and, if so, what proportion is related to these environmental factors, remains subject to speculation.

Cancer of the colon and rectum are treated together because substantial misclassification apparently exists between them on death certificates, and the frequency of misclassification has changed over time. Together, these cancers have the second highest incidence in the United States and throughout the developed world. In the 1940s, incidence rates for colon

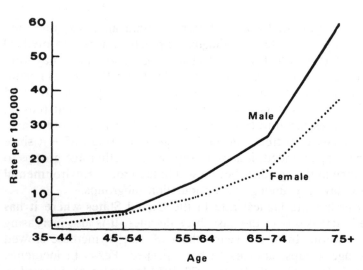

FIGURE 2-2 Lung cancer incidence mortality in nonsmokers by age (from Garfinkel, 1980).

cancer were generally higher among females, but male rates increased while female rates decreased, and males soon had the highest rates. The increasing trend is seen in males over age 55, with sharper increases in increases in older age groups. Rectal cancer incidence has remained relatively steady through the 1970s and early 1980s in all age groups. Colorectal cancer rates are, however, generally decreasing in many countries with high rates while increasing in developing countries which had the lowest rates. Dietary factors and alcohol consumption have been suspected as environmental agents. This may be a cancer associated with dietary changes of industrializing and urbanizing societies.

Breast cancer, although almost entirely a disease of women, is the third ranking cancer in the United States. Age-adjusted rates among females increased 31% between the late 1940s and 1983–1984, with the increase distributed primarily among women aged 35–74. Some age groups showed a higher increase in the mid-1970s followed by a decrease; it is speculated that this was due to early diagnosis resulting from an increased awareness of breast cancer. Increases in breast cancer have been associated with higher socioeconomic level, age at menarche, late age at menopause, and not having given birth or giving birth at a late age. Although obesity has been suggested to be related to postmenopausal breast cancer, the incidence rate among women aged 55–74 has increased despite a decline, beginning in the 1960s, of the proportion overweight.

Prostate cancer incidence increased 67% from the late 1940s to 1984, with the largest increases in 55–74 age group. Prostate cancer may remain asymptomatic for many years; its diagnosis may be incidental to a physical examination for routine or other reasons. Trends in mortality rates differed from incidenc trends; small decreases in mortality rates occurred from the early 1950s to the early 1970s, and small increases from then to 1984. It seems likely that some part of the increase in incidence is artifactual; what fraction, if any, may be related to causative factors is unknown.

Multiple myeloma has the highest rate of increase for the period from the late 1940s to 1984 of any cancer site, although large percentage increases must be considered together with the small initial rate. Increases in incidence were primarily in older age groups. In all age and sex groups, the bulk of the increases occurred between the late 1940s and 1970, most likely due to the introduction of improved diagnostic tools and their expanded use in the older population. International variation in incidence are likely due to differences in diagnostic capability. Other factors may also have had some part in the increase.

Bladder cancer is associated with smoking and has frequently been identified as associated with organic chemical exposure in occupational epidemiology. Bladder cancer incidence increased 72% in males and 24% in females from the late 1940s to 1983–1984. The increases appear in all age groups, although are more marked in the older ages. Part of the increase is likely to be artifactual because of the difficulty in differential diagnosis or differences in terminology among papillomas, carcinomas in situ, and malignant cancer. While incidence increased, mortality rates decreased; the contrast probably reflects diagnostic artifacts as well as improvements in treatment. As much as 40% to 50% of bladder cancer among males and 30% among females may be attributable to cigarette smoking, but even this does not fully explain the sex differential, suggesting a possible environmental exposure (Devesa et al., 1987).

Cutaneous malignant melanoma was among the most rapidly increasing cancers in terms of incidence and mortality in the period from the late 1940s to 1984. Most of the increase occurred during the 1970s. The increases are mostly among middle age groups rather than older ages. Sunlight is clearly involved in producing melanoma, but the relationship is not as clear as is the case for basal cell and squamous cell carcinoma. Unlike other skin cancers, outdoor workers do not have higher rates than people who are outdoors only intermittently and anatomic sites with lower (or more infrequent) sun exposure have higher melanoma rates. Cumulative hours of sun exposure apparently is not the appropriate measure of exposure. Frequency of exposure of sunlight to skin unprotected by suntan may be a better index. It is not clear whether changing patterns of exposure such as sunbathing or clothing style accounts entirely for the increasing trend or if other factors may have contributed to the trend.

Apportionment of Environmental Factors

In their seminal analysis of proportions of cancer deaths attributable to various causes, Doll and Peto (1981) attribute the largest fraction (35%) to dietary factors. They note that this figure is highly speculative and estimate acceptable estimates might range from 10% to 70%. They note that these dietary factors are not yet reliably identified, but suggest that the most likely causes are not traces of powerful carcinogens in food, but rather major components and characteristics of the food itself. This is supported by recent work by Ames et al. (1987).

The second, more specific and reliable cause of cancer is tobacco (30%). The range of acceptable estimates for the fraction of cancer deaths attributable to tobacco was given as 25–40%. Ten percent of cancer deaths were attribted to infection and seven percent to reproductive and sexual behavior.

The fraction of current cancer deaths attributed to occupational exposure, pollution, medicines, medical procedures, and industrial and commercial products was small; all of these combined were estimated to contribute less then 10% of cancer deaths. It is this 10% that is the focus of most cancer risk assessments. What of the massive introduction of synthetic organic chemicals into the environment? What of the acclaimed and predicted "cancer epidemic"? New chemical exposures could indeed add increments to the current cancer rate. Moreover, assessments of these exposures and their risks aid in planning technological development. Once recognized, many occupational and some public exposures can be reduced or eliminated by practicable means. But the increase in exposure to industrial chemicals began in the 1800s and has been rising rapidly since the middle of this century. Enough time has passed to expect to see the beginnings of the effect. Doll and Peto (1981) report that while "The human evidence that is currently available does not allow us to express any confident opinion about the extent of the harm that the introduction of these substances may or may not do in the future. The trends that are are being recorded do not, however, suggest that the United States (or Britain. . .) is beginning to experience an epidemic of cancer due to new factors."

ECONOMIC AND SOCIAL IMPACTS OF CANCER*

Cancer may produce pain, suffering, loss of a body part, impaired speech, disfigurement, disability, and death. It can bring personal catastrophy for the victims and their families either as a direct result of the disease or indirectly through its economic consequences. These may include social isolation, unwanted job changes, loss of promotion and educational opportunities, home relocation, and economic dependence. The environment surrounding a cancer case may create anxiety, reduced self-esteem, resentment, and emotional problems. Social costs fall on the victims, their families, friends, co-workers, and care givers. Most families with a member suffering from advanced cancer need help to maintain family stability. Social costs are difficult to quantify, particularly in monitary terms. Attempts to estimate these costs established a minimum social cost of cancer, excluding costs associated with death, of $2.5 billion in 1975.

Aside from its social aspects, cancer places a large economic burden on society. Neoplasms have been estimated to account for 8 to 9% of total costs associated with illness in the United States. Economic costs are divided into direct and indirect. Direct costs include costs of hospitalization, nursing home care, physicians' and nurses' services, and drugs. Indirect costs include costs of time lost from work. Costs of early death from cancer, including future earnings lost, are calculated based on age at death and normal expectation of life at that age. The total economic

TABLE 2-5 Estimated Direct Expenditures for Neoplasms, 1975

Type of expenditure	Amount in millions
Hospital care	$4,134
Physicians' services	671
Other professional services	50
Drugs and drug sundries	203
Nursing home care	221
Total	$5,279

Source: From Rice and Hodgson, 1981.

*Much of this section draws on Rice and Hodgson (1981).

TABLE 2-6 Estimated Indirect Costs of Neoplasms, 1975, by Patient Category

Patient category	Amount in millions
Morbidity	
Currently employed	$422
Keeping house	194
Unable to work	440
Institutionalized	49
Total	$1,105
Mortality (at 6% discount rate)	$15,974

Source: From Rice and Hodgson, 1981.

cost of cancer in 1975 was estimated to be between $19 and $28 billion, of which $5.3 billion were direct costs. Breakdowns of total direct and indirect costs are given in Tables 2-5 and 2-6. Different cancers involve different costs. Breakdowns of direct and indirect costs by cancer site are given in Tables 2-7 and 2-8. These are 1975 estimates; current values will vary not only due to inflation but due to increases in cancer incidence and changes in the mix of cancers.

TABLE 2-7 Estimated Direct Expenditures (in Millions of Dollars) for Hospital Costs and Physicians' Services Due to Neoplasm, 1975, by Cancer Site

Site of malignant neoplasms	Hospital	Physicians' visits
Digestive organs	$670	$114
Respiratory organs	494	78
Skin	84	46
Breast	344	84
Female genital organs	298	74
Male genital organs	169	51
Leukemia	131	24
Other malignant neoplasms	255	259
Benign and site unspecified	916	515

Source: From Rice and Hodgson, 1981.

TABLE 2-8 Person-Years Lost Per Death Due to Neoplasms and Estimated
Total Value of Earnings Lost Due to Cancer Deaths in 1975

Site of malignant neoplasms	Person-year lost/death	Total 1975 cost
Buccal cavity and pharynx	16.0	408
Stomach	13.4	487
Intestine and rectum	13.6	1,510
Other digestive organs	14.3	1,229
Trachea, lung, and bronchus	15.4	3,826
Other respiratory organs	15.5	226
Bone, connective, and other soft tissue	24.3	255
Skin	19.3	377
Breast	20.0	1,537
Cervix uteri	22.5	327
Other parts of uterus	16.2	163
Other female genital organs	19.3	489
Male genital organs	10.1	402
Urinary organs	13.3	522
Other and unspecified sites	17.8	1,807
Leukemia	21.2	898
Other lymphatic and hematopoietic tissues	17.7	1,068
Total malignant neoplasms	16.0	$15,530
Benign neoplasms and neoplasms of unspecified nature	23.2	$339

Source: From Rice and Hodgson, 1981.

REFERENCES

Ames, B.N., R. Magaw, and L.S. Gold. 1987. Ranking possible carcinogenic hazards. Science 236:271–280.

Ames, B.N. and L.S. Gold. 1988a. Letter. Science 238:1634.

Ames, B.N. and L.S. Gold. 1988b. (response). Science 240:1045–1047.

Anderson, M.W. 1987. Issues in biochemical applications to risk assessment: how do we evaluate individual components of multistage models? Environ. Health Perspect. 76:175–179.

Armenian, H.K. and A.M. Lilienfeld. 1974. The distribution of incubation periods of neoplastic diseases, Am. J Epidemiol. 99:92–100.

Barrett, J.C. and R.W. Wiseman. 1987. Cellular and molecular mechanisms of multistep carcinogenesis: relevance to carcinogenic risk assessment. *Environ. Health Perspect.* 76:65–70.

Bishop, J.M. 1987. The molecular genetics of cancer. *Science* 235:305–311.

Bos, J.L. 1988. The ras gene family and human carcinogenesis. *Mutation Res.* 195:255–271.

Cairns, J., J.L. Lyon, and M. Skolnick (eds.).1980. *Cancer Incidence in Defined Populations*, Banbury Report No. 4. Cold Spring Harbor Laboratory, Cold Spring Harbor, New York.

Davis, D.L. 1988. (letter). *Science* 238:1633–1634.

Devesa, S.S. and E.L. Diamond. 1983. Socioeconomic and racial differences in lung cancer incidence. *Am. J Epidemiol.* 118:818–831.

Devesa, S.S. and D.T. Silverman. 1978. Cancer incidence and mortality trends in the United States, 1935-74. *J. Natl. Cancer Inst.* 60:545–571.

Devesa, S.S. and D.T. Silverman. 1980. Trends in incidence and mortality in the United States. *J. Environ. Pathol. and Toxicol.* 3:127–155.

Devesa, S.S., D.T. Silverman, J.L. Young, Jr., E.S. Pollack, C.C. Brown, J.W. Horm, C.L. Percy, M.H. Myers, F.W. McKay, and J.F. Fraumeni, Jr. 1987. Cancer incidence and mortality trends among whites in the United States, 1947–1984. *J. Natl. Cancer Inst.* 79:701–770.

Doll, R. and R. Peto. 1981. The causes of cancer: quantitative estimates of avoidable risks of cancer in the United States today. *J. Natl. Cancer Inst.* 66:1192–1308.

Enstrom, J.E. and D.F. Austin. 1977. Interpreting cancer survival rates, *Science* 195:847–851.

Enstrom, J.E. 1979. Rising lung cancer mortality among nonsmokers. *J National Cancer Institute* 62:755–760.

Epstein, S.S., J.B. Swartz (and 15 co-signers). 1988. Carcinogenic risk estimation, *Science* 240:1043–1045.

Garfinkel, L. 1980. Cancer mortality in nonsmokers: prospective study by the American Cancer Society. *J. National Cancer Institute* 65:1169–1173.

Goldsmith, J.R. 1980. The "urban factor" in cancer: smoking, industrial exposures, and air pollutio as possible explanations. *J. Environ. Pathol. and Toxicol.* 3:205–217.

Guidelines. 1986. Guidelines on the use of mutagenicity tests in the toxicological evaluation of chemicals, a report of the environmental Contaminants Advisory Committee on Mutagenesis. Department of National Health and Welfare, Ottawa, Canada.

Horm, J.W., A.J. asire, J.L. Young, Jr., and E.S. Pollack. 1985. SEER Program: Cancer incidence and Mortality in the United States 1973–81 (NIH Publication No. 85-1837). National Cancer Institute, Bethesda, MD.

Hutter, R.W.P. 1988. Cancer prevention and detection: status report and future prospects. *Cancer* 61 (suppl): 2372–2378.

Klein, G. 1987. The approaching era of the tumor suppressor genes. *Science* 238:1539–1545.

Land, H., L.F. Parada, and R.A. Weinberg. 1983. Cellular oncogenes and multi-step carcinogenesis. *Science* 222:771–778.

Lyon, J.L., J.W. Gardner, and D.W. West. 1980. Cancer risk and life-style: cancer among Mormons from 1967 to 1975. In J. Cairns, J.L. Lyon, and M. Skolnick (eds.), *Cancer Incidence in Defined Populations*, Banbury Report No. 4. Cold Spring Harbor Laboratory, Cold Spring Harbor, New York, pp. 3–28.

Morris, S.C. 1982. Impact of energy and industrial pollution on public health, in R.R. Tice, D.L. Costa, and K.M. Schaich (eds.), *Genotoxic Effects of Airborne Agents*. Plenum Press, New York, pp. 555–574.

NCHS. 1984. Multiple causes of death in the United States. Final Data from the National Center for Health Statistics. *Monthly Vital Statistics Report* 32 (10), February 17. U.S. Department of Health and Human Services, Hyattsville, MD.

NCHS. 1987. Annual summary of births, marriages, divorces, and deaths: United States, 1986, National Center for Health Statistics. *Monthly Vital Statistics Report* 35 (13): 20, August 24, U.S. Department of Health and Human Services, Hyattsville, MD.

OTA. 1981. Assessment of Technologies for Determining Cancer Risks from the Environment. Office of Technology Assessment, Washington. D.C.

Parkin, D.M., E. Laara, and C.S. Muir. 1988. Estimates of the worldwide frequency of sixteen major cancers in 1980. *Int. J. Cancer* 41:184–197.

Pitot, H.C. and H.A. Campbell. 1987. An approach to the determination of the relative potencies of chemical agents during the stages of initiation and promotion in multistage hepatocarcinogenesis in the rat. *Environ. Health Perspect.* 76:49–56.

Pollack, C.S. and J.W. Horm. 1980. Trends in cancer incidence and mortality in the United States, 1969–76. *J. Natl. Cancer Inst.* 64:1091–1103.

Rice, D.P. and T.A. Hodgson. 1981. Social and economic implications of cancer in the United States (DHHS Publ No. PHS 81-1404). National Center for Health Statistics, Hyattsville, MD.

Ries, L.G., E.S. Pollack, and J.L. Young, Jr. 1983. Cancer patient survival: surveillance, epidemiology, and end results program, 1973–79. *J. Natl. Cancer Inst.* 70:693–707.

Robertson, L.S. 1980. Environmental correlates of intercity variation in age-adjusted cancer mortality rates, *Environ. Health Perspect.* 36:197–203.

Rous, P. and J.W. Beard. 1939. As cited by Klein, 1987.

Schneiderman, M.A. 1980. Reported in Toxic Chemicals and Public Protection, Toxic Substances Strategy Committee. U.S. Government Printing Office, Washington, D.C., pp. 161–165.

Sutherland, R.M. 1988. Cell and environment interactions in tumor microregions: the multicell spheroid model. *Science* 240:177–184.

Thomas, R.D. (ed). 1986. Mechanisms of carcinogenesis. In *Drinking Water and Health*, Volume 6. National Academy Press, Washington, D.C., pp. 139–167.

Vitetta, E.S., R.J. Fulton, R.D. May, M. Till, and J.W. Uhr. 1987. Redesigning nature's poisons to create anti-tumor reagents. *Science* 238:1098–1104.

Weinberg, R.A. 1988. The genetic origins of human cancer. *Cancer* 61:1963–1968.
WHO. 1977. *Manual of the International Statistical Classification of Diseases, Injuries, and Causes of Death* (ninth revision). World Health Organization, Geneva.

APPENDIX I   Major Cancer Categories of the International Classification of Diseases (WHO, 1977)

ICD Code	Classification
140	Malignant neoplasm of lip
141	Malignant neoplasm of tongue
142	Malignant neoplasm of major salivary glands
143	Malignant neoplasm of gum
144	Malignant neoplasm of floor of mouth
145	Malignant neoplasm of other and unspecified parts of mouth
146	Malignant neoplasm of oropharynx
147	Malignant neoplasm of nasopharynx
148	Malignant neoplasm of hypopharynx
149	Malignant neoplasm of other and ill-defined sites within the lip, oral cavity and pharynx
150	Malignant neoplasm of oesophagus
151	Malignant neoplasm of stomach
152	Malignant neoplasm of small intestine, including duodenum
153	Malignant neoplasm of colon
154	Malignant neoplasm of rectum, rectosigmoid junction and anus
155	Malignant neoplasm of liver and intrahepatic bile ducts
156	Malignant neoplasm of gallbladder and extrahepatic bile ducts
157	Malignant neoplasm of pancreas
158	Malignant neoplasm of retroperitoneum and peritoneum
159	Malignant neoplasm of other and ill-defined sites within the digestive organs and peritoneum
160	Malignant neoplasm of nasal cavities, middle ear and accessory sinuses
161	Malignant neoplasm of larynx
162	Malignant neoplasm of trachea, bronchus and lung
163	Malignant neoplasm of pleura
164	Malignant neoplasm of thymus, heart and mediastinum
165	Malignant neoplasm of other and ill-defined sites within the respiratory system and intrathoracic organs
170	Malignant neoplasm of bone and articular cartilage
171	Malignant neoplasm of connective and other soft tissue
172	Malignant melanoma of skin

APPENDIX I *Continued.*

ICD Code	Classification
173	Other malignant neoplasm of skin
174	Malignant neoplasm of female breast
175	Malignant neoplasm of male breast
179	Malignant neoplasm of uterus, part unspecified
180	Malignant neoplasm of cervix uteri
181	Malignant neoplasm of placenta
182	Malignant neoplasm of body of uterus
183	Malignant neoplasm of ovary and other uterine adnexa
184	Malignant neoplasm of other and unspecified female genital organs
185	Malignant neoplasm of prostate
186	Malignant neoplasm of testis
187	Malignant neoplasm of penis and other male genital organs
188	Malignant neoplasm of bladder
189	Malignant neoplasm of kidney and other and unspecified urinary organs
190	Malignant neoplasm of eye
191	Malignant neoplasm of brain
192	Malignant neoplasm of other and unspecified parts of nervous system
193	Malignant neoplasm of thyroid gland
194	Malignant neoplasm of other endocrine glands and related structures
195	Malignant neoplasm of other and ill-defined sites
196	Secondary and unspecified malignant neoplasm of lymph nodes
197	Secondary malignant neoplasm of respiratory and digestive systems
198	Secondary malignant neoplasm of other specified sites
199	Malignant neoplasm without specification of site
200	Lymphosarcoma and reticulosarcoma
201	Hodgkin's disease
202	Other malignant neoplasm of lymphoid and histiocytic tissue
203	Multiple myeloma and immunoproliferative neoplasm
204	Lymphoid leukaemia
205	Myeloid leukaemia
206	Monocytic leukaemia
207	Other specified leukaemia
208	Leukaemia of unspecified cell type
210	Benign neoplasm of lip, oral cavity and pharynx
211	Benign neoplasm of other parts of digestive system
212	Benign neoplasm of respiratory and intrathoracic organs
213	Benign neoplasm of bone and articular cartilage
214	Lipoma
215	Other benign neoplasm of connective and other soft tissue

APPENDIX I *Continued.*

ICD Code	Classification
216	Benign neoplasm of skin
217	Benign neoplasm of breast
218	Uterine leiomyoma
219	Other benign neoplams of uterus
220	Benign neoplasm of ovary
221	Benign neoplasm of other female genital organs
222	Benign neoplasm of male genital organs
223	Benign neoplasm of kidney and other urinary organs
224	Benign neoplasm of eye
225	Benign neoplasm of brain and other parts of nervous system
226	Benign neoplasm of thyroid gland
227	Benign neoplasm of other endocrine glands and related structures
228	Haemangioma and lymphangioma, any site
229	Benign neoplasm of other and unspecified sites
230	Carcinoma in situ of digestive organs
231	Carcinoma in situ of respiratory system
232	Carcinoma in situ of skin
233	Carcinoma in situ of breast and genitourinary system
234	Carcinoma in situ of other and unspecified sites
235	Neoplasm of uncertain behaviour of digestive and respiratory systems
236	Neoplasm of uncertain behaviour of genitourinary organs
237	Neoplasm of uncertain behaviour of endocrine glands and nervous system
238	Neoplasm of uncertain behaviour of other and unspecified sites and tissues
239	Neoplasm of unspecified nature

APPENDIX II Major Categories of Histological Type of Neoplasms (WHO, 1977)

Code	Type
M805-M808	Papillary and squamous cell neoplasms
M809-M811	Basal cell neoplasms
M812-M813	Transitial cell papillomas and carcinomas
M814-M838	Adenomas and adenocarcinomas
M839-M842	Adnexal and skin appendage neoplasms
M843	Mucoepidermoid neoplasms
M844-M849	Cystic, mucinous and serous neoplasms
M850-M854	Ductal, lobular and medullary neoplasms
M855	Acinar cell neoplasms
M856-M858	Complex epithelial neoplasms
M859-M867	Specialized gonadal neoplasms

APPENDIX II *Continued.*

ICD Code	Classification
M868-M871	Paragangliomas and glomus tumours
M872-M879	Naevi and melanomas
M880	Soft tissue tumours and sarcomas not otherwise specified
M881-M883	Fibromatous neoplasms
M884	Myxomatous neoplasms
M885-M888	Lipomatous neoplasms
M889-M892	Myomatous neoplasms
M893-M899	Complex mixed and stromal neoplasms
M900-M903	Fibroepithelial neoplasms
M904	Synovial neoplasms
M905	Mesothelial neoplasms
M906-M909	Germ cell neoplasms
M910	Trophoblastic neoplasms
M911	Mesonephromas
M912-M916	Blood vessel tumours
M917	Lymphatic vessel tumours
M918-M920	Osteomas and osteosarcomas
M921-M924	Chondromatous neoplasms
M925	Giant cell tumours
M926	Miscellaneous bone tumours
M927-M934	Odontogenic tumours
M935-M937	Miscellaneous tumors
M938-M948	Gliomas
M949-M952	Neuroepitheliomatous neoplasms
M953	Meningiomas
M954-M957	Nerve sheath tumour
M958	Granular cell tumours and alveolar soft part sarcoma
M959-M963	Lymophomas, not otherwise specified or diffuse
M964	Reticulosarcomas
M965-M966	Hodgkin's disease
M969	Lymphomas, nodular or follicular
M970	Mycosis fungoides
M971-M972	Miscellaneous reticuloendothelial neoplasms
M973	Plasma cell tumours
M974	Mast cell tumours
M975	Burkitt's tumour
M980-M994	Leukaemias
M995-M997	Miscellaneous myeloproliferative and lymphoproliferative disorders

3

Hazard Identification

Hazard identification is a qualitative evaluation of an agent's ability to produce cancer and the relevance of this to humans (OSTP, 1984). Most current bioassay work today is aimed at answering this qualitative question. The question is complex. Seldom is sufficient evidence avaliable to clearly demonstrate a cancer risk to humans. Epidemiological studies are always troubled by potentially confounding factors and seldom have adequate exposure estimates to associate observed effects with specific agents. Animal studies and short-term tests in simpler organisms are usually more definitive, but their applicability to humans can be questionable.

Hazard identification can be initiated in various ways and can include many different methods. Sometimes cancer hazards are identified quite by accident rather than in an activity organized for the purpose. Hazard identification is itself, however, a complex process. The NAS committee on risk assessment (1983) drew up 25 questions focused on cancer risks that needed to be addressed in the hazard assessment process (Table 3-1). These questions do not have single, correct answers. Some imply quantitative analysis. Hazard assessment ranges from an informal process to formal procedures established in regulations or in law. It requires interdisciplinary evaluation of a broad range of information (Interdisciplinary Panel, 1984). It is a crucial step, since if no hazard is identified, the risk assessment usually stops. In addition, hazard identification defines the character of the risk to be assessed in later stages; if it is misdirected, the entire process may go askew. Several government regulatory agencies have established their own criteria (e.g., OSHA, 1980; EPA, 1986a).

HAZARD IDENTIFICATION AS AN INDEPENDENT PROCESS

Hazard identification has a history on its own, and has been built into law, regulation, and practice as an independent activity. Many laws and regulations base cancer risk management entirely on hazard identification.

TABLE 3-1   Components in Hazard Identification

A. Epidemiologic Data

What relative weights should be given to studies with differing results? For example, should positive results outweigh negative results if the studies that yield them are comparable? Should a study be weighted in accord with its statistical power?

What relative weights should be given to results of different types of epidemiologic studies? For example, should the findings of a prospective study supersede those of a case-control study, or those of a case-control study of an ecologic study?

What statistical significance should be required for results to be considered positive?

Does a study have special characteristics (such as the questionable appropriateness of the control group) that lead one to question the validity of its results?

What is the significance of a positive finding in a study in which the route of exposure is different from that of a population at potential risk?

Should evidence on different types of responses be weighted or combined (e.g., data on different tumor sites and data on benign versus malignant tumors)?

B. Animal Bioassay Data

What degree of confirmation of positive results should be necessary? Is a positive result from a single animal study sufficient, or should positive results from two or more animal studies be required? Should negative results be disregarded or given less weight?

Should a study be weighted according to its quality and statistical power?

How should evidence of different metabolic pathways or vastly different metabolic rates between animals and humans be factored into a risk assessment?

How should the occurrence of rare tumors be treated? Should the appearance of rare tumors in a treated group be considered evidence of carcinogenicity even if the finding is not statistically significant?

How should experimental-animal data be used when the exposure routes in experimental animals and humans are different?

Should a dose-related increased in tumors be discounted when the tumors in question have high or extremely variable spontaneous rates?

What statistical significance should be required for results to be considered positive?

Does an experiment have special characteristics (e.g., the presence of carcinogenic contaminants in the test substance) that lead one to question the validity of its results?

How should findings of tissue damage or other toxic effects be used in the interpretation of tumor data? Should evidence that tumors may have resulted from these effects be taken to mean that they would not be expected to occur at lower doses?

TABLE 3-1 *Continued*

Should benign and malignant lesions be counted equally?

Into what categories should tumors be grouped for statistical purposes?

Should only increases in the numbers of tumors be considered, or should a decrease in the latent period for tumor occurrence also be used as evidence of carcinogenicity?

C. Short-Term Test Data

How much weight whould be placed on the results of various short-term tests?

What degree of confidence do short-term tests add to the results of animal bioassay in the evaluation of carcinogenic risks for humans?

Should in vitro transformation tests be accorded more weight than bacterial mutagenicity tests in seeking evidence of possible carcinogenic effect?

What statistical significance should be required for results to be considered positive?

How should different results of comparable tests be weighted? Should positive results be accorded greater weight than negative results?

D. Structural Similarity to Known Carcinogens

What additional weight does structural similarity add to the results of animal bioassays in the evaluation of carcinogenic risks for humans?

E. General

What is the overall weight of the evidence of carcinogenicity? (This determination must include a judgment of the *quality* of the data presented in the preceding sections.)

*F. National Toxicology Program Decision Criteria for Classification of Results of
    Animal Cancer Bioassay*

Clear evidence of carcinogenicity is demonstrated by studies that are interpreted as showing a chemically related increased incidence of malignant neoplasms, or studies that exhibit a substantially increased incidence of benign neoplasms with each increase with dose.

Some evidence of carcinogenicity is demonstrated by studies that are interpreted as showing a chemically related increased incidence of benign neoplasms, studies that exhibit marginal increases in neoplasms of several organs/tissues, or studies that exhibit a slight increase in uncommon malignant or benign neoplasms.

Equivocal evidence of carcinogenicity is demonstrated by studies that are interpreted as showing a chemically related marginal increase of neoplasms.

TABLE 3-1 *Continued*

No evidence of carcinogenicity is demonstrated by studies that are interpreted as showing no chemically related increases in malignant or benign neoplasms.

Inadequate study of carcinogenicity demonstrates that because of major qualitative or quantitative limitations, the studies cannot be interpreted as valid for showing either the presence or absence of a carcinogenic effect.

Source: From NAS, 1983.

There are great social, political, and economic consequences of a substance simply being named a carcinogen. It is not an action taken lightly.

Agencies define carefully the criteria by which they determine a material to be carcinogenic and the methods used to develop and analyse the data to which the criteria are applied. These policies are often expressed as guidelines. The political and scientific controversies involved in setting cancer policies and the ways in which those policies express attitudes toward risk are explored by Rushefsky (1986). Rushefsky defines these cancer policy guidelines as documents that

1. Guide decisions;
2. Inform both those inside and outside the agency how information on carcinogenesis will be treated;
3. Provide uniformity to the decision-making process rather than deal with each carcinogen on an ad hoc basis, developing all the rules from scratch; and
4. In some cases describe the state of the science.

Essentially, such policies provide answers to some or all of the NAS questions in Table 3-1.

The National Toxicology Program (NTP) established five "categories of interpretative conclusions" in 1983, by which the results of animal bioassays would be classified. The criteria used was that the decision would be made on the basis of the strength of the experimental evidence rather than potency level or mechanism (Table 3-2). These guidelines are defined for a rather narrow purpose dealing with the interpretation of animal studies. Guidelines such as those established by the Environmental Protection Agency (EPA, 1986b), the Occupational Safety and Health Administration (OSHA, 1980), the Interagency Regulatory Liaison Group (IRLG, 1979), or the Office of Science and Technology Policy (OSTP, 1984) tend to be broader. These directly address more fundamental questions such as the degree to which long-term animal studies or short-

TABLE 3-2 Sources of Biomedical Evidence Specifically Considered in EPA
Cancer Risk Assessment Guidelines

1.   Physical–chemical properties and routes and patterns of exposure
2.   Structure–activity relationships
3.   Metabolic and pharmacokinetic properties
4.   Toxicologic effects
5.   Short-term tests
6.   Long-term animal tests
7.   Human studies

Source: From EPA, 1986.

term in vitro studies may be relied on at all in determining a material's
carcinogenicity.

The IRLG was formed in 1977 specifically to coordinate cancer policy
among the four major regulatory agencies with jurisdiction (EPA, OSHA,
the Food and Drug Administration, and the Consumer Product Safety
Commission). Its report (IRLG, 1979) was influential in formulating later
policy, although its overall mission was unsuccessful and its mandate has
lapsed. Two important contributions made in this report were (1) to
provide a basis for quantitative risk analysis and quantitative extrapolation
of human risks from animals and (2) in quantitative estimation of risk, to
place equal emphasis on characterization of population exposure as on
the biomedical and statistical aspects of dose-response.

EPA (1986b) guidelines give hazard identification equal weight with
the combination of dose-response assessment, exposure assessment, and
risk characterization. They define hazard assessment as the review and
qualitative evaluation "of the relevant biological and chemical information
bearing on whether or not an agent may pose a carcinogenic hazard." All
sources of biomedical evidence are considered (Table 3-3). Attributes of
these sources of evidence are considered in later chapters in detail. The
decision on carcinogenecity is based on the "weight of evidence," but in
calculating this, EPA does not count all the sources of evidence equally.
The evidence from human and animal studies is characterized individually,
then a combined evaluation of the weight of evidence for human carcinogenicity considering both sources of data is made. Finally, this conclusion
is modified as appropriate based on evidence from all the other sources.

This process has been formalized by EPA (1986b), based on an approach of the International Agency for Research on Cancer. EPA makes

TABLE 3-3 Criteria and Supporting Factors for (A) Demonstration of a Causal Relationship in Human Data by EPA and (B) Increase Confidence in Inferring a Causal Association

---

A.
1. There is no identified bias that could explain the association
2. The possibility of confounding has been considered and ruled out as explaining the association
3. The association is unlikely to be due to chance

B.
1. Several independent studies are concordant in showing the association
2. The association is strong
3. There is a dose-response relationship
4. A reduction in exposure is followed by a reduction in the incidence of cancer

---

Source: From EPA, 1986.

clear that this procedure is not meant to be applied rigidly or mechanically as the scientific data usually has a complexity that cannot be captured by any classifiction scheme.

For human evidence, three criteria and four supporting factors are considered for demonstration of a causal relationship (Table 3-4). Given these criteria, the weight of evidence for carcinogenicity from studies in humans is classified into five categories (Table 3-5). For animal studies,

TABLE 3-4 EPA Weight of Evidence Categories for Human Data on Carcinogenicity

---

1. *Sufficient evidence of carcinogenicity*, which indicates that there is a causal relationship between the agent and human cancer
2. *Limited evidence of carcinogenicity*, which indicates that a causal interpretation is credible, but that alternative explanations, such as chance, bias or confounding could not adequately be excluded
3. *Inadequate evidence*, which indicates that one of two conditions prevailed:
    a. there were few pertinent data, or
    b. the available studies, while showing evidence of association, did not exclude chance, bias, or confounding and therefore a causal interpretation is not credible
4. *No data*, which indicates that data are not available
5. *No evidence*, which indicates that no association was found between exposure and an increased risk of cancer in well-designed and well-conducted independent analytical epidemiologic studies

---

Source: From EPA, 1986.

TABLE 3-5 EPA Weight of Evidence Categories for Animal Data on Carcinogenicity

---

1. *Sufficient evidence of carcinogenicity*, indicates that there is an increased incidence of malignant tumors or combined malignant and benign tumors:
   a. In multiple species or strains
   b. In multiple experiments (e.g., with different routes of administration or using different dose levels)
   c. To an unusual degree in a single experiment with regard to high incidence, unusual site or type of tumor, or early age at onset
   Additional evidence may be provided by data on dose-response effects, as well as information from short-term tests or on chemical structure
2. *Limited evidence of carcinogenicity* means that the data suggest a carcinogenic effect but are limited because
   a. The studies involve a single species, strain, or experiment and do not meet criteria for sufficient evidence
   b. The experiments are restricted by inadequate dosage levels, inadequate duration of exposure to the agent, inadequate period of follow-up, poor survival, too few animals, or inadequate reporting
   c. An increase in the incidence of benign tumors only
3. *Inadequate evidence* indicates that because of major qualitative or quantitative limitations, the studies cannot be interpreted as showing either the presence or absence of a carcinogenic effect
4. *No data* indicates that data are not available
5. *No evidence* indicates that there is no increased incidence of neoplasms in at least two well-designed and well conducted animal studies in different species

---

Source: From EPA, 1986.

weight of evidence is classified among the same five groups, although the criteria differ slightly. The classifications from human and animal studies are then combined to draw a conclusion as to the carcinogenic status of the material under study. The agent is put in one of five categories (Table 3-6). The guidelines illustrate the decision process. In the absence of strong evidence from one of the sources of information in Table 3-3, the conclusion appears to be rigidly directed. On the other hand, the classification of evidence for human and animal studies individually necessarily leaves considerable room for scientific judgment and interpretation.

TABLE 3-6 EPA Categories of Carcinogenic Status for Tested Agents

Group A: Human Carcinogen

This group is used only when there is sufficient evidence from epidemiologic studies to support a causal association between exposure to the agents and cancer.

Group B: Probable Human Carcinogen

This group includes agents for which the weight of evidence of human carcinogenicity based on epidemiologic studies is "limited" and also includes agents for which the weight of evidence of carcinogenicity based on animal studies is "sufficient." The group is divided into two subgroups. Usually, Group B1 is reserved for agents for which there is limited evidence of carcinogenicity from epidemiologic studies. It is reasonable, for practical purposes, to regard an agent for which there is "sufficient" evidence of carcinogenicity in animals as if it presented a carcinogenic risk to humans. Therefore, agents for which there is "sufficient" evidence from animal studies and for which there is "inadequate evidence" or "no data" from epidemiologic studies would usually be categorized under Group B2.

Group C: Possible Human Carcinogen

This group is used for agent with limited evidence of carcinogenicity in animals in the absence of human data. It includes a wide variety of evidence, e.g. (a) a malignant tumor response in a single well-conducted experiment that does not meet conditions for sufficient evidence, (b) tumor responses of marginal statistical significance in studies having inadequate design or reporting, (c) benign but not malignant tumors with an agent showing no response in a variety of short-term tests for mutagenicity, and (d) responses of marginal statistical significance in a tissue known to have a high or variable background rate.

Group D: Not Classifiable as to Human Carcinogenicity

This group is generally used for agents with inadequate human and animal evidence of carcinogenicity or for which no data are available.

Group E: Evidence of Noncarcinogenicity for Humans

This group is used for agents that show no evidence for carcinogenicity in at least two adequate animal tests in different species or in both adequate epidemiologic and animal studies

Source: From EPA, 1986b.

HAZARD IDENTIFICATION AS A STEP IN QUANTITATIVE CANCER RISK ASSESSMENT

As more emphasis is placed on the quantitative aspects of risk, the identi-fication of a substance as a carcinogen becomes only one stage in the entire risk assessment process. Thus, hazard identification itself comes to have less significance. The objective for hazard identification is reduced to a finding that there was sufficient evidence to warrent the effort of a further, quantitative, assessment, similar to the way a grand jury does not convict, but only determines if there is enough evidence to warrant a trial. This is not to say that hazard assessment becomes unimportant. It still remains the first step in the process. If the hazard is not identified, the assessment process stops, or gets off on the wrong track.

As it becomes part of a broader process, changes will occur in the definition of what constitutes it and in the methods used. The role of hazard assessment in quantitative cancer risk assessment is thus still de-veloping. This development, however, will reflect its prior, independent role. Consider the range of possibilities. In the current approach, The qualitative decision in hazard identification acts as a screening tool for a more extensive (and expensive) quantitative step. As an extreme alterna-tive, one could essentially bypass the qualitative question and focus im-mediately on quantitation. Any extensive hazard assessment requires the same basic kind of data that is needed in a quantitative assessment. The degree of uncertainty on this qualitative question, whether a substance is or is not a carcinogen, is also reflected in the degree of uncertainty on the quantitative estimate of potency. That is, if there is insufficient evidence to prove at the 95% level that a substance is a carcinogen, then the 95% confidence bounds on a calculated quantitative estimate will include zero—no effect. Regulations that could take into account the degree of uncertainty and the estimated quantitative impact might allow the limits of the two to be varied together. For example, given the same level of uncertainty, it might make sense to have increasingly stringent regulatory controls as the estimated quantitative impact increases and as the esti-mated uncertainty level decreases. Substances which can be "proven" to be carcinogens in the laboratory but which are estimated to have relatively inconsequential quantitative effects (say producing 1 cancer every 10 years), would be ignored by regulatory agencies. On the other hand, a substance which could not meet the necessary qualative "proof" for carcinogenicity, might be regulated if its potential effects were sufficiently high. This approach to regulation could be made as "conservative" as desired, in that it would lead to regulation of chemicals with a given probability that they might be carcinogenic. Risk is often defined as the probability of a bad event occurring (p) times the consequences given the bad event occurs (C given p). Usually, this concept is applied to accidents; if an accident sequence occurs, a release of y amount will result, leading to z cancers. If the probability of the accident is p, the risk is p.z. The same mathematical formulation can apply equally well to the uncertain quality of carcinogenicity: a continual exposure to y results in z cancers with uncertainty expressed as a probability, p. Here, also, the risk is p.z. Thus, changes in the role of hazard identification and movement toward quantitative assessment could lead to entirely different approaches to regulation than now used.

HAZARD ASSESSMENT

Hazard assessment is closely identified with risk assessment. The term is variously defined, but generally means something less than a full quantitative evaluation of risk and something more than hazard identification, which focuses almost entirely on dose–response properties of a material. It is often used in industrial environmental auditing where the focus is frequently on examination of hardware and of the probabilities of release of toxic agents (e.g., World Bank, 1985; Ozog and Benedixen, 1987).

A good example of a rather formal hazard assessment procedure which has its own legal implications, but which also can trigger a more detailed risk assessment is the procedure set up by EPA to deal with a requirement of the Comprehensive Environmental Response, Compensation, and Liability Act of 1980 (CERCLA). CERCLA establishes "reportable quantities" of hazardous materials; releases above the reportable quantity must be reported, leading to a chain of legal consequences. EPA can adjust the original reportable quantities based on an hazard assessment. Since there were over 700 CERCLA hazardous substances, many of which are potential carcinogens, a formal procedure was required to assure consistency in their treatment. The procedure proposed involved a double ranking system, one based on a qualitative evaluation and one on a quantitative evaluation (EPA, 1986a). In the first ranking, four literature sources were reviewed to determine if the substance was cited as a possible carcinogen. These sources were (1) the Annual Reports on Carcinogens of the National Toxicology Program; (2) the Monographs of the International Agency for Research on Cancer (IARC, 1972 et seq.); (3) final Agency determinations published in the *Federal Register* identifying substances as potential carcinogens; and (4) ongoing determinations by the Agency's Office of Health and Environmental Assessment that substances may be potential carcinogens. Then a "weight of evidence" approach similar to that described above was to be applied, ranking the evidence in the same categories as listed in Table 3-6. In the quantitative ranking scheme, the estimated dose of the substance which would be associated with a lifetime cancer risk of 10% (the ED_{10}) was calculated by extrapolating a dose-response function using EPA's linearized multistage model (see Chap. 9). A potency factor $F = 1/ED_{10}$ was then calculated. The substance was then placed in one of three potency groups based on whether the potency range factor F was over 100, between 1 and 100, or less than 1. A hazard ranking of high, medium, or low is then assigned based on the combination of the qualitative and quantitative rankings (Table 3-7). EPA describes this method as neither a risk assessment nor an absolute measure of harm, but simply a method for sorting a list of potentially carcinogenic substances into levels of relative potential carcinogenicity which may then be equated to reporting quantity levels. Once a notification is made, the Federal On-Scene Coordinator performs a more complete risk assessment. The hazard ranking does not directly result in a reportable quantity. The relationship between hazard rank and reportable quantity is shown in Table 3-8.

A number of screening methods used to identify pollutant emissions of importance or to set priorities for monitoring or regulatory action among many different pollutants from the same or different sources might also be considered a form of hazard assessment. One set of screening tools along these lines was developed for the Environmental Protection Agency (Cleland and Kingsbury, 1977; Kingsbury et al., 1979, 1980; Kingsbury and Chessin, 1983). These were intitially called Multimedia Environmental Goals (MEGs) and later Monitoring Trigger Levels (MTLs). They were not designed as a basis for regulation or risk analysis, but as a

TABLE 3-7 Hazard Ranking Scheme for Potential Carcinogens

Weight of evidence	Potency group		
	1	2	3
Group (from Table 3-6)	$F > 100$	$1 < F < 100$	$F < 1$
A	High	High	Medium
B	High	Low	
	Medium		
C	Medium	Low	Low
D	No hazard ranking		
E	No hazard ranking		

Source: From EPA, 1986a.

TABLE 3-8 Relationship Between Hazard
Rank and Reportable Quantity

Hazard rank	Reportable quantity (lbs)
High	1
Medium	10
Low	100
–	1000

Source: From EPA, 1986a.

practical approach to keeping regulatory requirements for monitoring in
bounds by screening emissions from industrial sources to help decide
which compounds must receive additional attention and which can be
quickly eliminated from further concern. They illustrate the difficulty with
hazard identification in the broad context. No risk assessment or regulatory process can reasonably deal with hundreds or even thousands of
individual chemical pollutants emitted from an industrial plant. A rational
approach to screening is necessary, but health effects potentially involved
are varied and available data on different diseases and on effects of
pollutants in different media (air or water) are often inconsistant. This
body of work by Kingsbury was an attempt to organize a database, which,
if not completely consistent, would be sufficient for practical engineering
decisions. Original toxicity rankings were drawn largely from occupational
threshold limit values or TLVs (ACGIH, 1985). Later, cancer risk estimates derived preferentially from EPA quantitative cancer risk assessments were included. The MTL value was defined as the level in ambient
air, drinking water, soil, or solid waste associated with a human risk of
developing cancer of 1×10^{-5}, assuming a linear dose–response curve at
low-dose levels. This is a case of going full circle, where results of quantitative assessments are used in later hazard identification. Unfortunately,
evaluating the comparability of the cancer risk levels with TLV-derived
toxicity rankings is difficult, although Spirtas et al. (1986) provides some
basis. Other considerations included in this database are implications of
short and long-term exposures, recognition of the various bases of ranking,
consideration of persistence and bioaccumulation of chemicals in the environment, environmental media through which the pollutant will move,
and degree of potential human ingestion. While the approach encourages
the exercise of judgment, there is a danger that such an institutionalized
data base will be misused in a rote manner by those not familiar with its
limitations. A limitation, inherent in almost all qualitative and quantitative analysis, is the so far intractable problem of complex mixtures. Hun-

TABLE 3-9   Criteria for Oncogenicity

1. Evidence of oncogenicity in humans by oral or inhalation route
2. Evidence of oncogenicity in humans by routes other than oral or inhalation
3. Evidence of oncogenicity in two or more animal species by any route of administration[a]
4. Evidence on oncogenicity in one animal species by any route of administration[a]
5. Compound scheduled for or currently undergoing oncogenicity testing
6. Negative or equivocal results from oncogenicity testing
7. No data

[a]If the data satisfy the criteria for Index 3 then Index 4 should not be considered.
Source: From Fingleton, 1985.

dreds of chemicals in a single emission stream are evaluated using toxicity information largely derived from tests of exposures to one compound at a time. The affect on risk of simultanious exposure to the entire mix is largely unknown. This problem is further discussed in later chapters.

While MEGs and MTLs use quantitative data as the source of rankings, a different approach to the development of a similar screening procedure constructs rankings from qualitative values. Fingleton et al.

TABLE 3-10   Criteria for Mutagenicity

1. Evidence of mutagenicity (in vivo) in at least on mammalian test species by the inhalation route
2. Evidence of mutagenicity (in vivo) in at least one mammalian test species by the noninhalation route
3. Evidence of mutagenicity (in vivo) in two or more mammalian test species
4. Evidence of mutagenicity (in vivo) in one mammalian test species[a]
5. Evidence of mutagenicity (in vivo) in two or more nonmammalian test species by any route of administration[b]
6. Evidence of mutagenicity (in vivo) in one nonmammalian test species by any route of administration[e]
7. Evidence of mutagenicity (in vitro) in two or more nonmammalian test species[c]
8. Evidence of mutagenicity (in vitro) in one nonmammalian test species[c]
9. Compound scheduled for or currently undergoing mutagenicity testing
10. Negative or equivocal results from mutagenicity testing
11. No data

[a]If the data satisfy the criteria for Index 3 then Index 4 should not be considered.
[b]If the data satisfy the criteria for Index 5 the Index 6 should not be considered.
[c]If the data satisfy the criteria in Index 7 then Index 8 should not be considered.
Source: From Smith and Fingleton, 1982.

(1985) developed a Multi-Attribute Hazard Assessment System (MAHAS). MAHAS is based on an earlier prioritization scheme (Smith and Fingleton, 1982), but includes the ability to deal with a waste stream containing many pollutants. MAHAS calculates a "degree of hazard" by scoring the waste stream on six factors: oncogenicity, mutagenicity, reproductive and developmental toxicity, acute lethality, other effects, and bioaccumulation. Each factor is made up of five to 13 criteria; oncogenicity criteria are shown in Table 3-9 and mutagenicity criteria in Table 3-10. The two are combined to form the carcinogenicity group.

INFORMATION SOURCES FOR HAZARD ASSESSMENT

Depending on its purpose, hazard assessment uses different methods which involve different levels of depth or effort. It can be a screening process, which relatively quickly screens out the chaff, allowing one to focus on areas more likely to be important. In a sense, the National Cancer Institute's "Cancer Atlas" (Mason et al., 1975) is a hazard identification tool. Its aim was to identify areas of the country with high cancer rates for more specific investigation. Indeed, a number of in-depth epidemiological studies were done in these areas. The "Cancer Atlas" has been updated by EPA (1987).

The "Cancer Atlas" takes the approach of identifying high incidences epidemiology. The more common approach in risk assessment is the reverse: a potential cause of disease is identified and subsequent analysis is done to determine if an increase in disease rate is likely to result.

Hazard assessment frequently focuses on the *possibility* of harm without regard to its *probability*. For example, EPA's guidelines on chemical emergencies (EPA, 1985) focus on a threshold level of hazardous material present at an industrial facility without regard to physical state, containment, or other factors. These are left to later, more detailed analysis. Thus, a hazard assessment may identify a *possible* hazard which on further study is shown to present no hazard at all, or a hazard which represents a small risk.

In addition to sources listed earlier, general references are often used to determine hazard (e.g., Sax, 1975; Clayton and Clayton, 1978). The National Research Council (e.g., NAS, 1972; 1980; 1981a; 1981b); and the World Health Organization (e.g., WHO, 1981) publish reviews of specific agents or groups of agents. Hazard analyses also may compare measured or estimated exposures to some standard: an environmental or occupational exposure standard (e.g., NIOSH/OSHA, 1978), for example, or may draw on existing epidemiological or toxicological literature and use findings for similar situations to make a first estimate of the potential

TABLE 3-11   Some Scientific and Professional
Journals Useful in Hazard Assessment

American Journal of Epidemiology
Archives of Environmental Health
Environmental Health Perspectives
Environment International
Environmental Mutagenesis
Environmental Research
Journal of the Air Pollution Control Association
Journal of Occupational Medicine
Mutation Research
Science
Risk Analysis

---

hazard in a new situation. Some scientific and professional journals which
have proved useful in this regard are listed in Table 3-11. Basically, any
and all sources of information should be drawn upon for a hazard analysis.

SUMMARY

Hazard identification is the primary focus of qualitative cancer assessment.
"Is this substance a carcinogen?" is a question currently of vital importance in regulatory practice. Designation as a carcinogen places a substance
in a different category, subject to different rules and regulations than
other substances. In an increasing number of situations, however, this is
not the end. Designation as a carcinogen is only the first step in a process
of risk assessment which ultimately estimates the quantitative cancer risk
to society.

REFERENCES

ACGIH. 1985. *Threshold Limit Values for Chemical Substances and Physical
     Agents in the Work Environment.* American Conference of Governmental
     Industrial Hygienists, Cincinnati, Ohio.
Clayton, G.D. and F.E. Clayton (eds.). 1978. *Patty's Industrial Hygiene and
     Toxicology.* John Wiley & Sons, New York.
Cleland, J.G. and G.L. Kingsbury. 1977. Multimedia environmental goals for
     environmental assessment (EPA-600/7-77-136a and b). Prepared for the U.S.
     Environmental Protection Agency by Research Triangle Institute, Research
     Triangle Park, N.C. .
EPA. 1985. Chemical emergency preparedness program interim guidance. En-
     vironmental Protection Agency, Washington, D.C.
EPA. 1986. Methodology for evaluating potential carcinogenicity in support of
     reportable quantity adjustments pursuant to CERCLA Section 102, Carcino-

gen Assessment Group, Office of Health and Environmental Assessment, U.S. Environmental Protection Agency, Washington, D.C.

EPA. 1986b. Guidlines for carcinogenic risk assessment. U.S. Environmental Protection Agency, *Fed. Reg.* 51:33992–34003.

EPA. 1987. U.S. Cancer Mortality Rates and Trends, 1950–1979 (EPA 600/1-83/015). U.S. Environmental Protection Agency, Research Triangle Park, N.C.

Fingleton, D.J., L.J. Habegger. S-Y. Chin, S.G. Barisas, and R.H. Petersen. 1985. Development of the multi-attribute hazard assessment system (MAHAS) and its application to energy-related waste streams. Presented at 78th Annual Meeting of the Air Pollution Control Association, Detroit, Mich. (preprint no. 85-33.6).

IARC. 1972 et seq. Monographs on the Evaluation of the Carcinogenic Risk of Chemicals to Humans. International Agency for Research on Cancer, Lyon, France.

Interdisciplinary Panel. 1984. Interdisciplinary Panel on Carcinogenicity, Criteria for evidence of chemical carcinogenicity. *Science* 225:682–687.

IRLG, 1979. Interagency Regulatory Liaison Group, Work Group on Risk Assessment, Scientific Bases for identifying potential carcinogens and estimating their risks.

Kingsbury, G.L., J.B. White, and J.S. Watson. 1980. Multimedia environmental goals for environmental assessment (EPA-600/7-80-041). Prepared for the Environmental Protection Agency by Research Triangle Institute, Research Triangle Park, N.C.

Kingsbury, G.L., R.C. Sims, and J.B. White. 1979. Multimedia environmental goals for environmental assessment (EPA-600/7-79-176a and b). Prepared for the Environmental Protection Agency by Research Triangle Institute, Research Triangle Park, N.C.

Kingsbury, G.L. and R.L. Chessin. 1983. Monitoring Trigger levels for process characterization studies (final draft). Prepared for the Environmental Protection Agency by Research Triangle Institute, Research Triangle Park, N.C.

Mason, T.J., F.W. McKay, R. Hoover, W.J. Blot, and J.F. Fraumeni, Jr. 1975. *Atlas of Cancer Mortality for U.S. Counties*: 1950–1970, DHEW Publication No. (NIH) 75-780. Washington, D.C., Government Printing Office.

NAS. 1972. Particulate polycyclic organic matter. Committee on Biologic Effects of Atmospheric Pollutants, National Research Council, National Academy of Sciences, Washington, D.C.

NAS. 1980. The effects on populations of exposure to low levels of ionizing radiation: 1980. Committee on the Biological Effects of Ionizing Radiation, National Research Council, National Academy Press, Washington, D.C.

NAS. 1981a. The health effects of nitrate, nitrite, and n-nitroso compounds. Committee on Nitrite and Alternative Curing Agents in Food, National Research Council. National Academy Press, Washington, D.C.

NAS. 1981b. Formaldehyde and other aldehydes, Committee on Aldehydes, National Research Council. National Academy Press, Washington, D.C.NIOSH/OSHA. 1978. Pocket guide to chemical hazards. National Institute for Occupational Safety and Health and Occupational Safety and Health Administration. U.S. Government Printing Office, Washington, D.C.

OSHA, 1980. Occupational Safety and Health Administration, Identification, classification and regulation of potential occupational carcinogens, *Fed. Reg.* 45:5002–5296.

OSTP, 1984. Office of Science and Technology Policy, Chemical carcinogens; notice of review of the science and its associated principles. *Federal Register* 49:21594–21661, May 22, 1984.

Ozog, H. and L.M. Benedixen. 1987. Hazard identification and quantification. *Chem. Eng. Progr.* 83(4):55–64.

Rushefsky, M.E. 1986. *Making Cancer Policy. State University of New York Press*, Albany.

Sax, N.I. 1975. *Dangerous Properties of Industrial Materials*, 4th ed. Van Nostrand Reinhold Company, New York.

Smith, A.E. and D.J. Fingleton. 1982. Hazardous air pollutant prioritization system (HAPPS) (EPA 450/5-82-008). Prepared for the Environmental Protection Agency by Argonne National Laboratory, Argonne, ILL.

Spirtas, R., M. Steinberg, R.C. Wands, and E.K. Weisburger. 1986. Identification and classification of carcinogens: procedures of the Chemical Substances Threshold Limit Value Committee, ACGIH. *American J. Public Health* 76: 1232-1235.

WHO. 1981. Environmental Health Criteria 18: Arsenic. World Health Organization, Geneva.

World Bank. 1985. *Manual for Industrial Hazard Assessment Techniques*, Office of Environment and Scientific Affairs, World Bank, Washington, D.C.

PART II

EXPOSURE AND DOSE ASSESSMENT

For there to be risk, there must be an exposure, or the chance of an exposure. If no one is or can be exposed, there is no risk. Exposure assessment stands on an equal footing with dose–response assessment. Both are needed to estimate risk. An important difference is that dose-response assessment can be generic: the dose-response function for arsenic, benzo[a]pyrene, or other toxic agents can be applied in a wide range of situations. Exposure assessment, on the other hand, is specific to a particular situation. The release of a chemical in one place will result in a different exposure than its release in another.

Most exposure assessments begin with source terms: where does the toxic material come from, how does it get into the environment, and how much gets into the environment. This oft-neglected area is discussed in Chapter 4. Exposure assessment is generally concerned with future exposures; the focus is thus on modeling rather than measuring. Understanding the models, however, requires some background in environmental measurements since the models must be developed and calibrated from measurement data. Some aspects of measurements are discussed in Chapter 5, while modeling is treated in greater detail in Chapter 6.

In reality, exposure assessment and dose–response assessment overlap in the translation from exposure to dose. Exposure is the environmental concentration to which people are exposed. Dose is the biologically effective impact on a tissue of concern. In many cases the effective dose is not even the same chemical as the exposure, but its metabolite. Since the processes that translate exposure to dose are simply a continuation of environmental transport, Chapter 7, on pharmacokinetics and metabolism, is included in this section. One should note that, from a disciplinary sense, the researchers who study transport and chemical transformation within the body are much closer to those who study dose-response than those who study environmental transport. Also, it should be recognized that, although ideally one estimates dose and then applies a dose–response function, often data are inadequate to do this. Instead, exposure assessment stops at exposure and dose-response assessment becomes exposure–response assessment.

4

Exposure Assessment: General Issues

INTRODUCTION

Exposure assessment is an integral part of the cancer risk assessment process. If no one is exposed, no cancers are induced. The most elaborate dose–response models are of little avail in the face of simplistic exposure data or models. Exposure assessment is a particularly case-specific process. Although "generic" exposure assessments are made, they are based on assumptions of a generic case or "reference environment." Moreover, it is well to keep in mind that cancer risk assessments are generally driven by exposure. Observations of high cancer rates prompt research, not assessments. Cancer risk assessments are initiated because of concern over an existing or potential exposure to a known or suspected carcinogen.

Exposure assessment may be based on measurements or models or both. It may involve one or several media: air, soil, water, food chains, direct contact. It includes "source term" assessment, environmental transport and transformation, and population exposure. Exposure assessment encompasses a broader range of disciplines than dose–response assessment and requires a greater variety of skills. Source term assessment requires engineers and chemists; environmental transport modeling requires meteorologists, hydrologists, chemists, biologists, and other scientists; population exposure requires demographers and psychologists who study population activity patterns. Finally, if exposure is extended to tissue or cellular-level dose, a range of biomedical disciplines come into play.

Estimating exposure for a study designed to develop dose–response functions, such as an epidemiology study, is different than exposure assessment for risk assessment, although the two have much in common. In the former, one needs information on both exposure and health measures on the study population. While individual exposure data is sometimes obtained with personal monitors or inferred from analysis of blood, urine, or exhaled breath, usually exposure estimates are made for groups based on more limited measures from area air sampling, routine sampling of community water supplies, etc. Sometimes exposure models are used to interpolate between sampling data or to estimate exposures retrospectively, but generally exposure estimates in dose-response studies are based on direct measurements. Particularly in epidemiological studies in which health data are collected on individuals, the objective is to estimate each individual's exposure as closely as possible. The researcher wants to link each person's exposure and health status. From this set of data pairs, overall dose-response patterns for the population are developed.

In cancer risk assessment, the order of the steps is changed. Population exposure is estimated and combined with dose-response information from other sources to predict risk in the population. Unlike a dose-response study, the aim is to assess the risk in the population, not to any individual. The population involved is generally much larger than the population typically used in epidemiological studies. The exposure of concern could be in the past, present, or future. For example, a risk assessment addressing the question, what is the cancer risk over the remainder of their lives, of a population occupationally exposed to asbestos over the last 30–40 years would deal principally with past exposures, for which no direct measurements are available. Similar exposure assessments are done following accidents which result in population exposure to carcinogens. The purpose of these assessments may be to estimate the overall impact of an accident or a prolonged past or existing exposure, or to determine liability for compensation. Most cancer risk assessments seek to predict the health effect of a change in exposure which a policy option might bring about in the future. These are stimulated by impending introduction of a new technology which may lead to exposures or even exposure to new chemicals, or by proposed regulations to limit existing exposures. The key exposure is usually the future exposure. Since neither future exposure nor past exposures can be measured, exposure assessment depends heavily on models.

EXPRESSION OF EXPOSURE

Exposure can be expressed in several different ways. An individual can be exposed to a certain amount of arsenic in water over a given period. This might be a day or a lifetime. If the concentration in the water is 0.1 mg/l, that might be taken as the exposure, or, if the individual consumes 2 liters of water per day, the *individual exposure* might be expressed as 0.2 mg/day. If 1000 people in a community have the same exposure, the *population exposure* might be expressed as the product, 200 person-mg/day. In the case of internally taken radioactive materials such as irradiates the body over a long period of time. This is called a *committed dose*, since, by ingesting the cesium, the person is committed to a continuing dose until all the cesium has decayed or been biologically removed. Like exposure, committed dose may also be expressed as either an individual or a population commitment. It may also be expressed as an *environmental commitment*. The Chernobyl accident, for example, released ^{137}Cs into the biosphere. With its 30-year half-life, it will remain available in the foodchain to be ingested by people for decades. This is an environmental commitment. A toxic chemical leaching from a hazardous waste dump into an aquifer presents a similar environmental commitment, sitting there waiting for someone to drink it.

While "exposure" and "dose" are often used as synonyms, there is an important difference. Specific definitions may vary, but exposure generally refers to an environmental concentration. A person might be exposed to a carcinogen at levels of 0.02 $\mu g/m^3$ in air or 20 ng/l in water. Dose, however, depends also on the amount of air breathed, water drunk, and the fraction of the total amount of the carcinogen consumed taken up by tissues. Dose sometimes refers to the total amount of material retained in the body for a significant time and sometimes to the total amount actually reaching a specific target tissue. In the latter case especially, exposure assessment must consider the metabolism and pharmacokinetic factors determining the delivery of the dose from entry to the body to the target tissue. A complicating factor here is that the chemical compound in the environment which constitutes the exposure may undergo change in the body and the biologically effective agent may then be its metabolite. Thus, exposure and dose may refer to different chemicals. Exposure assessment involves the environmental sciences primarily, while dose assessment carries the process further, into the body itself, thus involving the biomedical sciences.

While exposure and dose are usually considered in terms of an amount or concentration of a physical or chemical agent, at times they are measured by an index. This can take several different forms. When a quantitative estimate of exposure is not available, a surrogate is sometimes used. An example might be use of pollutant emissions as a crude approximation of environmental concentrations. This sort of analysis was frequently used in the past, but is generally no longer considered acceptable. Measurements and model results are not always what they appear, however, and sometimes such surrogates seem to work better than what would seem to be more definitive exposure estimates. Blood lead levels in children, for example, at one time seemed to be better correlated with gasoline consumption than with measurements of airborne lead concentrations. The crude surrogate may have captured more of the total exposure than the air measurements.

A similar surrogate approach is often used in the case of complex mixtures. Exposure to an index compound is used to represent the total exposure. Pitfalls involved in such an approach will be discussed later. A more common approach to assessing complex mixture exposure is to use an arbitrary sampling method which collects an aggregate. The simplest example is the common measure of total airborne respirable particles.

A final index is to use biological response as an index of dose. A number of relatively new biochemical methods are being explored. Many scientists feel that chromosome aberrations, for example may make a better index of exposure to a carcinogen or mutagen than an index of effect. Some biochemical measures may be appropriate as measures of both dose and effect, depending on the situation.

SOURCE TERMS

In some cases, a QCRA may not be concerned with a source but simply with an ambient level. One might ask what is the cancer risk of organic compounds in the air, without worrying about how they got there or how they might be removed. This might well be a question asked by EPA in considering an ambient air quality standard for a hazardous pollutant. More generally, and more practically, however, the concern is over exposure to a carcinogen from a particular source or class of sources, e.g., vinyl chloride or dioxin emissions from a specific plant or polycyclic aromatic hydrocarbons from coal combustion in general. In this case, exposure assessment begins with the source. What is the physical and chemical form of the release? Is it released to air, water, what? What is the release rate (kg/hour)? Is it a single point source like a factory smoke stack or a broad area source like many individual homes? Take arsenic as an example. Is the source a tall stack at a smelter releasing oxides of arsenic to the air or is it lead arsenate applied to the ground as a pesticide? The answers to these questions will determine the environmental pathways the material will follow, the route of exposure, and even whether the material is likely to be bioavailable at all. Exposure assessment need not flow linearly from source to transport to exposure. Sometimes the sources are known and the exposures are known, and the assessment must link the two together to provide a basis of risk management or regulation. Which sources are responsible for a specific exposure? Sometimes the link is indirect. Acid rain may mobilize toxic metals from the soil into the water supply. The "source" of the metals in the water might be considered, indirectly, to be the emissions of sulfur and nitrogen oxides from distant fossil fuel combustion.

One thinks of a "source" as an industrial stack spewing out pollutants on a regular basis. This is sometimes referred to as a "routine emission source." For cancer risk, it is generally the most important environmental emission source. Evaluation of such releases begins with a materials balance. What goes into an industrial process must come out somewhere; a materials balance will show where and may uncover unsuspected sources of release.

Intermittent and accidental releases can also be important. Occasional or intermittent releases of carcinogens may pose some cancer risk and indeed, in a highly industrialized region, the cumulation of many occasional releases from different sources may result in a substantial average dose to the population. In general, exposures from intermittent sources do not accumulate to sufficient doses to be significant cancer risks compared with routine releases. The same applies to accidental releases, although in some cases these can be sufficiently large to warrant assessment of the long-term cancer risk. In the case of nuclear power, for example, the *annualized* risk from large accidents is on a par with the annual risk from routine releases, even though the probability of such large accident releases is small. Because of accumulation in the environment, a sudden, one-time release may result in a long exposure period. The size and probability of accidental releases can be estimated using probabilistic risk analysis, a set of techniques developed to estimate risks of nuclear accidents which centers on fault-tree and event-tree construction and analysis. These techniques have also been applied to chemical accidents.

ENVIRONMENTAL TRANSPORT, DISPERSION, AND TRANSFORMATION

A carcinogen moves from the source through the environment to ultimately reach people. This may be instantaneous, as when a worker touches a leaky valve and gets a carcinogenic oil on his skin. It may be a long and complex route through air, water, soil, and food chains, exposing people thousands of miles from the source. The carcinogen may be temporarily bound in soil or bottom sediments in a lake and the time between emission from a source and population exposure measured in years or decades. The agent released from the source may be physically and chemically transformed enroute. Models for environmental transport and dispersion and their application to cancer risk assessment are treated in detail in Chapter 6.

EXPOSURE MEANS PEOPLE

Transport and dispersion models predict the levels of carcinogens at specific places in the environment, but if there are no people there, no cancers will result. Industrial hygienists have long recognized that the airborne concentration of an industrial toxin that concerned them was the concentration in the "breathing zone" of the worker. Too often, assessments of risk to the general population have assumed that the predicted concentration in the air was the population exposure. Surprisingly, it has only been recently recognized that people do not spend all their time sitting in their front yard just breathing the air. They spend part of their day at work, school, or other activity in a different place with a different exposure level. They spend most of their day indoors where the exposure levels can be quite different. A recent study, for example, has shown that exposures to volatile organic compounds are highly related to indoor home or occupational exposures rather than outdoor ambient air concentrations contributed by industrial emissions (Wallace, 1987).

The extreme example of this is assessment of the "fence-post" individual. This is a study of exposure to a hypothetical person who spends 24 hours per day, 365 days per year outdoors at the boundary of a plant site, and who relies for his entire diet on food produced at the same location. It was begun in the nuclear business as a way of estimating an "upper bound" level of radiation exposure to the public. It is possible to think up examples in which the fence-post individual would not be the maximally exposed person, but, in general, he or she is a good bet. It makes for good screening analysis when the objective of the exposure assessment is regulatory compliance rather than risk assessment. If the fence-post person is OK, then everyone is OK, and a lot of additional work is saved.

A problem with fence-post analysis is the difference between individual and collective risk. Some analysts calculated collective risks assuming the entire U.S. population would be exposed to the fence-post level. Even a negligibly small risk can yield a finite number of estimated tumors if multiplied by 200 million people. If the collective population effect is desired, then the exposure must be estimated appropriately.

Parts of the exposure assessment process are well developed disciplines in their own right. The practitioners of these disciplines frequently become so absorbed in their own area that they lose sight of the final objective of estimating population exposure. Of course, they may have other objectives than population exposure. The research meteorologist or air chemist is interested in describing how air pollution is transported and transformed in the atmosphere. The last thing they need are data from samplers which have been hooked on people who are moving around all the time. The cancer risk analyst must beware of accepting blindly exposure estimates made by others for different purposes. These estimates may ignore parts of the exposure route outside the discipline of the investigator or may introduce potential mismatches between exposure models and dose-response models. It is the people side of exposure assessment which is most often ignored. How many people are exposed, at what concentrations, in what way?

When exposure estimates involve past or future time periods, ramifications of population change over time must be considered. For small areas or for long time projections, a wide range of uncertainty can be introduced and is often neglected. Since cancer risk can depend on age at exposure, changes in the age structure can also be important. Once the number and structure of the population is decided, these people must be placed in time and space corresponding to environmental concentration estimates. This includes consideration of daily activity patterns and concentrations on the microenvironment level for the short term and migration rates in the long term.

At times, however, the size of the population is not an important aspect of the analysis. In extreme cases, risks of technological development may be projected decades or even centuries into the future. Examples are radon emissions from uranium mill tailings, high level radioactive waste repositories, and chemically contaminated aquifers. It makes no sense to complicate these assessments with large uncertainties or impossibilities of predicting population dynamics that far into the future. If there are more people, there will be more cancers, but that has little to do with the issue of concern in these cases. The key points are (1) what is the individual level of risk and (2) can we reasonably expect that there will be a large enough population at risk to make the population risk of social concern?

In considering the people factors, it is important to consider the dose-response characteristics which determine the specifications of exposure estimates needed. The kinds of exposure estimates needed are different for a cancer risk assessment than for an assessment of acute effects of carbon monoxide exposure. Acute exposures to carcinogens are not generally important. Predicting the long-term effects of another Hiroshima or its chemical equivalent might be an exception and, from a dose-response view, there may be important differences between effects of long-term averages and shorter exposures. If a short exposure is the concern, it should not be simply averaged into the lifetime exposure, but its time characteristics maintained (duration, age at exposure). In general, however, it is the long-term average or cumulative exposure which is usually more important in most cases. This simplifies matters a great deal. Dealing with averages is much easier than having to account for every minor excursion above the norm. It is important to be sure that the average includes those occasional short-term peaks. The possibility that frequent acute doses make a significant contribution to cumulative exposure should not be overlooked.

Often, dose-response functions are derived from occupational studies. To apply these to general populations the exposure must be translated from 8-hours/day, 5-days/week for a working life of perhaps 40 years to

24-hours/day, 365-days/year over an entire lifetime. The simplest approach falls back on equating total lifetime exposure (or average daily lifetime exposure). A more refined treatment will consider a lifetable approach, taking into account the effect of latency periods. Often more difficult to take into account is the possible difference in susceptibility to exposures in childhood which are not included in the occupational data and the possible effect of dose fractionation (that respite during evenings and weekends).

BACKGROUND EXPOSURE

Some synthetic chemicals may have a unique source so that the exposure from that source is the total exposure. In most cases, however, the exposure of interest is an increment which adds to a pre-existing background exposure to the same agent. In many cases, this incremental exposure is very small and cannot even be measured against the background exposure. The linear model assumes the affect of an increment is unchanged by the presence of a background exposure. In some cases, this assumption is actually an approximation limited to the "low dose" region. Even with a nonlinear dose-response function, linearity can be assumed for a small incremental dose, although the linear coefficient may vary with background level.

A problem which is not generally considered, but of considerable potential importance, is to what degree each exposure is independent. People are exposed to many carcinogens. Some act with similar or identical mechanisms, others act entirely differently. What then, is the appropriate background level? Is it the dose due to other sources of the specific agent under consideration? Or does it also include the background exposure to other similarly acting agents? Exposures from inhalation, ingestion, and skin adsorption may result in doses to different organs of the body. To what extent should route of exposure be included in the background?

Very few exposures are to a single agent; almost all real exposures are complex mixtures. A complex mixture is one in which there is no possibility of exploring all possible interactions among each individual constituent. It may not be possible to even identify all the constituents. Methods to quantify effects of exposure to complex mixtures generally focus on index compounds or less specific index measures (e.g., total particles, benzene soluble material) for ambient air or water samples. For a long time, the most common index compound for organic pollutants from combustion or processing of coal was benzo[a]pyrene (BaP). BaP was the most studied of the polycyclic aromatic compounds and, as Gammage (1979) points out, the practice of using BaP as an index of complex organic mixture was more for reasons of familiarity than sound reasoning. Reasons against the use of BaP as an index include (Gammage, 1979):

1. BaP may be a minor constitute in the mixture and the parent mixture's chemical profile may differ considerably from one sample to another or from one situation to another;
2. The biological activity of a sample may be associated primarily with other compounds;
3. BaP may be chemically less stable than other compounds in the mixture.

These reasons, of course, hold for many potential indices. The only "solid" justification for using an index is in an industrial situation with a stable mix, so the index is roughly representative of the mix on a day-to-day basis. Indices are particularly dangerous when used to transfer dose-response information from one situation to another, for example, from cigarette smoke or coke-oven pollutants to residential coal combustion products or diesel engine exhaust. Another situation in which indices are potential trouble is in an emissions plume (either in air or water) where the character of the mix is constantly changing due to chemical and photochemical processes. Here the relationship between the index and the total mix which it presumes to represent is constantly changing.

Having thus demolished the concept of index compounds, only one reason remains to justify their use: there is generally no practical alternative. Complete characterization of the mixture with gas chromatography/-mass spectrometry (GC/MS) is time-consuming, expensive, and, perhaps most importantly, produces a result as complex as the mixture itself, thus defying the comparison of different mixtures. The only practical solution appears to be to use an index, but when comparing different mixes, to fall-back on an ad hoc comparison of the GC/MS scan as a means of tempering the use of the index with some idea of uncertainty. Current thinking would seem to tend toward use of the aggregate indices such as benzene soluble organics for this purpose. Perhaps this might be coupled with additional information from short-term bioassays (see Chap. 10) and a quantitative factor developed to modify the index value. This remains an area open to both long-term basic research and to development of practical solutions.

Recently, direct biologic indices have become common, such as measuring mutagenicity of environmental samples, as well as biochemical measures of dose or effect, such as chromosome aberrations in peripheral blood or mutagenicity in urine. Toxicological applications involve primarily short-term tests and are discussed in Chapter 10. General background on complex mixtures is discussed in NAS (1988), which focuses primarily on testing their toxicity. Techniques of chemical fractionation combined with mutagenicity testing (e.g., Austin et al., 1985) provide the means to determine which components of the complex mixture are the major contributors to overall mutagenicity. Epidemiological applications are discussed in NAS (1985). Many useful examples of exposure applications are given in the symposium proceedings edited by Gray et al. (1987).

SUMMARY

A key consideration is that the exposure and dose-response parts of the equation must fit together. If the dose-response function is nonlinear in dose, is based on dose to the target tissue, and depends on age at exposure, than the exposure estimate must strive to provide those details. If they cannot be reasonably estimated, then the effect of a range of different possible values might be investigated. If, on the other hand, the best dose-response function available is in the form of x lifetime cancers per y milligrams lifetime intake, than great detail in exposure estimates is wasted. Thus, while exposure assessment and dose-response assessment are separate subjects and can be carried out by different people at different times, they are not independent. The two must be carefully matched so that they fit together properly in the risk characterization stage.

Keep in mind all potential routes of exposure. Some "back of the envelope" calculations can help to set priorities on how much emphasis should be placed on each route. Beware the assessment which focuses on air exposures because a sophisticated air dispersion model was available rather than because preliminary calculations showed the air route to be the most important. Most problems involve multimedia exposures; most solutions wrongly ignore one or more media.

REFERENCES

Austin, A.C., L.D. Claxton, and J. Lewtas. 1985. Mutagenicity of the fractionated organic emissions from diesel, cigarette smoke condensate, coke oven, and roofing tar in the Ames assay. *Environ. Mutagen.* 7:471–487.

Gammage, R.B. 1979. Preliminary thoughts on proxy PNA compounds in the vapor and solid phase. in O. White (ed.), *Proceedings of the Symposium on Assessing the Industrial Hygiene Monitoring Needs for the Coal Conversion and Oil Shale Industries* (BNL 51002). Brookhaven National Laboratory, Upton, NY, pp. 173–188.

Gray, R.H., E.K. Chess, P.J. Mellinger, R.G. Riley, and D.L. Springer (eds). 1987. Health and Environmental Research on Complex Organic Mixtures (CONF-851027). Pacific Northwest Laboratory, Richland, Wa.

NAS. 1985. *Epidemiology and Air Pollution*, report of the National Research Council Committee on the Epidemiology of Air Pollutants. National Academy Press, Washington, D.C.

NAS. 1988. *Complex Mixtures, Methods for In Vivo Toxicity Testing*. National Research Council. National Academy Press, Washington D.C.

Wallace, L.A. 1987. The total exposure assessment methodology (TEAM) study: summary and analysis; Vol I. (EPA/600/6-87/002a). U.S. Environmental Protection Agency, Washington, D.C.

5

Measurement of Exposure and Dose

WHY BE CONCERNED ABOUT MEASUREMENT?

Exposure assessment may be entirely based on direct measurements of exposure. The measurements themselves may be part of a single study to assess cancer risk. Even here, maintaining close coordination between the measurement team and the health effects and assessment team can be difficult. It is easy for each group to become absorbed in their own work, resulting in the tasks not being well meshed. Equally as important, insights into cross-disciplinary problems may be missed.

More frequently, risk assessment is performed completely independent from any measurement effort and relies on either measurements taken at an earlier time and for a different purpose, or on model predictions of exposure. In such a case, exposure assessment may consist entirely of selecting data from established databases and manipulating it in models. But, the data in the database were obtained originally by measurement; since the measurements were made for a different purpose, the design of the measurement scheme, the methods used, and the quality of the data may not be entirely appropriate for exposure assessment and may be completely unsuitable. The analyst must be able to evaluate the measurement data to determine their suitability for the exposure assessment. To what extent an exposure assessment is based on preexisting data, includes a direct exposure measurement phase, or relies on exposure models, depends on the nature of the assessment and the time and resources available.

Cancer risk assessment must put exposure estimates together with a dose–response function. The latter includes its own, independent exposure measures. Ideally, measurements made for the exposure assessment will be compatible with the exposure measurements made in the development of the dose–response function. If the dose–response function is in terms of increased cancers per unit exposure to benzo[a]pyrene as an index of a complex organic mixture, then developing an exposure assessment using total benzene-soluble particles as the index of a complex mixture exposure would create difficulties in assessing the cancer risk. Mismatching the actual substance measured is an obvious problem, but more subtle differences may also create inconsistencies. Examples include differences in the location of sampling sites relative to the population; the duration and frequency of sampling; and the sampling and analysis methods used. At times, inconsistencies of this sort cannot be avoided, especially if one must rely on existing exposure data, but they should be introduced with full knowledge of their implications, not blundered into mistakenly. The analyst must therefore have an understanding of the exposure measurement process in the exposure assessment, and also of the exposure measurements made as part of epidemiological or toxicological studies from which the dose–response function is drawn.

This chapter is not a tutorial on sampling or analysis of environmental media. Experts in these areas must be employed in the exposure assessment task. The health effects expert and the risk analyst should, if possible, be active participants in the design of any environmental sampling programs which are part of the risk assessment. To perform effectively, they must have an understanding of the steps involved in environmental measurement. If drawing on existing data or models, analysts should have some understanding of what lies behind the data and the ability to recognize and evaluate potential inconsistencies in exposure estimates in different parts of the study. They must know that the quantities reported by the atmospheric or water chemist are not absolute, but that these results are dependent on sampling and analytical methods and the presence of interfering chemicals as well as on the actual quantity present of the chemical of interest. They must be able to understand and collaborate with chemists and others with expertise in sampling and laboratory analysis. Two excellent reviews on measurements for exposure assessment which include detail beyond the scope of this chapter are Hushon and Clerman (1981) and Lave and Upton (1987).

MEASUREMENT APPROACHES AND DESIGN CHARACTERISTICS

Environmental media are complicated, heterogeneous systems that rarely lend themselves to simple chemical or physical analysis. Sampling design is important not only to ensure that the sample is representative of the environment being sampled, but because sampling techniques may alter the physical and chemical characteristics of the contaminants. Examples include indoor air sampling at too high an air flow rate, which may alter the atmospheric dynamics in the building; sampling particles without presize selection, forever eliminating the possibility of identifying particle size distribution in the sample; and choosing a sample medium that allows chemical interaction of the sampled contaminant with other chemicals, changing the chemical character of the sample from that in the environment. Potential interfering substances must always be considered during sampling and analysis. The chemist and the risk analyst must have a keen insight into the nature of such interferences and other problems associated with the sampling and analysis techniques. These interferences may be unique to a particular situation and can lead to inaccurate data and cause misleading conclusions. Results must be interpreted in light of field observations and the history of the sample (Mancy, 1971).

The field of exposure measurements is subdivided into a number of categories, generally identified by environmental media since each presents its particular problems. The development of sampling and analysis methods has progressed along relatively independent lines for air, water, food, tissues, and body fluids. Air and water measurements have generally focused on either monitoring trends in pollution levels over time or on assurance of regulatory compliance. Unfortunately, neither of these aims is especially compatible with assessing population exposure.

Air

Air pollution monitoring began in the 1930s and routine monitoring was firmly established in the United States in the 1960s. Most air sampling is done at fixed locations selected for convenience, as representative of an area, or appropriate for monitoring the impact of a particular point-source emission. Focus is on criteria pollutants established under the Clean Air Act. The Environmental Protection Agency establishes guidelines and criteria for monitoring site selection and sampling equipment design. During the 1970s, this type of data was the basis of exposure assessment. To obtain finer grain exposure estimates for epidemiological studies, fixed monitors were established in local communities being studied. Study designs might, for example, require that the monitor be within half a mile of the residence of each study participant. Not until the late 1970s was there common recognition that exposures might vary significantly depending on personal activities such as commuting to work on crowded streets or the percentage of time spent indoors or outdoors. This introduced two new air sampling designs: personal exposure monitoring and microenvironment monitoring.

Personal exposure monitoring involves attaching an air-sampling device to a person. This provides a measure of that person's exposure over the time the sampler is worn. The approach was borrowed from industrial hygiene and health physics where personal monitoring pumps and film badges had long been in use. Three types of personal monitors are used: (1) battery-powered analytical instruments which make pollutant measurements on the spot and either provide the user with a digital readout or store the results for later statistical analysis, (2) battery-powered collection devices using air pumps, which accumulate the pollutant for later analysis in the laboratory, and (3) passive devices that do not require power sources and which usually include a chemical substance that reacts with the pollutant and is then later analyzed in the laboratory (Morgan and Morris, 1977; Mage and Wallace, 1979; WHO, 1982; Spengler and Soczek, 1984). Passive monitors provide an exposure measure integrated over the period of use, while active monitors more easily measure short duration exposures and resolve peaks. Unlike pollutants with acute effects, long-term average exposure estimates are acceptable for carcinogens from the dose–response viewpoint, but a daily average exposure estimate does not identify when or where the exposure was received, limiting the ability to link the exposure to its source. Passive monitors which did not require pumps and their associated battery packs proved more acceptable because they were lighter, less bulky, and quiet. The whirring of an air pump, unnoticeable on the factory floor, proved bothersome in the home and unacceptable in the school or office. Even passive monitoring proved less practicable for general populations than for workers, however, because of the greater numbers of people involved, the reduced control over the handling of the monitors, and the cost of collecting the resulting samples from many people. It must generally be limited to small sample populations and used for specific purposes, including verification of exposure estimates developed from microenvironmental monitoring.

Monitoring of microenvironments is a more practical approach, linking the results with population activity patterns to estimate population exposure (described more fully in Chap. 6). The most widely adopted microenvironmental monitoring has been for indoor monitoring. Most people spend the majority of their time indoors, and it is now widely recognized that indoor concentrations of many pollutants are different from outdoor concentrations. A building forms a protection against many reactive outdoor pollutants which are adsorbed on surfaces as they enter or after entering the building. Fine particles ($<1\mu$m) are not impaired, however, and these are more likely to contain toxic components (Natusch et al., 1974). In addition, indoor sources have been shown to be important. Kerosene heaters, gas stoves, household chemicals, evaporative emissions of gasoline components from automobiles in attached garages, and off-gassing from building materials and furnishings are examples (NAS, 1981). Indoor sampling poses problems not faced in outdoor sampling; high-volume pumps, needed to obtain samples of sufficient size for chemical analysis, cannot be used indoors because their flow volume disrupts air circulation in the building and their noise level is often objectionable (Howes et al., 1986). Measurements must be representative of exposures within the microenvironment. Radon measurements, for example, are often made in basements where the highest levels in the building are likely to be found but these are hardly representative of the exposure people receive in the building.

Sampling and Analysis Techniques

Sampling techniques include filtration, inertial separation, and sorption; analysis techniques include atomic absorption and atomic emission spectrometry, neutron activation analysis, x-ray fluorescence spectrometry, gas chromatography (GC), mass spectrometry (MS), Fourier transform infrared (FTIR) spectrometry, liquid chromatography, soxhlet extraction, and surface-enhanced Raman spectroscopic (SERS) techniques). Detailed discussion of these techniques is beyond the scope of this book; several recent reviews are available (Stevens, 1986; Schroeder et al 1987; Davis et al., 1987).

Measuring Exposure: An Example

Some flavor for the design and conduct of a sampling study can be gained from an example that has been reported in detail (Wallace, 1987). EPA's Total Exposure Assessment Methodology (TEAM) Study was designed to develop methods to measure individual exposures to pollutants through air, food, and water and to apply these methods in several U.S. cities. In a preliminary study, 30 sampling and analytical protocols were tested for 15 volatile organics, 8 semivolatile organics, 3 metals, and 6 polyaromatic hydrocarbons. The main TEAM study then measured personal exposures of 600 people to 20 target chemicals selected from the initial 30 (Table 5-1). These people were selected to be representative of a total population of 700,000 in seven cities in four states.

Each participant carried a personal air sampler throughout a normal 24-hour day, collecting two 12-h samples (a daytime sample and an overnight sample). Identical samplers were run in fixed locations in the backyard of one participant's home in each of over 100 "clusters" to measure ambient air concentrations. At the end of the 24-h period, a sample of exhaled breath was collected from each participant. The study was conducted during three seasons (summer, fall, and winter), although samples were not taken in all cities during all three seasons. The air

TABLE 5-1 Target compounds
for air monitoring in the
TEAM study

Vinylidene chloride
Chloroform
1,2-Dichloroethane
1,1,1-Trichloroethane
Benzene
Carbon tetrachloride
Trichloroethylene
Bromodichloromethane
Dibromochloromethane
Tetrachloroethylene
Chlorobenzene
Bromoform
Dibromochloropropane
Styrene
p-Dichlorobenzene
Ethylbenzene
o-Xylene
p-Xylene
o-Dichlorobenzene

Source: From Wallace, 1987.

sampler was a glass cartridge containing a granular sorbent called Tenax-GC. The sampler was attached to a vest to hold it near the person's breathing zone and air was pulled through the cartridge at 30 ml per minute by a small pump. Roughly 20 liters of air was pulled through the cartridge for each 12 h sample. The samples were analyzed by capillary gas chromatography mass spectrometry (GC-MS) techniques followed by a combination of manual and automated spectra analyses.

Several pollutants of interest could not be included in the study because they were not amenable to collection on Tenax. Highly volatile chemicals such as vinyl chloride and methylene chloride would "break through" the Tenax cartridge before the sampling period was over. Any sorbent can hold only a given amount of a particular chemical; when that limit is exceeded, the chemical "breaks through" and some of the sample is lost. To assure no break through occurred or to enable the amount of material that breaks through to be estimated, a second cartridge is often put in the sampling train following the first. Formaldehyde is reactive and cannot be collected on Tenax, nor can any other substances such as phenols.

About 30% of all samples taken were either blanks, spikes, or duplicates. Blanks are extra cartridges carried into the field and treated like the samples, except they are not exposed. They indicate how much, if any, of the pollutant collected in the samples was due to contamination during handling rather than during sampling. Blanks were generally low (less than 10 ng of all chemicals) but, on one TEAM sampling campaign, blank values were high. Estimated concentrations are calculated by subtracting the blank values from the sampled values so high blanks do not necessarily invalidate the data, but result in lower precision and indicate unwanted contamination. The high blanks were attributed to recent renovations in the hotel where the sampling team stayed. Recent construction and new materials in the hotel apparently led to higher indoor pollutant levels which contaminated the cartridges even though they were in sealed cans. Following this incident, all Tenax cartridges in the field were kept under a helium bath during storage. Benzene had chronically high and variable levels on the blanks. Toluene had such high levels on blanks, presumably due to contamination of air in the laboratory, that results were considered too unreliable and were not reported.

Spikes are cartridges that have had a known amount of pollutant sorbed on them. They serve as a check to see how much of the pollutant sorbed on the Tenax is recovered in the laboratory and, if they are spiked in the field, can indicate the existence of degradation or loss of sampled material through chemical reaction in the cartridge or from off-gassing. Recovery efficiencies for the spikes ranged from 80 to 110%. A recovery of over 100% is obviously wrong, but is not uncommon. It indicates the inherent error in the analysis. Recoveries for most chemicals were higher for laboratory spikes than for field spikes, indicating a greater loss of material during storage and transport in the field than under laboratory conditions. Duplicates are two samples taken together and sent to different laboratories for analysis as a quality control check.

Measurements were classified as nondetectable, trace, and measurable. The limit of detection (LOD) is based on the total quantity of the substance in the sample; it is thus a function of the analytical method, the particular substance, and the amount collected which, in turn, depends on the sampling time, the air flow rate in the sampler, and the concentration in air. Lower concentrations in air can be measured by using longer sampling times or higher sampling rates. Most methods of analysis cannot demonstrate a chemical is not present, only that it cannot be detected with the methods used. These methods include the sampling and analysis methods, since a chemical present in the air may degrade, react, or off gas during transport and storage of the sample and no longer be in the sample at the time of analysis. There is a range above the LOD in which the presence of the chemical can be identified, but the amount cannot be quantified accurately. The top of that range is the quantifiable limit (QL), above which quantitative results can be obtained. In the TEAM study, the QL was taken to be four times the LOD.

Another air sampling study for which extensive information has been published and which might serve as a further case example is the Airborne Toxic Elements and Organic Substances (ATEOS) project which was designed to measure atmospheric levels of over 50 toxic and carcinogenic chemicals in three urban centers and one rural area in New Jersey (Lioy and Daisey, 1986).

Emission Rates

Emissions are the drivers of environmental transport models, but often more emphasis is placed on evaluation of the credibility of the models than of the emission rates used with them. Air emission rates are determined either by mass balance (e.g., the amount of carbon in the fuel less the amount remaining in the ash is the amount that went out the stack) or by stack measurements. Stack sampling is a demanding task. Effluents are usually at high concentrations and high temperatures and may be corrosive. Sampling locations which avoid turbulent flow may be hard to find. Timing is vital, and an understanding of the process generating the emissions is important to scheduling sampling, as emission rates may be highly nonuniform in time. Basic technical background information on stack sampling techniques can be found in Paulus and Thron (1976) and Nader (1976), although these cover primarily conventional pollutants. More recently, emissions of potentially carcinogenic substances have become of greater concern; this has led to development of new analytical methods specific to volatile and semivolatile organic emissions (Johnson, 1986; Jayanty and Hochheiser, 1987; Margeson et al., 1987). Even more difficult than stack emissions, however, are measurement of diffuse emissions from industrial facilities (fugitive emissions) or gaseous and volatile emissions from land treatment facilities and waste ponds. These include volatile organics from hazardous waste sites (Dupont, 1987) and radon from uranium mill tailings (NAS, 1987).

Occupational Exposures

Many occupational exposures are through the air route, and sampling techniques generally use personal exposure monitoring supplemented by fixed monitors. Unlike ambient air measurements, industrial hygienists monitoring the work environment have always focused on measuring what the worker actually breathes. Many of the techniques developed for industrial hygiene have been adapted in the new approaches to estimating exposures in the general population more realistically. The data still must be interpreted with care, however, because, while the aim may be to represent an individual's exposure, the individual measured may have been selected because he was at greater risk and not because he was representative of a class of workers. Occupational exposure measurements are often made for purposes of exposure management or regulatory compliance. Selection of workplaces and workers included in the measurement design may be biased toward high-exposure workers; care must be taken in using results of these measurements to represent the general exposure levels in an industry or job classification.

Occupational exposure also follows other routes. Skin contact has proved a difficult exposure for which to develop quantitative estimates. Some carcinogenic substances may be absorbed directly through the skin; others, deposited on the hands, may be ingested through hand-to-mouth contact or though contact with food. There are currently no widely accepted methods for sampling or analysis that can provide quantitative estimates of skin exposure (DOE, 1984). Although good industrial hygiene practice separates eating places from work places and avoids the problem of workers carrying contaminants home on their clothes or bodies by requiring showering and changing of clothing, these are potential routes of occupationally related exposure.

Frequently it is necessary to estimate occupational exposures retrospectively. An occupational exposure history is much like a medical history; it involves a probing interview and evaluation of the information previously obtained and recorded by industrial hygienists and chemists (Gerin et al., 1985). Exposure histories are generally limited to the worker's current job or company. Recognize, however, that many workers worked somewhere else previously, or hold a second job, or run a small shop out of their garage. All of these contribute to the occupational exposure history and, if unrecorded, may confound the results.

An understanding of the measurement of occupational exposures is obviously important in assessing occupational cancer risks, but the impact of occupational data go far beyond that. Because of the higher exposure levels and the better medical monitoring of workers, dose–response functions can be derived from occupational epidemiology when data on the general population are insufficient. Because they are based on people directly, these dose–response functions are generally preferred to those derived from animal experiments. The Environmental Protection Agency, for example, bases their dose–response functions for benzene exposure on occupational data. When using occupationally derived dose–response functions, it is important to understand the differences represented in the exposure measurements. Workers begin their exposures as adults and then are generally exposed 8-hours per day, 5-days per week. Exposures may even be concentrated in shorter periods of the work day. Seldom are workers exposed to one substance only; they are exposed to a complex mixture which is likely to be different from that to which the general public is exposed. Uranium miners, for example, are exposed to numerous dust and gaseous pollutants in the mines, but a dose–response function linking their radon gas exposure to lung cancer is often casually applied to the general public exposed to radon in their homes without considering that the public dose not have the same concurrent exposures. Moreover, occupational exposures are not total exposures. They do not include those hours (roughly 75% of the time) during which the worker has unmeasured exposures received in the course of hobbies, a second job, or other activities.

Water

The number of contaminants in water is limited only by the analytical techniques used for measurement (Shackelford and Cline, 1986). Most water samples are analyzed for a limited number of specific substances which are regulated or have been identified as potential carcinogens or priority pollutants. More rarely, samples are analyzed more extensively in an attempt to characterize the water quality. There are many contaminants in water, however, which cannot be adequately identified or quantified.

Measurement errors of physical and chemical properties of water contaminants are generally well within 25% of observed mean values; natural variations over time or space are much larger, typically 100% to 400% (Mar et al., 1986). This illustrates the importance of sampling design, an area sometimes given less attention than laboratory analysis.

Waters sampled for analysis of carcinogenic compounds include drinking water, surface waters, ground waters, and waste waters. Direct exposure measurements focus on drinking water. The standard approach is to sample from well-flushed taps to assure that, while the measurements reflect the water at the point of use, they are not affected by lead and other contaminants the water may pick up while lying stagnant in the household plumbing. Concern with indirect effects of acid rain, however, has led to flushing consistent with typical use patterns so that exposures are accurately represented.

Contaminant concentrations in surface waters are sometimes related to exposures during swimming, but this is usually not a significant source. Measurements in surface water, ground water, and municipal and industrial waste waters provide data to drive or verify environmental models used to predict exposure rather than direct exposure data. Sampling and analysis methods are detailed in Standard Methods for the Examination of Water and Wastewaters (APHA/AWWA/WPCA, 1985) and various Environmental Protection Agency reports (e.g., EPA, 1979, 1982a; Summers and Gherini, 1987).

Sampling groundwater presents special problems. The essential elements of effective groundwater sampling are (Barcelona et al., 1986):

Evaluation of the hydrogeologic setting and program information needs
Proper placement and construction of the sampling well
Evaluation of performance of the sampling well and purging strategies
Design and execution of appropriate sampling mechanisms and materials, and sample collection, handling, and analysis procedures

Soil

Contaminated soil poses risks in several ways: direct contact, especially to children; entrainment of soil into the air and subsequent inhalation; leaching of contaminants into groundwater; volatilization of contaminants from the soil into the air; and transfer of contaminants from the soil into the food chain through uptake through the roots of plants. Soil may be contaminated by deposition from the air, direct spills or dumping of contaminants, movement of contaminants from nearby contaminated soil, and volatilization of contaminant gases in ground water. Measurement of soil contamination is probably more closely tied to the contamination source than is the case for other environmental media. Spatial sampling design is also especially important in soil sampling. Geological and hydrologic factors, soil characterization, and location of potential sources of contamination must be considered. Contamination must be measured as a function of soil depth. The depth of concern depends upon the circumstances of contamination and potential exposure. For hand-to-mouth exposure in children, the first few centimeter are important; for uptake to plants, the depth will depend on the local species and how deep their roots penetrate; for potential groundwater contamination, a profile of soil contamination with depth will be useful to trace the penetration of contaminants through the unsaturated zone.

Analysis of polycyclic aromatic hydrocarbons and other solid-phase contaminants in soil samples, including those sorbed on soil particles, is similar to their analyses in particulate matter filtered from air (e.g., Blumer and Youngblood, 1975; Kitumen et al., 1987; Vogt et al., 1987). Recently, measurement of gas-phase volatile organic compounds in the air filling the space between soil particles has become important as a preliminary screening tool, planning more detailed sampling designs using groundwater monitoring wells or soil borings, and defining boundaries of contaminant plumes (Marrin and Kerfoot, 1988). Soil gas sampling methods require drilling of shallow boreholes or installation of sampling probes. Choice of a sampling technique is site-specific. Jowise et al. (1987) evaluate the attributes of five different techniques considering field effectiveness, analytical limitations, data validity, and cost.

Food

More than any other biological media, research has focused on developing analytical methods for detecting carcinogens in foods (Wogan and Tannen- baum, 1987). The methods developed for sampling and analysis of food in the Food and Drug Administration's Total Diet Study (Lombardo, 1986) might form the basis of any direct measurements of exposure via food in an exposure assessment. Consistent with a philosophy of population exposure, foods are not analyzed as purchased, but as eaten. The Total Diet Study includes 234 foods such as "beef and vegetable stew" and "apple pie." Washing, cooking, and other preparation steps can considerably reduce contaminant residues on food.

Each food was selected to represent a class of foods in the American diet and various weighted combinations among them represent the dietary intake of eight age-sex groups. Each food is then analyzed for industrial chemicals (e.g., polychlorinated biphenyls), heavy metals (e.g., cadmium, lead, mercury), pesticide residues, and radionuclides. Dietary intakes are calculated for each age-sex group. The 16–19-year-old male group is considered to have the highest dietary intake of chemical residues because of the kinds and quantities of foods consumed (Travis and Arms, 1987). Assessments which focus on particular ethnic groups or other subpopulations with distinctive food preparation or dietary habits must consider the sources and treatment of food eaten by the population of concern.

Biological Monitoring

Biological monitoring refers to measurements of contaminants or their indicators in body tissues and fluids. What better measure of a person's actual intake of a contaminant than the accumulation of that contaminant in the body? Measures of carboxyhemoglobin in blood, or carbon monoxide in alveolar air has always been accepted as a better measure of exposure to carbon monoxide than air samples. Lead content of blood is the standard approach to measuring lead exposure. Biological monitoring can provide an accurate and integrated measure of body intake of a contaminant from all sources and all exposure routes. It thus overcomes the problem of an unsuspected and unmeasured route of exposure. It automatically takes into account the various factors influencing uptake and absorption of the chemical such as individual variability, work load, hygiene habits or work practices (Bernard and Lauwerys, 1986). Recent increased emphasis on biological modeling and the development of new techniques stems from an increased focus on risk assessment (Dowd, 1984). Biological monitoring is not a panacea, however; it has its problems. For example, it is more expensive and more intrusive on peoples' lives than ambient monitoring; not all contaminants accumulate in the body and the biological half-life of those that do varies among chemicals; chemicals with short-lived metabolites (e.g., vinyl chloride) may not be adequately represented if sampled far from the target tissue. Nonetheless, biological monitoring is a powerful tool for measuring exposure that is rapidly becoming more important.

Some relationships between exposure and concentrations in blood or urine are sufficiently well established that index levels have been recommended. The American Conference of Governmental Industrial Hygienist, which propagates threshold limit values (TLVs) for occupational exposure to various substances, has developed biological exposure indices (BEIs) which correspond to TLVs. They are defined as "an index chemical that appears in a biological fluid or expired air following an exposure to a workplace chemical" (Lowry, 1986).

The measure of exposure is one which most closely approximates or correlates with the biologically effective dose, i.e., the dose to the target cell or tissue. Measuring contaminants in exhaled breath, in blood, or in urine is generally a better method of measuring exposure from this perspective than measuring concentrations in ambient air, food, or drinking water. Measures known to represent concentrations in the target tissue are yet better, and measures of the specific exposure to the DNA of the target cell (possibly achieved by measuring DNA adducts) the best. Of course, while these may be progressively better measures of total exposure, they are not useful in identifying the source of the exposure. If the purpose of the risk assessment is to determine the link between a specific exposure to cancer risk, environmental measures will be necessary to determine the contributions of various routes to the total and modeling may be necessary to bring this home to a specific source. Nonetheless, knowing the total exposure avoids the problem of attempting to assign the total cancer burden in a population to one source of exposure among many.

The biological measure may represent different things depending on the character of the pollutant and the kind of biological marker selected.

These include: the amount of chemical recently absorbed, the amount of chemical stored in one or more body compartments (e.g., bone or fatty tissue) over a considerable time, the amount of metabolic products of the chemical stored in the body, the amount of chemical interacting with the target site, or some measure of biological effect which is indicative of the exposure. Some of these may be more specifically linked to environmental exposures than others. Blood lead content is specific for environmental exposure to lead, but some fraction of carboxyhemoglobin is endogenously generated and carboxyhemoglobin may also be produced by exposure to methylene chloride, a common paint stripper. Several organic compounds may have the same metabolite. The amount of that metabolite in blood or urine is, then, not specific to any one exposure. Moreover, the quantitative relationship of a metabolite with its initial compound may depend on dose rate and individual variation in metabolism. Despite these limitations, metabolites are an important class of markers for compound-specific and chemical-class exposures. Diazopositive metabolites in urine have been proposed to monitor exposure to aromatic amines, and thioesters in urine to indicate exposure to electrophilic substances which include many carcinogens (Bernard and Lauwerys, 1986). Radioimmunoassay is a rapidly developing approach for measuring metabolites which can detect extremely small concentrations; for example, as little as 1 ng of 4-acetamidobiphenyl, a metabolite of the carcinogen 4-aminobiphenyl, can be detected in urine by this method (Wogan and Gorelick, 1985).

Smoking is such an important confounding factor in epidemiological studies of environmental carcinogenesis and self-reporting is so often inaccurate (perhaps the product of self-deception on the part of smokers), that a biomarker which can provide a definite and quantitative measure of smoking is highly desirable. Moreover, a marker that could provide a quantitative measure of passive smoking—the involuntary exposure of nearby people to side-stream cigarette smoke—would also be of use. Some nicotine is excreted in the urine; it can be measured in the saliva, also. The rate of nicotine metabolism varies as much as fourfold among smokers, however, so nicotine levels in urine, while specific, do not provide an accurate quantitative indicator unless calibrated in each individual. Levels of cotinine, the major metabolite of nicotine, vary much less than residual nicotine levels; measured in urine, cotinine provides both a specific and relatively accurate quantitative measure of exposure to tobacco smoke. Thiocyanate, a metabolite of hydrogen cyanide (a component of cigarette smoke) has also been suggested as a biomarker for exposure to tobacco smoke; but cyanide is also a component of leafy vegetables, some nuts, and beer, so its metabolite is not specific to cigarette smoke (HHS, 1986).

The Ames test for mutagenicity has demonstrated its usefulness in identifying mutagenic substances in urine, the direct or metabolic products of carcinogenic exposures (Yamasaki and Ames, 1977; Everson, 1986; Fatiadi, 1984). It is completely nonspecific in that it simply identifies the presence of mutagenic substances, not any specific chemical. This may be looked upon as an advantage for a screening assay, in which the exposure or its metabolites are unknown. It can be followed with more detailed chemical fractionation to identify the chemical source of the mutagenic action. While the Ames test is discussed in greater detail in a later chapter, some further comment must be added here. In testing environmental samples, enzymes may be added to metabolize the environmental contaminant, simulating the metabolic action taking place in the body. These are reported as estimates of direct and indirect mutagenicity. When the sample taken is from urine, presence of an indirect acting mutagen is of less biological significance since the exposure has already gone through the metabolic process and the active metabolite has not appeared. Everson (1986) noted inconsistency in the results of Ames testing of urine among occupational studies. He attributed this to (1) variation in the exposure mix, (2) differences among unstudied confounding factors, (3) differences in assay technique among researchers, (4) confounding effects of toxic or growth-promoting substances in the extracts tested, (5) inadequate or inappropriate statistical analysis. Nonetheless, he concluded that they should continue to have a significant role in detection of mutagenic exposures in situations that can capitalize on their advantages.

Markers of effect can also indicate exposure and dose. Like mutagenicity in urine, effects markers are generally not specific. Hydroxyproline in urine or its ratio to creatinine may indicate break-down of lung tissue and has been suggested as an indicator of nitrogen dioxide exposure to the lung, but other pollutants and even diet can affect this measure. Smoking status is an important confounding factor in studies using nonspecific tests for mutagens and carcinogens since many of these tests are, of course, affected by the carcinogenic nature of tobacco smoke exposure. Because of the importance of smoking, it is advisable to include in the study measurement of tobacco-specific indicators rather than relying on statements of whether people are smokers or nonsmokers or on how much they smoke.

Some biochemical indicators may serve either as a measure of exposure or effect. Chromosome aberrations, for example, are an effect, but their meaningfulness as an earlier indicator of a carcinogenic effect is unclear. Their best purpose at present may be as a nonspecific measure of exposure to mutagenic agents. Even here, however, it must be recognized that the results may be influenced by infection or processes other than chemical exposure.

Most tests rely on the determination of the chemical or its metabolites in urine, blood, and alveolar air; sputum, saliva, and nasal mucosa are also readily accessible for noninvasive sampling for biochemical indicators of respiratory system exposure. Analytical methods to identify and quantify chemical contaminants in human fat, skin, nails, hair, blood, urine, and breath were evaluated by Sheldon et al. (1986) to determine their accuracy, precision, ease, speed, and cost. Contaminant concentrations in or on hair have frequently been used as a biological sampling site but have proved not to be satisfactory because of variations due to washing. Concentrations in urine, when collected at an appropriate time, are generally better than alveolar air. The metabolism of the chemical in humans must have been sufficiently investigated to provide a basis for deciding the best source of the sample, the specific metabolite for which to sample, and the appropriate time of day or lag following exposure (Bernard and Lauwerys, 1986).

DNA Adducts

Especially exciting opportunities for biomarkers of exposure are found in DNA adducts. The active forms of many chemical carcinogens are metabolites which bind to cellular macromolecules, including nucleic acids and proteins; the product of these bindings are called adducts. The formation of DNA adducts are thought by many to be cancer-initiating events (Wogan and Tannenbaum, 1987). What better index of the biologically effective dose than the actual dose causing the initiating event itself. As discussed earlier (Chap. 2), in addition to initiation, the progression step in carcinogenesis may also require a DNA-damaging event. Thus, DNA adducts may be indicators of exposure affecting both early and late steps in cancer development (Harris, 1985). Much work has been done to build an understanding of the relationship between exposure or, in experimental animals, administered dose, and the levels of DNA adducts. A linear relationship is often, but not always, found (Perera, 1987; Belinsky et al., 1987; Adriaenssens et al., 1983; Dunn, 1983). Pharmacokinetics, discussed in a later chapter, rules this relationship.

The relationship between DNA adducts and tumor formation is not as well understood. Perera (1987) points out three lines of evidence: (1) correlation between the ability of polyaromatic hydrocarbons and alkylating agents to form adducts and their carcinogenic potency in animal bioassay; (2) in vitro studies linking adduct formation to cell transformation; and (3) elevated adduct formation in sensitive animal species. The last has also been shown in presumed cancer-sensitive individuals among humans (Rudiger et al, 1985) and suggests the possible use of DNA adduct measurements as a screening tool for detecting sensitivity as well as exposure. The variability introduced by sensitivity also may be a confounding factor in interpreting DNA adduct measurements as a marker of dose. A particularly strong bit of evidence is provided by Swenberg et al. (1985). They found that two classes of carcinogens, methylating hepatocarcinogens and ethylating agents produced a predominance of DNA adducts in rat livers with the same specificity in cell type as they were known to produce tumors.

The measurement of DNA adducts is not as simple as might appear, however. DNA adducts can be measured in white blood cells or, since some adducts are removed from cellular DNA and excreted, the measurement can be made in urine. Initially, DNA adducts were measured using experimental exposure to radiotagged carcinogens, but it has become possible to quantify DNA adducts from specific environmental exposures using monoclonal antibodies with highly sensitive immunoassays (Santella et al., 1985). If the chemical nature and stability of the adducts and their excretion rates have been fully characterized (not a simple task), qualitative and quantitative identification of adduct levels can, *in principle*, provide an estimate of recent exposure history and biologically effective dose. There are complexities in interpretation and practical application, however (Wogan and Tannenbaum, 1987): carcinogens vary in structural complexity and form covalent bonds at a variety of nucleophilic sites on all four DNA bases as well as on the phosphate backbone of DNA, and adducts are removed from DNA at different rates for each tissue or even for the same adduct in different types of cells in the same tissue. The amount of DNA adduct also depends on the dynamic metabolic balance between carcinogen activation and deactivation and DNA repair rates. This varies by individual; a 50- to 150-fold variation in adduct formation and several-fold variation in repair has been measured in cultured human tissues (Harris, 1985). While the promise is great, much work is still needed before DNA adducts are a fully useful and practical tool for exposure assessment.

COMPLEX MIXTURES

Exposures via all environmental media involve complex mixtures, i.e., collections of so many chemicals that estimating risk or toxicity based on some combination of the toxicities of the individual components of the mixture is impossible or involves too much uncertainty to be useful. In this chapter, the concern is not with the toxicity of the mixture, but with sampling measurement and chemical characterization. This cannot be done independent from consideration of the toxicology and health effects; it must provide sufficient detail to allow factors which influence the exposure-response relationship to be considered. For example, SO_2 gas alone does not penetrate deep into the respiratory system, but when fine particles are available to which it may adsorb, it can be carried there. The exposure characterization must include information on the presence of fine particles.

Chemical interferences pose difficulties with complex mixtures. Methods developed and tested in a relatively clean laboratory environment may suffer from unexpected interferences in a complex mixture. Field testing, e.g., with spiked field samples, is essential. Methods to fractionate complex mixtures into component groupings using extraction, concentration, and separation are discussed in NAS (1988). Additional work in this area may be found in Wright et al. (1983) and Gray et al. (1987).

It is not possible to measure the concentrations of all the constituents of an exposure environment or bodily tissues or fluids. Indicators or surrogate compounds must be used; these might be a subset of key components, one predominant compound, a commonly used indicator compound for a class of chemicals (such as benzo[a]pyrene), or other chemical or biological markers such as "benzene soluble substances" or mutagenic activity on the Ames test. None of these is ideal, but they must serve until something better is found. Correlation between index compounds and effect in different mixes has often proved to be poor; there is great need for better methods of characterizing exposures to complex mixtures. Given the use of an index, comparisons among different exposures may be improved by modifications based on more detailed characterization. Detailed characterization is expensive and time-consuming. One approach is to carry out detailed characterization on a small number of samples which, while not fully representative of the exposure, may provide some basis for going beyond the index measurements. Moreover, an initial detailed characterization can help to select appropriate index compounds or to determine the validity of commonly used indices for a particular exposure. Another approach is the use of target monitoring of human tissues or sentinel animals using biological markers of effect such as chromosome aberrations or sister chromotid exchange (Falco, 1984; Galloway and Tice, 1982).

PRE-COMPILED MEASUREMENTS: ENVIRONMENTAL DATABASES

Exposure assessments often are forced to rely on information gleaned from available databases rather than direct measurements. There is certain basic information that must be available in a database for the data to be even minimally acceptable for exposure assessment; these include: the location, date and time of the sampling; the sampling protocol; the analytical method used. In addition, there must be some stated measure of quality assurance associated with the maintenance of the database and minimum quality requirements for allowing data to be entered in the database. Because the data were generally collected for a different purpose than exposure assessment, much important information cannot be expected. This generally involves data on individuals that confound or modify exposure such as cigarette smoking and occupational exposure. Some of the potential pitfalls in using pre-existing databases are discussed by Gann (1986).

Drinking Water

There are over 200,000 public water systems in the United States. The Federal Reporting Data System (FRDS), established by EPA under the Safe Drinking Water Act, contains water quality data only for measurements which exceed National Interim Primary Drinking Water Regulations. It is not a useful source of water quality data for exposure assessments. Files of State agencies charged with monitoring drinking water quality more often contain complete analytical results, not simply exceedences. State data also generally cover a longer time period. Unfortunately, much of the state data are not computerized, making retrieval difficult. Data may also be available from individual water suppliers, but again is unlikely to be in computerized form (Wentworth et al., 1986).

Ambient Water Sources

The Environmental Protection Agency maintains a massive database of water quality measurements called STORET (EPA, 1982b). STORET currently holds over 80 million data points, including measurements of organic and inorganic pollutants in water and some additional measurements of sediment and tissue (Shackelford and Cline, 1986). Each measurement is associated with identifying information such as sampling location, date, and weather conditions. STORET can be a powerful resource, but the size and complexity of the STORET database and lack of uniform quality control on the data result in a requirement for the investment of considerable time and effort to extract useful and meaningful information.

About 500,000 ground and surface water sites for which water quality data are available are listed in the U.S. Geological Survey's Master Water

Data Index (MWDI). This can be searched by geographical area, type of site, and longitude/latitude.

Food

Since the early 1960s, the Food and Drug Administration has conducted the Total Diet Study, also known as the Market Basket Study (Lombardo, 1986). Currently, 234 food items are selected to represent 5,000 different foods identified in a national diet survey. Four times a year the foods are purchased retail in three cities within one of four geographical areas of the country. The foods are prepared as for consumption and each of the 234 prepared foods is analyzed individually. Analyses include over 100 pesticide, many industrial chemicals, heavy metals, radionuclides, and essential elements. Based on dietary survey information, intakes are then calculated for eight age–sex groups. While these data provide a general picture of pollutant levels in food, they are not directly useful as exposure measures in any particular exposure assessment (except a general exposure assessment of total exposure from all sources of one of the contaminants included). They might be used as measures of background exposure levels, forming a base to which exposures from a particular source might be added.

Biological

The National Human Adipose Tissue Database contains approximately 22,000 measurements of 20 chemicals in human adipose tissue. It is maintained by the EPA Office of Toxic Substances (OTS). Additional information is maintained by OTS in the Chemicals Identified in Human Biological Media Database which contains human body burden data on 1,000 chemicals. The EPA Office of Pesticide Program's National Human Milk Monitoring Program contains measurements of chlorinated hydrocarbon insecticides and PCB residues found in human milk samples from 3,000 volunteers randomly selected from the entire United States.

SUMMARY

Environmental measurements may be the basis of exposure assessment, part of the basis of a dose–response function, or the source of information in an exposure database. No matter what their role in the analysis, or how far removed from the current study the measurements were made, an understanding of the implications the sampling and chemical and biochemical analysis have for the rest of the risk assessment is vital knowledge which the analyst must have. While some characteristics of sampling design and chemical analysis are similar, measurement techniques have generally been developed independently for the various environmental media. Many of these measurement methods are designed for establishing trends, for assuring regulatory compliance, or other purposes. The analyst must recognize that many of these purposes are not entirely compatible with the needs of exposure assessment. Exposure estimates must often draw entirely on available databases; these are introduced.

REFERENCES

Adriaenssens, P.I., C.M. White, and M.W. Anderson. 1983. Dose-response relationships for the binding of benzo[a]pyrene metabolites to DNA and protein in lung, liver, and forestomach of control and butylated hydroxyanisole-treated mice. *Cancer Res.* 43: 3712-3719.

APHA/AWWA.WPCA. 1985. *Standard Methods for the Examination of Water and Wastewaters*, 16th ed. American Public Health Associate, American Water Works Association, Water Pollution Control Federation, Washington, D.C.

Barcelona, M.J., J.P. Gibb, J.A. Helfrich, and E.E. Garske. 1986. Practical guide for ground-water sampling (EPA/600-85/104). U.S. Environmental Protection Agency, Robert S. Kerr Environmental Research Laboratory, Ada, OK.

Belinsky, S.A., C.M. White, T.R. Devereux, and M.W. Anderson. 1987. DNA adducts as a dosimeter for risk estimation. *Environ. Health Perspect.* 76:3-8.

Bernard, A. and R. Lauwerys. 1986. Present status and trends in biological monitoring of exposure to industrial chemicals. *J. Occupat. Med.* 28:558-562.

Blumer, M. and W.W. Youngblood. 1975. Polycyclic aromatic hydrocarbons in soils and recent sediments. *Science* 188:53-55.

Davis, C.S., P. Fellin, and R. Otson. 1987. A review of sampling methods for polyaromatic hydrocarbons in air. *J. Air Pollution Control Assoc.* 37:1397-1408.

Dunn. B.P. 1983. Wide-range linear dose–response curve for DNA binding of orally administered benzo[a]pyrene in mice. *Cancer Res.* 43:2654-2658.

DOE. 1984. Proceedings of the DOE-OHER Workshop on Monitoring and Dosimetry in an Occupational Health Research Program for Synfuel Technologies (CONF-8403150). U.S. Department of Energy, Washington, D.C.

Dowd, R.M. 1984. Biological monitoring. *Environ. Sci. Technol.* 18:215A.

Dupont, R.R. 1987. Measurement of volatile hazardous organic emissions from land treatment facilities. *J. Air Pollution Control Assoc.* 37:168-176.

EPA. 1979. Methods for chemical analysis of water and wastes (EPA-600/4-79-020). U.S. Environmental Protection Agency, Cincinnati, OH.

EPA. 1982a. Handbook for sampling and sample preservation of water and wastewater (EPA-600/4-82-029). U.S. Environmental Protection Agency, Cincinnati, OH.

EPA. 1982b. STORET User Handbook, Office of Information and Resources Management. U.S. Environmental Protection Agency, Washington, D.C.

Everson, R.B. 1986. Detection of occupational and environmental exposures by bacterial mutagenesis assays of human body fluids. *J. Occupat. Med.* 28:647-655.

Falco, J. 1984. Assessment of exposures. In J.F. Stara and L.S. Erdreich (eds.), Approaches to Risk Assessment for Multiple Chemical Exposures (EPA 600/9-84-008), U.S. Environmental Protection Agency, Cincinnati, OH, pp. 184-185.

Fatiadi, A.J. 1984. Priority toxic pollutants in human urine: their occurrence and analysis. *Environ. Int.* 10:175-205.

Galloway, S.M. and R.R. Tice. 1982. Cytogenetic monitoring of human populations, in R.R. Tice, D.L. Costa, and K.M. Schaich, (eds.), *Genotoxic Effects of Airborne Agents*. Plenum Press, New York., pp. 463-488.

Gann. P. 1986. Use and misuse of existing data bases in environmental epidemiology: the case of air pollution, in F.C. Kopfler and G.F. Craun (eds.), *Environmental Epidemiology: The Importance of Exposure Assessment* (EPA 600/9-86/030), U.S. Environmental Protection Agency, Health Effects Research Laboratory, Cincinnati, OH, pp. 105-118.

Gerin, M., J. Siemiatycki, H. Kemper, and D. Begin. 1985. obtaining occupational exposure histories in epidemiologic case-control studies. *J. Occupat Med.* 27:420-426.

Gray, R.H., E.K. Chess, P.J. Mellinger, R.G. Riley, and D.L. Springer. 1987. *Health & Environmental Research on Complex Organic Mixtures* (CONF-851027). Pacific Northwest Laboratory, Richland, WA.

Harris, C.C. 1985. Future directions in the use of DNA adducts as internal dosimeters for monitoring human exposure to environmental mutagens and carcinogens. *Environ. Health Perspectives* 62: 185-191.

HHS. 1986. the Health Consequences of Involuntary Smoking, A Report of the Surgeon General. U.S. Department of Health and Human Services, Rockville, MD.

Howes, J.E., T.L. Merriman, C.A. Oritz, A.R. McFarland, and M.R. Kuhlman. 1986. Development of a sampler for particulate-associated and low volatility organic pollutants in residential air (EPA/600/4-85/079). U.S. Environmental Protection Agency, Research Triangle Park, NC.

Hushon, J.M. and R.J. Clerman. 1981. Estimation of exposure to hazardous chemicals. In J. Saxena and F. Fisher (eds.), *Hazard Assessment of Chemicals*. Academic Press, New York, pp. 323-388.

Jayanty, R.K.M. and S. Hochheiser. 1987. Summary of the 1987 EPA/APCA symposium on measurement of toxic and related air pollutants. *J. Air Pollution Control Assoc.* 37:898-905.

Johnson, L.D. 1986. Detecting waste combustion emissions. *Environ. Sci. Technol.* 20:223-227.

Jowise, P.P., J.D. Villnow, L.I. Gorelik, and R.M. Ryding. 1987. Comparative analysis of soil gas sampling techniques. In *Proceedings, National Conference on Hazardous Wastes and Hazardous Materials*. Hazardous Materials Control Research Institute, Silver Spring, MD, pp. 193-199.

Kitumen, V.H., R.J. Valo, and M.S. Salkinoj-Salonen. 1987. Contamination of soil around wood-preserving facilities by polychlorinated aromatic compounds. *Environ. Sci. Technol.* 21:96-101.

Lave, L.B. and A.C. Upton (eds.). 1987. *Toxic Chemicals, Health, and the Environment.* The Johns Hopkins University Press, Baltimore.

Lioy, P.J. and J.M. Daisey. 1986. Airborne toxic elements and organic substances. *Environ. Sci. Technol.* 20:8-14.

Lombardo, P. 1986. The FDA Total Diet Study program. In F.C. Kopfler (ed.), *Environmental Epidemiology: The Importance of Exposure Assessment* (EPA/600/9-86/030). U.S. Environmental Protection Agency, Research Triangle Park, NC, pp. 136-143.

Lowry, L.K. 1986. Biological exposure index as a complement to the TLV. *J. Occupat. Med.* 28:578-582.

Mage, D.T. and L.A. Wallace (eds.). 1979. *Proceedings of the symposium on the Development and Usage of Personal Monitors for Exposure and Health Effect Studies* (EPA-600/0-79-032). U.S. Environmental Protection Agency, Research Triangle Park, NC.

Mancy, K.H. (ed.). 1971. *Instrumental Analysis for Water Pollution Control.* Ann Arbor Science Publishers, Ann Arbor, MI.

Mar, B.W., R.R. Horner, J.S. Richey, R.N. Palmer, and D.P. Lettenmaier. 1986. Data acquisition, cost-effective methods for obtaining data on water quality. *Environ. Sci. Technol.* 20:545-551.

Margeson, J.H., J.E. Knoll, M.R. Midgett, D.E. Wagoner, J. Rice, and J.B. Homolya. 1987. An evaluation of the semi-VOST method for determining emissions from hazardous waste incinerators. *JAPCA* 37:1067-1074.

Marrin, D.L. and H.B. Kerfoot. 1988. Soil-gas surveying techniques. *Environ. Sci. Technol.* 22:740745.

Morgan, M.G. and S.C. Morris. 1977. Needed: a national R&D effort to develop individual air pollution monitors. *J. Air Pollution Control Assoc.* 27:670-673.

Nader, J.S. 1976. Source monitoring. In A.C. Stern (ed.), *Air Pollution* 3d Ed, Vol III. Academic Press, New York, pp. 589-645.

NAS. 1981. *Indoor Pollutants.* Committee on Indoor Pollutants, National Research Council. National Academy Press, Washington, D.C.

NAS. 1988. *Complex Mixtures, Methods for In Vivo Toxicity Testing.* Committee on Methods for the In Vivo Toxicity Testing of Complex Mixtures. National Academy Press, Washington, D.C.

NAS. 1986. Scientific Basis for Risk Assessment and Management of Uranium Mill Tailings. Uranium Mill Tailings Study Panel, National Research Council. National Academy Press, Washington, D.C.

Natusch, D.F.S., J.R. Wallace, and C.A. Evans. 1974. Toxic trace elements: preferential concentration in respirable particles. *Science* 183:202-204.

Paulus, H.J. and R.W. Thron. 1976. Stack Sampling. In A.C. Stern (ed.), *Air Pollution*, (3d Ed) Vol III. Academic Press, New York, pp. 525-587.

Perera, F. 1987. The potential usefulness of biological markers in risk assessment. *Environ. Health Perspec.* 76:141-145.

Rudiger, H.W., D. Nowak, K. Hartmann, and P. Cerutti. 1985. Enhanced formation of benzo[a]pyrene: DNA adducts in monocytes of patients with a presumed predisposition to lung cancer. *Cancer Res.* 45:5890-5894.

Santella, R.M., L-L. Hsieh, C-D. Lin, S. Viet, and I.B. Weinstein. 1985. Quantitation of exposure to benzo[a]pyrene with monoclonal antibodies. *Environ. Health Perspect.* 62:95-99.

Schroeder, W.H., M. Dobson, D.M. Kane, N.D. Johnson. 1987. Toxic trace elements associated with airborne particulate matter: a review. *J. Air Pollution Control Assoc.* 37:1267-1285.

Shackelford, W.M and D.M. Cline. 1986. Organic compounds in water. *Environ. Sci. Technol.* 20:652-657.   ·

Sheldon, L., M. Umana, J. Bursey, W. Gutknecht, R. Handy, P. Hyldburg, L. Michael, A. Moseley, J. Raymer, D. Smith, C. Sparacino, and M. Warner. 1986. Evaluation of methods for analysis of human fat, skin, nails, hair, blood, urine, and breath (EPA 600/8-85/020). U.S. Environmental Protection Agency, Washington, D.C.

Spengler, J.D. and M.L. Soczek. 1984. Evidence for improved ambient air quality and the need for personal exposure research. *Environ. Sci. Technol.* 18:269A-280A.

Stevens, R.K. 1986. Modern methods to measure air pollutants. In S.D. Lee, T. Schneider, L.D. Grant, and P.J. Verkerk (eds.), *Aerosols: Research, Risk Assessment, and Control Strategies.* Lewis Publishers, Chelsea, MI, pp. 69-95.

Summers, K.V. and S.A. Gherini. 1987. Sampling guidelines for groundwater quality (EA-4952). Electric Power Research Institute, Palo Alto, CA.

Swenberg, J. A., F. C. Richardson, J. A. Boucheron, and M. C. Dyroff. 1985. Relationships between DNA adduct formation and carcinogenesis. *Environmental Health Perspectives* 62:177-183.

Travis, C.C. and A.D. Arms. 1987. The food chain as a source of toxic chemical exposure. In L.B. Lave and A.C. Upton, (eds.), *Toxic Chemicals, Health, and the Environment.* The Johns Hopkins University Press, Baltimore, pp. 95-113.

Vogt, N.B., F.Brakstad, K. Thrane, S. Nordenson, J. Krane, E. Aamot, K. Koiset, K. Esbensen, and E. Steinnes. 1987. Polycyclic aromatic hydrocarbons in soil and air: statistical analysis and classification by the SIMCA method. *Environ. Sci. Technol.* 21:35-44.

Wallace, L.A. 1987. The Total Exposure Assessment Methodology (TEAM) Study: Summary and Analysis: volume I (EPA/600/6-87/002a). U.S Environmental Protection Agency, Washington, D.C.

Wentworth, N.W., K.K. Wang, and J.J. Westrick. 1986. Drinking water quality data bases. In F.C. Kopfler (ed.), *Environmental Epidemiology: The Importance of Exposure Assessment* (EPA/600/9-86/030). U.S. Environmental Protection Agency, Research Triangle Park, NC, pp. 127-135.

WHO. 1982. *Estimating Human Exposure to Air Pollutants* (WHO Offset Publ. No. 69). World Health Organization, Geneva.

Wogan, G.N. and N.J. Gorelick. 1985. Chemical and biochemical dosimetry of exposure to genotoxic chemicals. *Environ. Health Perspect.* 62:5-18.

Wogan, G.N. and S.R. Tannenbaum. 1987. Biological monitoring of environmental toxic chemicals. In L.B. Lave and A.C. Upton. (eds.), *Toxic Chemicals, Health, and the Environment.* The Johns Hopkins University Press, Baltimore, MD., pp 142-169..

Wright, C.W., W.C. Weimer, and W.D. Felix (eds.). 1983. *Advanced Techniques in Synthetic Fuels Analysis* (PNL-SA-11552). Technical Information Center, U.S. Department of Energy, Washington, D.C.

Yamasaki, E. and B.N. Ames. 1977. Concentration of mutgens from urine by adsorption with nonpolar resin XAD-2: cigarette smokers have mutagenic urine. *Proc. Natl. Acad. Sci.* 74:3555-3559.

6

Modeling Exposure

Although it would be nice to base all exposure assessments on measurements, it is more usual to find few or none are available and the assessment must be based on environmental models. Moreover, assessments often are concerned with future possibilities or the comparison of different options. Exposure models are the only way of doing these assessments. Environmental transport and dispersion modeling is a highly developed field of study; in fact, it is several highly developed fields of study, since transport in each of the different environmental media (air, water, food chains) is the realm of a different discipline. Several interdisciplinary efforts have created integrated multimedia sets of compatible models.

There is no unifying theory of environmental transport models. The processes involved and the methods of treating those processes differ among the environmental media. This makes multimedia modeling particularly difficult, especially when models must interact with each other.

Preliminary exposure assessments for hazard assessments or preliminary risk assessments may focus on the single largest or most probable route of exposure. Even in more detailed exposure assessments, a given route of exposure may, at some level of analysis, be judged insignificant and not pursued further (EPA, 1986a). Pathways that form the major routes of human exposure are called principal exposure pathways. Analysis to identify principal exposure pathways should evaluate sources, locations, and types of environmental releases as well as the characteristics of the substance itself which determine its behavior in the environment.

A difficulty for exposure assessment is that environmental transport models have not, in general, been developed to estimate human exposure, but to estimate environmental concentrations at some distance from the source, often for regulatory analysis. One or more steps must be added, therefore, to carry the exposure to the population who breathe indoor, not outdoor, air, who drink treated water, and eat processed food not grown in their neighborhood. Since most models were designed for regulatory purposes, "conservative" assumptions are built-in to assure concentrations are overestimated rather than underestimated. These overestimates then carry through the risk assessment. Investigation of the model and its basic assumptions can sometimes reveal the sources of the overestimates, but their size is usually difficult or impossible to determine.

Models are, of course, simplifications of reality and often include substantial uncertainty.

Transport models can range from simple calculations done on hand calculators to complex models involving the solution of hundreds of coupled partial differential equations which can only be run on modern supercomputer systems. Most models used for risk assessment are somewhere in between. Models were originally designed to operate on mainframe computers. Until the 1980s, access to computers spelled the difference between sophisticated risk assessment and "back of the envelope"-based assessment. The advent of microcomputers has made fairly sophisticated models widely available. The EPA EXAMS model (Burns et al., 1982, 1985), for example, is now available in a version suitable for the IBM-XT with 5 megabytes of hard disk storage.

It must be remembered, however, that modeling capability is only partly in the computer; the knowledge of the analyst in using and interpreting the results of the model is a key component. Also, no matter how sophisticated the model, the results can be no better than the data used to drive the model. Depending on the situation, data can be more or less important. All models require data, but most computer codes have "default" data built-in. In some cases, for example for new chemicals, data may have to be "borrowed" from other, presumably similar, substances and exposure analysis based on analogy (EPA, 1986). The use of poor or inappropriate data with a sophisticated model may obscure the uncertainty in exposure calculations by making them appear to be more credible than the data would justify. Proper data selection and handling is one of the most important tasks requiring the knowledge, skill, experience, and judgment of the expert modeler.

Assessment sometimes focuses on potential effects of an existing or proposed plant at a particular spot. At other times, an entire industry or national or global use of a particular chemical might be the subject of the assessment with estimation of exposures from many different sources. Another approach is the generic assessment, in which a typical or reference facility is examined which represents a large class of existing or proposed facilities. Risk assessments of the development of a new synthetic fuels industry were based on scenarios of how and where the industry might develop and included not just reference facilities; entire "reference environments" were developed to allow standardized situations in which to compare the effects of different proposed technologies (Travis et al., 1983).

In addition to different media, environmental transport includes many different processes. These can be divided into three main categories: (1) transport (e.g., advection and dispersion), (2) transfer (e.g., sorption and volatilization, and (3) transformation (e.g., photolysis and biodegradation). In general, the importance of the processes, and current understanding are in the order given (Donigian and Brown, 1983). Transport is considered first since transport processes are the best understood and data are more likely to be available to support models of these processes. Also, contaminants must move from their source to expose people and transport processes define the range of movement and the scope of potential exposure. Transfer processes involve movement from one media to another. Assessments focusing on a single media often consider transfers to other media (e.g., deposition of air pollutions to soil or water) to be losses, but these are in fact source terms for other environmental pathways. In many cases, these secondary sources may be much less important than primary sources; this should not be assumed, however, without justification. Transformation also is often considered to be a loss, but the analyst should be aware that transformation products may be pollutants also. The need to follow multiple transformation products can substantially complicate exposure assessments since changes in chemical form can change transport parameters. This is most important in following radioactive pollutants where decay products are sometimes more important than the initial substance; radon gas is an example.

This chapter begins with a brief discussion of considerations in evaluating and selecting models. It then describes emission scenarios and source terms, the initiators of the transport process. This is followed by a discussion of models for each of the major transport pathways: air, water, soil, and food chains. A useful further reference on these models, although focused on modeling of radiological exposure, is Till and Meyer (1982). Pathway models generally end with estimates of concentrations in the media (air, water, food) to which people might be exposed. Since there is no exposure without people, the role of exposed populations in exposure assessment is then described. The chapter concludes with a discussion of integrated population exposure modeling. This takes the focus off the environmental models and puts it on population exposure by carrying the exposure pathway calculations through from concentrations in environmental media to which people could be exposed to estimates of the levels to which people actually are exposed.

EVALUATION OF ENVIRONMENTAL MODELS

There are a number of general considerations in selecting environmental transport and exposure models for use in an exposure assessment (Table 6-1). Models are based on known physical concepts such as conservation of mass or continuity, or on empirical observations. These concepts are generally implemented in a computer code with mathematical algorithms. Some algorithms may better represent the theory than others. In addition, various assumptions are often built into transport models. The theory, algorithms, and assumptions can all affect the accuracy and uncertainty of model results and these implications should be understood by the analyst. Since risk assessments frequently involve low-dose exposures, the extent to which the theory and assumptions of the model are applicable and the equations used well-behaved at the expected exposure levels are important considerations. The very approach taken in the model may be designed to determine regulatory compliance and be inappropriate for risk assessment.

Many environmental carcinogens undergo chemical changes during environmental transport due to exposure to sunlight or interaction with other chemicals in the ambient environment. Radioactive pollutants undergo decay. Some of these changes may inactivate them, making them no longer of interest in the assessment. Other changes may activate previously benign materials or increase the potency of toxins (e.g., biological formation of methyl mercury from mercury depositing in sediments). Complex chemical processes may be involved such as in the formation of photochemical smog. The degree to which the model can handle these processes is a factor in model selection.

TABLE 6-1   General Evaluation Criteria for Environmental Transport and Exposure Models

Theory on which the model is based
Algorithm(s) used in implementing the model
Applicability of the model to the site and/or scenario
Ability of the model to treat chemical or physical transformations of pollutants
Extent to which the model has been verified and validated
Extent to which the model has been subjected to sensitivity and uncertainty analysis
Compatibility of the model input and output with available data and with other models used

Source: Adapted from Morris et al., 1986.

Validation, Calibration, and Verification

Validation is a comparison of the model predictions with actual laboratory or field experimental results, or with results of other "validated" or accepted models. Validation may range from a rigorous experimental protocol and statistical performance evaluation to "insightful groping" for clues to model improvements. The latter involves experience and intuition; the former, protocols to measure the absence of bias, gross error, correlation between residuals and observed values, and correlation between residuals and exogenous variables. Validation at one site or under one set of circumstances does not necessarily imply validation for different sites or circumstances. For example, a model might be validated between one and three kilometers from the source, but not at 30 km from the source, where it is to be applied. Models are usually *calibrated* or tuned with an actual data set to fix all the coefficients. Almost all models are in this sense partly empirically based. Models cannot be validated with the same data with which they were calibrated. Ideally, they should be validated in an entirely different locale. Validation is discussed in more detail in Chapter 15. Environmental transport models are often poorly validated except for those which predict nearby concentrations. Validation is expensive, difficult, and sometimes essentially impossible. Much more common are studies which compare the results of two or more models for specific test situations. These indicate potential errors and highlight the implications of differences among models. Comparison of results with an existing standard model might be considered similar to validation against a secondary standard.

Verification is different than validation. It is a test of whether the equations were properly coded in the computer model and that the computer code does, in fact, compute what it was intended to. Verification tests can be made by hand calculations or comparisons with previously verified results.

Input/Output Compatibility

Environmental transport models are often used in "chains" to link transport from one environmental media to another. For example, an air transport model may estimate deposition of material on the ground which is then washed into waterways and becomes an input component of a water transport model. The output of the one model must be compatible with the input of the other. This does not mean they must match exactly; it is often necessary to perform some operation to modify the output of one model so it can be fed into the next. The extent of this linkage is important in model selection. The source terms required to drive the models must be compatible with available data. A model that requires detailed, precise input data cannot be used if such data are not available or cannot be obtained.

Relationship to Dose–Response

Similarly, the final results of the environmental assessment must be compatible to the dose–response function to be used in the overall risk assessment. Indeed, the requirements of the dose–response function should be the first consideration in selecting exposure models. The state-of-the-art of environmental transport modeling is, in general, more advanced than that of dose–response modeling. It is a frequently stated axiom that the various steps in a risk assessment should be conducted at comparable levels; that a highly sophisticated exposure model should not be used in conjunction with a simple dose–response model. The sophistication of the the dose–response model clearly should be considered in selecting the exposure models. However, it should be kept in mind that the understanding of dose–response often exceeds the ability to quantify that understanding in models and, in fact, development of dose–response models may depend in some degree on the sophistication and detail of available exposure information. It thus may prove valuable to have the exposure assessment at a somewhat more sophisticated level than the dose–response assessment.

SOURCE TERMS

Environmental transport models are driven by source terms. Examples are emissions from factory smokestacks, fugitive emissions from leaky valves at process plants, treated process wastewaters discharged to lakes or rivers, and solid wastes or sludges placed in landfills from which, in turn, pollutants leach into groundwater. A material is released and moves through environmental pathways to expose human populations. How much is released, the rate at which it is released, where it is released, and its chemical and physical form all affect its transport and ultimately population exposure. Surprisingly, source terms can be one of the largest sources of uncertainty in an exposure assessment.

The source is usually the subject of the risk assessment. One might assess, for example, the risk posed by an incinerator emitting dioxin to the air, or the combined releases to air of polycyclic aromatic hydrocarbons from all fossil fuel combustion sources in the country. The source term in the former might be based on actual measurements of emissions. In the latter, a complex array of source terms is necessary; emissions from large sources (e.g., large power plants) might be based on measurements; those of intermediate sources (e.g., industrial heating plants) calculated from "emission factors" based on data from the literature on fuel and technology characteristics of similar technologies, and small dispersed sources (e.g., home furnaces, automobiles) based on emission factors combined with census data on the number of homes and fuel types used and with available data on the ages and models of automobiles in service with estimates of mileage driven in different areas. This set of source terms is called a source scenario. An assessment might evaluate the comparative risk of several source scenarios. A scenario represents a pattern held together by one or more assumptions. For example, one emissions scenario might be based on a "business as usual" assumption of continued industrial growth combined with continuation of current pollution control regulations. Risk associated with this scenario might be compared with that of two or more different scenarios assuming lower or higher growth rates across the board or in particular sectors of the economy and more stringent, less stringent, or simply different approaches to pollution control requirements. Scenarios may be based on proposed regulations or legislation. The development of scenarios of this kind is an art in itself. It can involve economics, political science, engineering, and other disciplines, but also requires imagination.

"Emission factors" are coefficients developed from measurements which take the form of mass of a particular pollutant emitted from a given process or technology per unit production. They can be quite specific. For example, kilograms of particles emitted from bituminous coal-fired electric power production in tangentially fired boilers per thousand joules of heat energy used. EPA developed emission factors of this type for a wide variety of industrial and combustion processes (EPA, 1977). Emission factors are often based on a small number of studies which might be very limited in scope. Despite their specificity, measurements from one, or a few sources may not be adequate to accurately represent emissions from an entire category of sources which may have physical differences, be operated in different ways and under different conditions, with a variety of feedstocks. The degree of uncertainty introduced from this source has never adequately been evaluated.

Pollution control is especially difficult to include in emissions factors. Different methods of pollution control can lead to considerable differences in emissions. For this reason, emission factors are often given in terms of "uncontrolled" and "controlled" so that if specific rates of control are known they can be included. Care must be taken in this, however, since "uncontrolled" often does not mean no control, but some base level of control commonly in place before imposition of emission standards.

Moreover, "controlled" emission rates generally are not based on the effectiveness of control technologies, but simply on the allowable emissions under some standard such as the EPA New Source Performance Standards. Actual sources, of course, may exceed or outperform such standards. It is especially important to distinguish the difference between technology-based emission factors and standards-based emissions factors when applying these factors to a different time or legal structure from which they were developed. An example might be using U.S. emission factors to estimate European or African emissions. Compendiums of emissions standards in different countries are available (WHO, 1983; OECD, 1984).

Materials balance is another approach to emissions (Conway et al., 1982). What goes into a process must come out. Materials balances, particularly on an elemental level, can be helpful in determining emissions and in allocating them to air, water, and solids discharges. In one case, for example, computer codes were developed to combine data available on the concentration of 20 different trace elements in coal from various seams and mines with information on specific coal technologies and limited measurements of trace element emission patterns to partition these 20 trace elements among air, water, and solid-waste emissions (Crowther et al., 1980).

Emissions from smoke stacks and wastewater outfalls can be measured and databases established which can be drawn upon for modeling. Some source terms, however, are difficult to quantify. Fugitive emissions, such as leaks from faulty valves or from cracks in processing vessels, are difficult to measure. Detailed atmospheric measurements within a plant site may form the basis for estimating fugitive emission rates. In some cases they may be sufficiently large that mass balance approaches may be useful.

Source terms under accident conditions can be estimated crudely based on knowledge of the quantity of each substance present and the conditions in which it was stored or undergoing processing (Kayes, 1985).

More difficult are emissions to soil and groundwater through seepage from waste ponds or leachate from hazardous waste landfills. Everything occurs underground where it cannot be seen. The volume of leachate can be estimated from a water-balancing calculation; precipitation which does not runoff or become lost to evapotranspiration percolates through the waste site, leaching contaminants, and eventually exits into the ground (Dass et al., 1977). Estimation of the mass or concentration of contaminants leached during percolation and present in the leachate is highly dependent on the characteristics of the site, its contents, and their physical and chemical state (EPA, 1988).

While the chemical and physical form of emissions can be important for various processes associated with transport, they are often not well known, even when measurements are available. Measurements are often "total particles," or elemental analysis (e.g., so much cadmium) without specification of the chemical form. Also, emissions are often complex mixtures of chemicals that have not been, or cannot be, fully defined. Only the principal components are given or, sometimes, only an index chemical. For example, polycyclic aromatic hydrocarbon emissions might be represented only by benzo[a]pyrene or total organic fraction.

Risk assessments often deal with the future. What would the risk of cancer in the population be if a certain kind of development were to take place? It might be possible to only estimate emissions from preliminary designs of the technology or from measurements made at pilot plants which may not include all processes in a commercial facility. What pollution control processes will be included may not even be determined at the time of the assessment. Estimates must be made using "best engineering judgment." These estimates are best made in cooperation with engineers familiar with the processes to be used and with pollution control technologies.

TRANSPORT THROUGH AIR

Air is the most common pathway seen in risk assessments. There are several reasons for special concern with the air route: a variety of different kinds of sources emit toxic materials to the air; once in the air, these materials can be carried quickly to human populations; and exposure is difficult or impossible to avoid. Methods of analysis for population exposure to air pollution in the vicinity of emissions have been in common use for nearly 40 years. Concern for long distance transport stems back to early studies of fallout from atomic bomb tests, but routine application of source to receptor models over long distances are more recent.

Local Air Exposure

Essentially all local (up to 80 km) air pollution exposure assessments use a Gaussian plume model. Some of the reasons for its widespread use are (Hanna et al., 1982):

It produces results that agree with experimental data as well as any model
It is fairly easy to perform mathematical operations on the Gaussian
    equation;
It is conceptually appealing
It is consistent with the random nature of turbulence

It is a solution to the Fickian diffusion equation for constants K and u

Other so-called theoretical formulas contain large amounts of empiricism in their final stages

As a result of the above, it has found its way into most government guidebooks and some government regulation

Simple descriptions of this model are available (Slade, 1968; Turner, 1970; Hanna et al., 1982). A continuous plume from a point source travels downwind (along the x axis on a three-dimensional coordinate system) while it disperses (spreads) in a Gaussian (or normal) distribution both vertically (z axis) and horizontally (y axis) at right angles to the direction of air flow (Fig. 6-1). The basic Gaussian equation for the concentration at any point downwind, where y and z are zero along the axis of the plume, is:

$$C_{(x,y,z)} = \frac{Q}{2\pi\sigma_y\sigma_z u} \exp\left(-\frac{1}{2}\right)\left(\frac{y^2}{\sigma_y^2} + \frac{z^2}{\sigma_z^2}\right)$$

where

$C_{(x,y,z)}$ = pollutant concentration (mass per volume) at coordinates x,y,z
$\quad$ Q = source emission rate (mass per time)

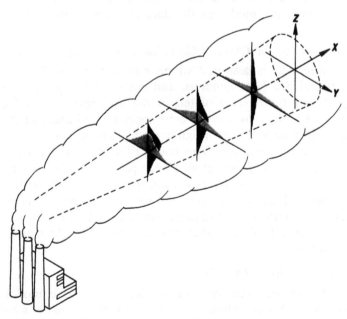

FIGURE 6-1 Gaussian dispersion of air pollution plume in y and z directions with transport in x direction.

σ_y = the standard deviation of the Gaussian in the y axis
σ_z = the standard deviation of the Gaussian in the z axis
u = wind speed
h = effective stack height (actual stack height plus a "plume rise factor" accounting for effects of temperature and inertia in the plume as it leaves the stack.

The two standard deviations (σ) are a function of the distance downwind (x axis) and of the stability or "gustiness" of the air. The latter is defined by empirically derived atmospheric stability factors designated by terms such as "extremely unstable," "slightly unstable," and "moderately stable." The most commonly used classification system includes six stability categories. As it moves downwind, the plume disperses at a rate that depends on the atmospheric conditions.

Although all Gaussian plume models have basically the same structure, there are dozens (perhaps hundreds) of different versions (e.g., EPA, 1986b), each handling various things about the model in different ways. Some of these make little difference in result, some lead to greater differences. The risk analyst should understand the basic properties all Gaussian plume models share, which have implications for interpreting exposure assessment results based on the entire model class, as well as the ways in which either the model or the data inputs vary in different versions.

Assumptions Common to the Class of Gaussian Plume Models

Wind speed and direction is assumed to be constant, wind shear to be insignificant, turbulence homogeneous, and eddy diffusivity constant (Hosker, 1980). All of these are violated in the atmosphere, but for long-term averages the effect does not seem important. Diffusion in the downwind direction is assumed to be insignificant in comparison to transport and omitted from the equation. This could affect results at zero or very low wind speeds, but as Hanna et al. (1982) point out, while anemometers near the surface may register zero wind speed, the winds seldom stop entirely. The ground is assumed to be flat with a uniform surface so as not to interfere with uniform atmospheric conditions. This is a matter of considerable concern and substantial efforts have gone into developing complex terrain models.

Variations in Gaussian Plume Models

Factors which differ in different versions of Gaussian plume models include the way they calculate plume rise, the way they handle what happens when the plume hits the ground or an inversion layer (absorbed, bounces off), and the number of stability categories used and how they are treated. A plume coming out of a smokestack rises due to its high temperature and the inertia of its current movement. The point of origin of the plume dispersion model is not the top of the stack, but the point to which the plume rises. This is called the "virtual stack height" and there are differing ideas on how it should be calculated. This is an important parameter since it, combined with the dispersion characteristics, will define where the plume will first hit the ground. The simplest versions assume the plume is 100% reflected off the ground like a mirror. A similar phenomenon is often assumed when the plume hits an inversion layer which acts as a lid on the mixing zone. Pollutants hitting the ground, however, in actuality are often adsorbed rather than reflected, especially if they are chemically reactive. Loss to the ground is called deposition. More sophisticated versions take this into account by allowing a percentage "loss" to the ground with the rest reflected. In some versions deposition is determined by assigning a "deposition velocity." Some versions account for this "dry deposition" through one mechanism and for "wet deposition," contaminants washed out by rain and snow, by a separate mechanism. Predicted concentrations in air are not especially sensitive to differences in accounting for deposition or in errors in deposition rate. At times, however, concern is with the material deposited rather than the air concentration. The amount of material deposited is sensitive to the method of determining deposition and to errors in deposition parameters. Unfortunately, the ability to predict deposition includes numerous uncertainties.

Using the Gaussian Plume Model to Assess Exposure

Most exposure assessments estimate average air pollution concentration in a polar grid surrounding a point source. The grid has a radius of 80 km and consists of 16 sectors, corresponding to the points of the compass. These are further divided by a series of concentric circles around the source (Fig. 6-2). The concentric circles are sometimes evenly spaced (e.g., 10 km apart), but sometimes are more closely spaced near the source to give greater definition.

The Gaussian plume model is driven by an emission source term (characterized by an emission rate, stack height, stack diameter, velocity, and temperature) and an array of meteorological data providing the joint probability distribution of wind speed, direction and stability class. These data provide the percentage of time the wind blows at each combination of direction, speed, and stability class. Climatology data organized in this way (called STAR data after the computer program which generates them) are available for many sites in the country from the National Climatic Center in Asheville, North Carolina. This is generally produced as six wind speed classes, five stability classes, and 16 wind directions, for a total of 480 numbers (each the probability of the given combination).

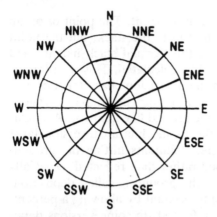

FIGURE 6-2 Polar grid used for air pollution exposure assessment around a point source using Gaussian plume model.

The model then calculates concentrations at ground level (or sometimes 2 m) for incremental distances from the source for each pie-wedge-shaped sector downwind for each direction–speed–stability combination and accumulates them on a time-weighted basis to annual average concentrations in each prescribed subsector. There are several implications of this approach. Steady-state conditions are assumed; a whole year's experience of a direction–speed–stability category is done at once independently from each other category. Wind speed is constant for the entire 80 km. With a wind speed of, say 1 to 4 m/s, that assumes as much as 20 hours of undeviating wind speed. In reality, of course, wind speed and stability changes more frequently so that typically the areas more distant from the source would see pollution that has experienced a variety of wind speed, stability, and even directional changes rather than a uniform pattern. For annual average concentrations (usually suitable for cancer risk assessment), many of these vagaries of the wind "average out."

If population data have been compiled on the same polar grid pattern, cumulative population exposure is often calculated in the same computer code by multiplying the predicted concentration by the population in each cell and adding all the results. Too often, this is as far as "population exposure" goes, with no attempt made to estimate if and how people are actually exposed to the pollutants. Methods to consider population movement, indoor-outdoor differences, and other factors affecting actual population exposure from air and other pathways are described in the last section of this chapter.

Complex Terrain

While the standard Gaussian plume model is usually adequate for risk assessment, applications in areas of complex terrain are often questionable. Complex terrain is often described tautologically as settings in which the behavior of airflow and pollutant dispersion is different from that which occurs over flat ground. The complex terrain problem can be appreciated by considering the effects complex terrain can have on air flow. Yocke et al. (1984) describe four ways that complex terrain can affect atmospheric motion, all of which may occur simultaneously:

1. Wind flow can be channeled by such topographic features as valleys, canyons, promontories, and gaps
2. Thermal effects can be created by vertical and spatial temperature gradients (drainage flows, upslope winds, down-canyon flows, land/sea breezes)
3. Dynamic effects can be created by the blocking of airflow, spatial temperature gradients, and gravity oscillations (e.g., lee waves)
4. Boundary-layer effects can be enhanced by surface friction and vegetation as well as local pressure gradients

A number of detailed studies have been done in complex terrain and several models have been developed. Some of these are essentially modifications of Gaussian models and are limited in their ability to treat three-dimensional, time-varying characteristics of airflow over complex terrain. The EPA Valley model is an example of this type (Burt, 1977). More advanced models take a more fundamental approach to atmospheric dispersion. The Lawrence Livermore Laboratory's ADPIC model is an example (Lange, 1973).

Some important considerations in selecting and evaluating complex terrain models are (Yocke et al., 1984):

Expert consultation in the selection and use of models is much more important in complex terrain than in flat terrain.

Models with more sophisticated physics are intuitively expected to perform better than simple Gaussian models.

Establishment of appropriate transport trajectories is a crucial modeling problem.

Transferability of dispersion rates from one location to another is more restricted than in flat-terrain situations.

Current modeling capabilities in complex terrain are most appropriate in the 1–20 km range. The greatest uncertainty is in the 20–200 km range. Above 200 km, complex terrain is usually not an issue.

Air Transport Modeling of Organic Carcinogens and
Complex Mixtures

Cancer risk assessment involves particular concerns in air transport modeling relating to the pollutants that are modeled. Much air modeling has focused on criteria air pollutants rather than toxic or carcinogenic materials. Moreover, cancer risk assessment must continually be cognizant of the complex mixture of pollutants in the air, and not attempt to treat single compounds in isolation. A recent workshop concluded that modeling of toxic organics did not require any special treatment of atmospheric transport and dispersion; the difficulty was that frequently little was known about their chemical reaction steps or the reaction rates important to decay or formation processes (Yocke et al., 1985). Compounds were divided into three groups: (1) those that have been well studied, (2) those for which limited information is available and for which relatively simple approaches were recommended, and (3) those which have been included in photochemical models. Most compounds fell in the second group and a first-order chemical reaction model was recommended. While this model is often used to describe simple chemical systems, it is also used for very complex systems that are poorly understood or too difficult to model comprehensively.

The first order chemical reaction model is stated as:

$$C = C_0 \exp[-kt] \quad \text{or} \quad C = C_0 \exp[-t/T]$$

where

C is the concentration at the point of interest
C_0 is the concentration at time zero
t is the reaction time between C_0 and C
k is a reaction rate constant
T is a time constant equal to 1/k, sometimes called the half-life.

This chemical model is easily embedded in a Gaussian plume model since, with a constant wind speed for each calculation, distance is a function of time. Conservative concentrations can be calculated from conservative transport (no loss) and then the first-order chemical model applied based on the known time of travel. Compounds recommended for this approach include polycyclic aromatic hydrocarbons (PAH), aza arenes, epoxides, and benzene. In most cases, application of the first-order chemistry is only applied to daytime conditions.

Although some carcinogenic substances are included in photochemical models, treatment of these species has not been the focus of these models and nothing "off the shelf" is available for exposure assessment of these chemicals.

Long-Range Air Transport

If a mass balance is carried out on a Gaussian plume model dispersion analysis, one finds that a substantial portion of the pollutant is carried beyond the 80–100 km range of the model. The focus of long-range transport model development has been regional studies of acid-rain related pollutants and regional transport of photochemical smog. In these cases, modeling has demonstrated that a substantial fraction of air pollutants, especially in rural areas, can be contributed by long-range transport from outside the area. The contribution of any single source to the pollution level hundreds or thousands of kilometers distant is infinitesimally small, but, in principal, it might be held accountable for its share of the risk of that distant pollution. The cumulative effect of these infinitesimally small contributions to population exposure can be substantial. In addition to this, a strict interpretation of the no-threshold dose–response function commonly used in cancer risk assessment leads to the assumption that each increment, no matter how small, contributes an additional increment of risk. It would thus seem incumbent on an exposure assessment, as part of a cancer risk assessment, to consider long range transport, since the bulk of the exposure may be beyond the local area.

Long-range transport models are controversial, however. It is clearly difficult to predict with any degree of certainty where the winds will carry pollution over 1000 km or more. As the distance downwind increases, errors in transport and dispersion factors and in loss rates multiply. Seiler (1987) notes that, "although sizeable contributions to the population exposure may be calculated, their errors will eventually become so large as to make the contribution meaningless." On this basis, he argues that there should be a cut-off distance for each model based on its predictive power and the characteristics of the contaminant. There is no question that the error increases with distance. While for long-term average exposures the error associated with transport and dispersion may tend to "average out" to some degree, errors on loss rates will not. If the chemical is removed from the atmosphere through reaction with the ground or with other pollutants in the air more quickly than expected, it may never actually reach those far distant points where the model is predicting contributions to population exposure. Unfortunately, setting cut-off distances based on model and contaminant characteristics could lead to an unevenness in exposure assessment which often happens in risk assessment: exposure to contaminants which are better understood will be modeled over longer distances than contaminants that are not well understood, leading to an artifactual difference in estimated exposure.

Two Approaches to Long-Range Transport Modeling

Although there have been several approaches to modeling long-range transport of air pollutants, they are exemplified by two: (1) a trajectory model which follows "puffs" from a continuous emission source where ever the winds blow them and numerically integrates the exposure at different locations and (2) a simplified analytical model which bears some resemblance to the Gaussian plume model.

Most versions of the trajectory model are modifications of what is called the Heffter model (Heffter et al., 1975). Typically, the continuous source is lumped into four puffs per day, one every six hours. Transport is modeled based on actual meteorologic patterns, e.g., wind speed and direction from stations across the country reported at 6-h intervals for an actual period of a month or a year. Based on this national meteorological data base, wind speed and direction at the source is determined at the time a puff is released and off it goes. Six hours later, it is off at a new speed and direction based on actual meteorological information for the place it has reached. This pattern continues for perhaps five or ten days, during which time the puff describes a path or "trajectory" across the country. As it travels, the plume disperses horizontally and vertically; the methods used to describe dispersion vary among several versions of trajectory models. Meanwhile, every six hours, a new puff leaves the source and begins a new trajectory. Exposure to each cell of a grid on the ground is accumulated as they are crossed by trajectories. Some detailed examples of this type of modeling are given by Meyers et al. (1979). Trajectory models can be very computer-intensive. For representative exposures, trajectories (four per day) must be accumulated from months or years of detailed meteorological data. For ease in assessment, model results were determined for transport of sulfur dioxide and respirable particles from each of 243 Air Quality Control Region to every other region under a fixed set of conditions, producing a 243×243 "transfer matrix" (Eadie and Davis, 1979; Rowe, 1980; 1981). This allowed evaluation of the effects of different power plant siting patterns, for example, but assessments requiring evaluation of the effects of varying stack height, or examining the effect of different loss rates, had to rerun the original transport models.

For long averaging times (e.g., annual average exposure), many of the details of transport and diffusion processes become unimportant at ranges over 250 km (Hosker, 1980). Fay and Rosenzweig (1979) proposed a model in which infinitely many puffs averaged over a long time reduce to a steady-state diffusion problem with an appropriately determined horizontal diffusion coefficient. The long-term average wind speed and direction was used for the direction of transport and each receptor considered an offset from this direction. Sensitivity analysis indicated the model was not sensitive to the spatial distribution of mixing height in the atmosphere, so a uniform mixing height could be used. Comparison runs against the Heffter model showed reasonable correlation and suggest that a simple analytical model such as this would be adequate for many cancer risk assessments.

TRANSPORT THROUGH WATER AND SOIL

A variety of models are necessary to follow pollutant transport through different soil and water routes. Although surface and groundwater systems are connected, transport, dispersion, and degradation processes such as biological breakdown of the toxic chemicals differ between the two media. Direct discharges from industrial and municipal outfalls are the principal sources to surface water bodies. Toxic contaminants also wash into surface waters from the land. Although there have been direct injection wells to dispose of wastes in groundwater, most groundwater contamination is leachate, which percolates through soils from land deposits.

The following sections consider surface runoff, surface water transport, groundwater transport, and movement through the unsaturated zone.

Surface Runoff

Deposition from atmospheric transport models puts contaminants on the ground. Here they can be re-entrained into the air, percolate into the soil, or washed by surface runoff into surface waters. Such an intermedia transport is usually of only secondary importance, but in some cases it can be significant. Surface runoff also carries contaminants from sources other than air deposition into surface waters. For example, road tar dust can contain up to 0.5 g of carcinogenic substances per kilogram, and surface runoff from city streets is one of the main sources of PAH in surface water (Borneff, 1977).

Methods to estimate the quantity of storm water runoff based on precipitation data and surface characteristics have long been available in engineering hydrology (Linsley and Franzini, 1979). The addition of methods to estimate contaminant loading for surface waters from this source has been the subject of considerable EPA-sponsored research and model development. For accuracy in site-specific applications, these models demand vast amounts of data and extensive calibration by experienced modelers (Freeman et al., 1986). Improvements to these highly empirical models, leading toward more physically based models, are needed. One new model applicable to impervious surfaces was proposed by Akan (1987).

Surface Water Transport

It is somewhat of a paradox that it is generally more difficult to model exposures via the water route than the air route although rivers move in defined channels while the air might go anywhere. The reason is that generalized models can be used for air without much error due to local differences in meteorology except in the case of complex terrain, while for water, detailed local data are required in every case. Generic assessments require development of specific reference environments. Surface water models encompass lakes, streams, rivers, canals, estuaries, and even oceans. Each has its own characteristics which must be included in models.

Contaminants may enter water bodies from direct discharges at point sources, overland runoff, or from the groundwater aquifer. The latter two are nonpoint sources. The discharge rate from point sources is usually defined directly as part of the source scenario. In most cases, it is assumed to be a continuous, uniform discharge. Nonpoint source discharges are generally the output of another model rather than part of the input data. These discharges are generally nonuniform. Overland runoff, as an example, varies with rainfall patterns. Since long-term exposure is usually sufficient for cancer risk assessment and short-term variations are of lesser importance, even this nonuniform source can usually be averaged over the year. One must do some sensitivity analysis to assure that the actual variation in time does not result in significant changes in loss rates (e.g., that biodegradation is not a function of concentration). Since a nonpoint source might be considered as a series of point sources, models which must deal with nonpoint sources are naturally more complex. When the point of interest is sufficiently far downstream, however, a nonpoint source can often be considered as a single point source.

Water Quality Models Vary in Sophistication

The simplest analysis considers only dilution; the pollutant load is divided by the waterbody or streamflow volume to obtain concentrations. The next level of sophistication has been called screening or simplified fate models (Donigian and Brown, 1983). These add partitioning of contaminants between water and sediment and degradation processes such as volatilization, photolysis, and biodegradation. Some models account for sediment moving at different rates than water and even consider various classes of sediment. One model, for example, can consider as many as 12 size classes of sediment in three compartments: sediment resident on the stream bed, sediment in transit on the stream bed, and sediment in transit as suspended solids (Baes et al., 1975). Volatilization, photolysis (transformation of chemical compounds by absorption of light or through photosensitized chemical reactions) and hydrolysis (adding a hydroxyl group to the compound), and biodegradation (chemical changes caused by microorganisms) are usually treated as loss processes since they usually (but not always) yield a more benign compound than the original. More detailed discussion of these loss processes may be found in Southworth et al. (1982) and Lee (1982). They are especially important in modeling the environmental transport of carcinogens since many carcinogens are highly affected by these processes. Ignoring these loss processes can usually be considered a worst-case analysis, particularly in the long-term (in the short term, release of material accumulated in sediments can cause peak exposures). In addition to greater model sophistication, these models have much greater data requirements, as coefficients for partitioning, volatilization, etc., are all compound-specific and some degradation coefficients may differ between dissolved and adsorbed phases of the same compound. The EPA EXAMS model is at this level (Burns et al., 1982; 1985).

The background quality of the water body may also be considered in a model (or in the selection of model parameters). Sediment load affects chemical adsorption and pH affects the hydrolysis rate (Lee, 1982). Other background quality factors of possible importance include temperature, transparency, and alkalinity.

The highest level of analysis adds a dynamic aspect. While simpler models assume steady-state conditions, dynamic models include time-varying hydrologic, hydrodynamic, and sediment transport processes (Donigian and Brown, 1983). An example of a dynamic model suitable for a detailed exposure assessment is TOXIWASP (Ambrose et al., 1983). An example application of TOXIWASP is given in Ambrose (1986).

Example of a Simple Model

A rudimentary river flow model, with a point-source, one-dimensional, steady state, uniform flow serves as an illustration for discussion of simplified fate models:

$$C(x) = C_0 \, e^{jx}$$
$$C_0 = [11.6 \text{ W}]/[Q*\text{TERM}]$$

$$j = (V/2E)*(1 - TERM)$$
$$TERM = [1 - (4KE/V^2)]^{1/2}$$

where

x is the distance downstream from the point source

$C(x)$ is the concentration at x in $\mu g/l$

C_0 is the stream concentration $(\mu g/l)$ at the point source (11.6 is a unit conversion)

W is the point-source discharge rate (kg/s)

Q is the stream flow rate (m³/s)

V is the stream velocity (m/day)

E is a longitudinal dispersion coefficient (m²/day)

K is a first-order pollutant decay coefficient (L/d) which combines all loss rates (Table 6-2)

This simple model does not treat sediments except as a loss to the system and combines all losses into one rate. Thus, it does not allow different loss processes to be made dependent on different environmental characteristics such as temperature or pH. The cross-sectional area of the stream is contained in the combination of flow quantity (m³/s) and velocity (m/s) and is assumed constant. The model is thus not able to distinguish between a stream 50 m across and 1 m deep and one 10 m across and 5 m deep, although the character of the flow and loss processes are apt to be quite different under these different conditions. To account for changes in flow or cross-section from, for example, the confluence with a tributary stream, modeling is usually done sequentially by "reaches" where physical

TABLE 6-2   First-Order Pollutant Decay Rate for Common Pollutants

Pollutant	K (l/day)	Principal loss process
Benzene	0.55	Sorption, volatilization
Chloroform	0.55	Volatilization
Ethylbenzene	0.61	Volatilization
Methylene chloride	0.55	Volatilization
Toluene	0.65	Sorption, volatilization
Phenol	0.25	Volatilization, photolysis, biodegradation
Di-*n*-butyl phthalate	0.25	Sorption, biodegradation, bioaccumulation

Source: From Warwick and Cale, 1986.

conditions can be defined separately for each reach. Uncertainties associated with this model are analyzed by Jaffe and Parker (1984) and Warwick and Cale (1986).

Models for estuaries are considerably more complicated because tidal motion affects flow and concentration distribution. The difference in density between salt and fresh water creates additional complicating circulation in an estuary, as do wind-driven currents (Jirka, 1982).

Using Water Quality Models for Exposure Assessment

Exposure assessment currently relies primarily on screening or simplified fate models. Data availability and time and funding constraints usually prevent the application of more detailed models. Often data are inadequate to sufficiently characterize degradation of the pollutant. Simplified fate models suitable for many risk assessment purposes but more sophisticated than the simple one illustrated above are in the public domain and available from the EPA Environmental Research Laboratory in Athens, Georgia (e.g., Burns et al., 1985; Brown and Barnwell, 1985).

Modeling for regulatory purposes usually focuses on the near-field where concentrations are highest. For risk assessment, however, the focus is on human exposure. Principal exposure pathways usually require concentrations to be determined at water supply intakes, points of irrigation water withdrawal (for input to a food-chain model), and at bathing beaches. If the aquatic food chain is important, concentrations will be required throughout areas which have fisheries. The near-field, which requires the most rigorous modeling due to transient conditions, is not as important for risk assessment and usually can be neglected. This tends to simplify the models (usually one-dimensional models are adequate) and eliminate some data requirements. On the other hand, degradation rates such as volatilization, photolysis, and biodegradation, which, especially at low concentrations, are poorly known, become much more important because these loss processes, rather than dilution, soon begin to dominate the estimated concentrations. This is particularly true in the very far-field, e.g., estimates of organic pollutants in New Orleans resulting from discharges more than 1,000 km upstream in the Ohio River. Estimates of this kind, which can be important in risk assessments, are generally unheard of among aquatic modelers involved in regulatory work.

Detailed models of well-known water bodies may achieve accuracy within a factor of two to four while the screening level and simplified fate models have uncertainty of factors of 10-100 (Freeman et al., 1986; Donigian and Brown, 1983).

Groundwater Transport

Models designed to analyze groundwater flow to assess aquifer yields and assist in wellfield design and management have been used for over 100 years (Linsley and Franzini 1979). Their modification to include analysis of pollutant transport in groundwater is much more recent, however. Applications were relatively limited until the late 1970s, when national concern with potential leaching of toxic materials from hazardous waste sites into groundwater led to the Comprehensive Environmental Response, Compensation, and Liability Act of 1980 (Superfund). This brought groundwater modeling to the fore (see EPA, 1988).

The most difficult problem with groundwater modeling is the limited data availability. The geologic media and the characteristics of the groundwater must be estimated based on a few test wells. Even the source term, e.g., leachate from a waste site, must be inferred.

Groundwater modeling is at a reasonably high level of sophistication, but the more advanced models are seldom suitable for exposure assessment as a part of risk assessment. On the other hand, the simple, worst case analysis sometimes used for regulatory screening is to assume no attenuation or delay in the groundwater system; the entire mass of contaminant in a leachate release is diluted only by the amount of drinking water drawn from the aquifer. This is unsatisfactory for even the most rudimentary exposure analysis. The simplest realistic exposure analysis is to assume the release is diluted by the uncontaminated ground water. Unlike a river, however, the amount of groundwater available for dilution is not immediately available or easily obtainable information. Some level of modeling of the flow field in the ground-water system is necessary. Key mechanisms of pollutant mobility typically included in models are advection, hydrodynamic dispersion, adsorption and desorption, and degradation or decay. While the simplest models assume contaminants do not sorb or otherwise interact with the soil media and, thus, travel at the same rate as the groundwater, even the more sophisticated screening-level models include sorption. Groundwater is obviously in much more intimate contact with soil than surface water with the result being much greater importance of sorption. The contaminant sorption process is usually described by a constant, K_d, representing the ratio between the contaminant adsorbed to the soil matrix and the contaminant dissolved in solution.

It is sometimes necessary to reconstruct the exposure history when groundwater contamination is discovered in wells. Freni and Phillips (1987) describe an empirical approach to this problem, estimating the time exposure started and the change in concentration of volatile organic chemicals in the groundwater over time for several wells affected by a plume from a leaking underground tank.

A compilation of one-dimensional groundwater transport models with analytical solutions is available (Van Genuchten and Alves, 1982). Most two- and three-dimensional groundwater transport models are not suitable for analytic solutions; approximate numerical methods such as finite-element and finite differences are necessary (Pinder and Gray, 1977; Huyakoin and Pinder, 1983). Mercer et al. (1983) describe the application of a two-dimensional groundwater model in the Love Canal area. Codell et al. (1982) describe various groundwater models. Information on available groundwater models can be obtained from the Model Annotation Retrieval System (MARS) at the International Ground Water Modeling Center* or the EPA Kerr Environmental Research Laboratory.[†]

Unsaturated Zone

Before reaching the groundwater aquifer, a zone completely saturated with water, pollutants must migrate through unsaturated or partially saturated soil. The distance from the surface to the saturated zone may range from virtually zero to several thousand meters. For screening assessments, migration of contaminants in the unsaturated zone is usually neglected if the depth to the groundwater aquifer is less than 50 m (Donigian and Brown, 1983). The flow of water and solutes in the unsaturated zone is based on the same principles as in groundwater models, but since the soil pores or voids are only partially filled with water, the remainder being filled with air, the cross sectional area available for water flow is reduced and modeling water flow is more complex. Hydraulic conductivity becomes a function of moisture content rather than a constant as it is in the saturated aquifer. Characterization of the geologic media in the unsaturated zone is especially important, and, again unlike the saturated aquifer, climatological factors are important. Rainfall is responsible for the movement of contaminants through the unsaturated zone; it infiltrates through the land surface and transports contaminants vertically downward. At the same time, rainfall and evaporation rate affect the moisture content of the

---

*International Ground Water Modeling Center, Holcomb Research Institute, Butler University, Indianapolis, IN 46208.
[†]Ground Water Research Branch, R.S. Kerr Environmental Research Laboratory, P.O. Box 1198, Ada, OK 74820.

unsaturated zone, influencing hydraulic conductivity and pore distribution. Modeling is much more difficult. For greater detail see Oster (1982).

FOOD CHAINS

Air and water pathways to human exposure are, for the most part, fairly direct and governed by straightforward physical and chemical processes. Food chains are initiated by air and water transport and involve biological processes by which pollutants are incorporated in the human food supply. Food chains may draw on more than one route; for example, a plant may incorporate contaminants from polluted irrigation water and also from pollutants deposited from the air. In both cases, part of the contamination may be due to direct contamination of plant surfaces and part due to uptake through the roots of contaminated soil. Food chains may involve more than one step; contaminants taken up from the soil by forage crops may be eaten by cows and incorporated in meat and milk. The most striking feature of food chains is the ability of some plants and animals to accumulate or "bioconcentrate" certain contaminants. Partly for this reason, food chains can be a significant contributor to human exposure.

Terrestrial food chains are linked primarily with agricultural production, although some natural environments may be important for some population subgroups (e.g., the case of game animals). Aquatic food chains are, by necessity, tied closely to specific aquatic environments and aquatic food chain models are frequently closely linked to location-specific aquatic transport and dispersion models. Although aquatic food chains can be important in certain circumstances, terrestrial food chains are more usually the primary focus of attention. This is because (1) most of the human diet derives from terrestrial agriculture and (2) the air is more frequently the primary environmental pathway and terrestrial food chains are generally more closely linked to deposition from the air than are aquatic food chains. Most work in food chain model development has focused on either radioactive materials or certain toxic trace metals such as cadmium.

Most food chain models used in exposure assessment are quasi-equilibrium models. They follow an approach defined as the concentration factor (CF) method (ICRP, 1979) and many follow detailed requirements set forth by the Nuclear Regulatory Commission (NRC, 1977). They divide the food chain into "compartments." Quasiequilibrium models assume that the concentrations of pollutants are at steady state in some compartments and change with time in others. For those compartments at steady state, a compartment's concentration is simply the concentration in the previous compartment multiplied by a concentration factor. As described by Kaye et al. (1984):

$$C_B^* = C_A^* \times P_{AB}$$

where

C_B^* = the equilibrium concentration of a pollutant in a receptor food-chain compartment B,

C_A^* = the steady-state concentration in a donor food chain compartment A, and

P_{AB} = the equilibrium concentration factor for the flow of pollutants between compartments A and B.

Compartments not in equilibrium must be corrected for the differences between the value at equilibrium and the value attained at harvest:

$$C_B(t) = C_A^* \times P_{AB} (1 - e^{-K_2 t}),$$

where

$C_B(t)$ = the concentration of a pollutant in compartment B at time t subsequent to a continuous exposure to the pollutant,

K_2 = the effective first order rate constant for the loss of pollutants from compartment B (time^{-1}), and

t = the time between initial exposure to the pollutant and harvest (or the end of the exposure period).

When the reciprocal of the effective rate constant (K_2^{-1}) is large with respect to t, the correction factor $(1 - e^{-K_2 t})$ becomes simply $K_2 t$. When K_2^{-1} is small with respect to t, $C_B(t) = C_B^*$. The model thus reduces to a series of multiplicative chains. More sophisticated versions may contain other factors, e.g., a factor to account for loss through metabolism.

The quasiequilibrium models are simple in structure but highly data dependent. Concentration factors are estimated in laboratory studies or are derived from ratios of average concentrations of pollutants in the different "compartments" in the field, sometimes taken from unrelated references in the literature (Kaye et al., 1984). Even given this liberal approach to derivation of the parameters for food chain models, the necessary data are often not available for specific chemical contaminants. In these cases, parameters are estimated from correlations with physicochemical properties. One such property is the octanol/water partition coefficient (K_{ow}). This is the ratio of a chemical's concentration in the octanol phase to its concentration in the aqueous phase of a two-phase octanol/water system. Travis et al. (1986) report relationships between K_{ow} and several food chain parameters, based on regression analysis, which they derive from various sources. The distribution coefficient (K_d), the ratio of the concentration in the soil to the concentration in the solute at equilibrium (similar to the K_d in groundwater models), is used in estimating soil concentrations which, in turn, are used to determine plant uptake from soil. It is related to K_{ow} as:

$$K_d = -99 + 0.53 \,(\log K_{ow})$$

Root uptake of organic chemicals distributed in soils to the vegetative portion of food crops (B_v) was related to K_{ow} as:

$$\log B_v = 2.71 - 0.62 \,(\log K_{ow}).$$

The concentration of organic chemical in the nonvegetative portion of food crops was assumed to be 10% of that in the vegetative portion. Finally the bioconcentration factors in beef fat (F_f) and milk (F_m) relative to the concentrations in the animal's feed were given as:

$$\log F_f = -5.15 + 0.50 \,(\log K_{ow}) \qquad \log F_m = -6.13 + 0.5 \,(\log K_{ow})$$

These are mean values from regression analysis of many compounds; they are only crude estimates for general use when specific data are not available and may not be suitable for all organic compounds. Only experimental measurements can provide reasonably reliable estimates, and even these are difficult to field test. The octanol/water partition coefficient has been shown, at least in some cases, not to be appropriate for fish (Vaughn, 1984).

In addition to chemical-specific parameters, site-specific data are needed to describe agricultural production in the exposed area. Such data have been tabulated at the county level for selected products (Shor et al., 1982). This tabulation includes beef cattle, milk cows, and seven vegetable and food crops: (1) leafy vegetables presenting a broad flat leaf surface for atmospheric deposition and for which the leafy part is generally the edible part; (2) exposed produce (e.g., snap beans, tomatoes, apples) which are available for atmospheric deposition but who's surface area is small compared to leafy vegetables; (3) protected produce (e.g., potatoes, peanuts, citrus fruits) in which edible portions are not directly exposed to atmospheric deposition; (4) grains which are similar to protected produce but which are used as feed for animals as well as their direct contribution to the human diet; (5) pasture; (6) hay; and (7) silage.

Assessment models often aggregate several underlying processes and mechanisms into general transfer coefficients that relate the concentration of a pollutant in one compartment of a food chain to that in another. Freeman et al. (1986) estimate that site-specific predictions from food chain models are likely to include two or three orders of magnitude uncertainty. Although some of this will tend to cancel out for national level assessments, uncertainty remains at the order of magnitude level. In addition to uncertainty, food chain models may introduce a deliberate bias. In many cases, assessment models have been developed for regulatory screening purposes and contain "an intentional degree of conservative bias to reduce the probability of underestimation" (Kaye et al., 1984). Models commonly do not indicate the degree of conservatism used or provide guidance for interpreting predictions (Hoffman et al., 1984).

Quasiequilibrium models do not handle short-term releases well, especially when exposures are limited to particular phases of the growth cycle of plants. For this situation, dynamic models which are based on system kinetics are needed. These models, however, can be even more demanding of data.

POPULATION AT RISK

The theme of this entire section on exposure assessment is that exposure involves people; if no one is exposed, there is no exposure. Assessments for regulatory purposes often examine hypothetical exposure situations which are quite unrealistic. An example is exposure to the "fence-post individual," a fictitious person who spends 100% of his time outdoors at the boundary of a facility where he presumably receives the highest air pollution exposure, and also derives all of his food and water from the same location. Such worst-case modeling can be useful as a simple screening tool. Occasionally, individual risk levels of people in different situations may be sufficient for an assessment, but more often exposure assessment for cancer risk assessment demands more. The size of the population exposed, the level of their exposure, and other characteristics such as age and sex distribution; eating, drinking, smoking, and other habits; and socioeconomic characteristics must be estimated.

Defining the exposed population involves a combination of exposure pathway modeling and demographic information. The methods vary. For example, the pattern of air pollutant concentrations may be described on a map together with the pattern of population distribution or a similar process conducted entirely by computer. Depending on the nature of the assessment, estimates of current, past, or future populations may be necessary.

Gridding Population Data

Population data are available at several levels of detail: state (50), county (over 3000), cities and towns, census tracts or enumeration districts (over

30,000), and in urban areas at even finer levels. For national level exposure
assessments, county level data are generally the most appropriate (Morris
et al., 1979). States are too coarse a grid, and enumeration districts too
fine and, because of their small size, do not include as much information
as county data. Other related data, such as environmental, social, agricultural, or economic data are often available on the county level. Data
which are self-reported such as migration must be at the county level since
it is a unit that is recognized by the majority of the population. It must
be remembered, however, that the variation of population characteristics
within a county is often as great or greater than the variation among
counties. Moreover, the size of counties vary widely and the within-county
variation can be particularly important in the very large western counties
which include relatively small high-density urban areas but the rest of
the county is almost unpopulated; this distorts population density and
environmental exposure estimates made at the county level. County
boundaries are, of course, politically based, and are not related to boundaries of airsheds, watersheds, aquifers, and other natural regions which
might influence environmental exposure. Even more directly important
for assessment, most environmental pathway exposure models produce
exposures based on some kind of a grid. Mapping population data from
irregular shaped counties to a uniform grid introduces uncertainty due to
the assumption of uniform population density in the county. Area to area
mapping is a more difficult problem than mapping a set of data at discrete
points. An example of an area to area transformation procedure is RE-
GRID (Mashburn et al., 1976).

Population Projection

For assessment of current exposure, data from the most recent census is
often adequate. If rapidly changing population distribution is a factor,
these data must be projected to the present year. Frequently, exposure
assessment must project 10 to 20 years into the future or longer. Population projections for small areas are highly uncertain. The analyst must
consider carefully if adding this additional uncertainty is warranted. Sometimes use of population projections can be avoided if they do not directly
contribute to the objectives of the assessment. For example, the individual
risk level in an area as a result of a technological development may be
expected to remain constant over the next 30 years, but the number of
cancers induced are expected to triple because the population size is
expected to triple. Which answer is appropriate? In some cases, the
increasing effects due to an increasing population may be important, in

others, the population increase may obscure, rather than illuminate, the impact.

Some examples of different kinds of population projection models include: SEAM (Stenehjem, 1978), a social and economic assessment model designed to predict future population and socioeconomic indicators at the county level in areas of large energy development; EFFECTS (Wenzel and Gallegos, 1985), a life-table model designed for cancer risk assessment which tracks population dynamics of a stable population and does not include in- or out-migration; BREAM (Mountain West Research, Inc., 1981) is not a population forecast model, but a tool to examine systematically the economic and demographic implications of explicit assumptions about an area's future. It may be useful for describing different implications for future population based on different scenarios.

Activity and Mobility

People do not simply stay in one place and absorb what pollutants the environment brings their way. They go to work, to school, to stores. They spend time indoors and outdoors, in homes, office buildings, malls, parking garages, automobiles, buses, trains, and on city streets. Only in the past decade has the importance of these movements for environmental exposure been fully recognized. Sociologists are interested in how people spend their day, and research on activity patterns can be useful in exposure assessment. The principal concern for exposure, however, is not how, but where people spend their day. The use of activity pattern information and models to combine it with estimates of microenvironmental exposure levels are discussed below in the section on integrated population exposure. Information on commuting patterns can be inferred from census data and, sometimes, is available in greater detail from regional planning agencies or local highway and transportation departments. More detailed movements, if not measured by surveys of the population at risk, must be taken from reports of surveys of other populations (Szalai, 1972; Chapin, 1974).

Migration

Cancer risk analysis deals with long-term effects. The interval between first exposure and appearance of a tumor is frequently 20 years or more. In epidemiological studies of cancer, this lag period is very important because exposure levels at current place of residence may not reflect long-term exposure. Some individuals in the current high-exposure population, for example, may have only recently migrated from other areas with different exposure levels.

In risk assessments, the problem of migration may not be as great. The concern is generally not with who specifically gets cancer, but the individual risk of cancer, how many cancers are produced over a given time frame or the overall rate of increase in cancer expected. Risk can be expressed in terms of length of residence in an exposed area. For example, the risk of cancer from radon exposure in homes is often expressed in terms of the number of years one lives in the house. If a linear dose–response function is used, it does not matter for estimating total numbers of cancers whether the population is stable or there is a constant flux of people moving through. The cumulative population exposure (person-rem or person-$\mu g/m^3$) is the same, it is simply distributed among a larger population. The analyst must be aware of this, however, if an attempt is to be made to predict relative risk.

Population and Uncertainty

Too frequently, population estimation is relegated a comparatively minor role in the assessment; this is a mistake. The outcome of many assessments is directly dependent on the population estimates and the results more sensitive to changes in population than to changes in concentration. One might at first think that the population is what it is and the numbers are simply extracted from census data. That is seldom the case. Even if it were, census data themselves contain some level of error and possible sources of bias, but beyond that, some level of manipulation is usually necessary. Population can prove to be a major source of uncertainty in an assessment. When estimating exposure uncertainties, it is important to include contributions from the population estimates.

High-Risk Groups

Some subgroups of the population are often at substantially higher risk than the average because of higher exposure or higher sensitivity. While insufficient data are available in many exposure assessments to even determine the existence of these subgroups in the population, let alone their size and exposure level, all exposure assessments should consider their possibility and implications. It is often the case that only in these high-risk groups is there any significant risk; if their risk were diluted among the entire population by not recognizing the existence of the high-risk group, the hazard of the substance being evaluated might be disregarded.

When high-risk results from unusually high exposure, its identification falls within the exposure assessment itself. For example, if the principal exposure pathway is through aquatic food chains, people who eat more than an average amount of fish or shellfish may be at high risk. The analyst must consider if such subgroups exist within areas which might have high concentrations of the pollutant. People with occupational exposures or who live near sources may be at higher risk.

Subgroups with high-risk because they are especially sensitive to the pollutant are generally harder to identify. Including these subgroups in the exposure assessment also requires close coordination with dose–response assessment; it is in the latter that the sources of increased susceptibility will generally be identified. One reason for increased susceptibility might be an enzyme problem which results in a greater than average fraction of the exposure being metabolized into a carcinogenic form.

INTEGRATED POPULATION EXPOSURE ASSESSMENT

Environmental transport models get pollutants to where people can be exposed to them, but seldom take them right to the people. Exposure assessment involves more than just estimating environmental concentrations of pollutants in air and water; it involves determining the population exposed and the magnitude of the exposure. Integrated population exposure assessment also recognizes that people are exposed from multiple sources and through multiple routes. It takes the ambient concentrations in the various environmental media produced by transport models and combines them with population-related data to estimate total population exposure.

The last step in exposure calculations from source through an environmental pathway to man is sometimes the most uncertain. The uncertainty stems primarily from individual variability. Everyone has a unique exposure based on their individual movements in time and space relative to the distribution of ambient concentrations, on their own actions, and on the rate their body interacts with ambient conditions. Reference values are published and used in risk assessments to represent these factors which affect exposure (e.g., ICRP, 1975), but the actual values vary considerably among different groups of people and among individuals. The reference values may not be averages at all and in some cases may be drawn from limited data which could be unrepresentative. The calculations generally tend to be rather simple. They are discussed below by route of exposure. Since such calculations are frequently more ad hoc than previous transport modeling, some examples from actual assessments are given. These calculations are intermediate between exposure and dose. The concentration of a pollutant in the air one breaths is an exposure. Here we calculate this exposure to a person integrated over his day as he moves from place to place experiencing different ambient levels. We then go on, however, to calculate how much air is actually taken into the lung, and of that how much of the pollutant of interest is retained in the body (much is simply exhaled). The next step, how much of that pollutant moves within the body to the various organs and whether in the process it is metabolized to other substances is the subject of the next chapter.

Inhalation

Most risk assessments estimate the average pollutant concentration in a given area or "cell" with an air dispersion model, estimate the population residing in that cell directly from census data or from population projection models, and multiply the two to obtain population exposure in units of person-μg/m^3 (e.g., Travis et al., 1986; Moskowitz et al., 1985). Better methods are possible, but not yet simple to use. Ott and Mage (1975) proposed an approach which summed time-weighted average concentrations. Horie and Chaplin (1977) implemented a partial application of this approach, joining population and employment statistics to estimate population exposure by summing the time-weighted products of the air pollution concentrations in the business section of the city with the numbers employed and the pollution concentrations in the residential section with the numbers assumed to be there at various times. This was proposed as an alternative indicator of changes in air quality and not for risk assessment, but was part of a trend toward greater appreciation of the need to more accurately estimate population exposure. Fugas (1975) estimated total exposure by measuring concentrations outdoors, in homes, offices and on the street; hers was the first consistent data set to allow total air-pollution exposure estimates. Morgan and Morris (1977a, 1977b) used Fugas' Zagreb data, combined with data on residential and commuting patterns in the United States, to simulate exposure patterns in an urban population. Duan (1980) and Ott (1980) formalized the concept of microenvironments in which an individual's total exposure is computed as the weighted average of his exposures in each microenvironment:

$$E_{i,j} = \sum_{k=1}^{K} c_{i,j,k} \, t_{i,j,k}$$

where

$E_{i,j}$ = integrated exposure of the i-th individual during the j-th time period
$c_{i,j,k}$ = average concentration in the k-th microenvironment during the j-th time period
$t_{i,j,k}$ = activity pattern coefficient denoting the time the i-th individual spent in the k-th microenvironment during the j-th time period.

This concept has been most effectively applied to measuring exposure to carbon monoxide. Two computer models have been developed. The first, the NAAQS Exposure Model (NEM) generates hour-by-hour movements of representative population groups through selected microenvironments in each district of a city; the second, Simulation of Human Air Pollution Exposures (SHAPE), used Monte Carlo simulation to combine data on activity patterns with statistical descriptions of pollutant concentrations in 14 microenvironments (Ott, 1981, 1985). SHAPE, as designed for carbon monoxide exposures, is available from EPA in a form that can be run on an IBM-XT microcomputer. These models could be redesigned to estimate total exposure to carcinogens, the microenvironments must be chosen to be appropriate for each pollutant. Microenvironments used in SHAPE for carbon monoxide are listed in Table 6-3; typical microenvironments that might be used for volatile organics are gas stations, dry cleaning stores, freshly painted rooms, and households with solvents stored indoors (Ott, 1985). The difficulty in implementing such models is the data intensity required. Sufficient data must be available to characterize pollutant concentrations in the microenvironments and the population's activity patterns to estimate the time spent in each microenvironment by each population subgroup of concern.

In some cases, simplified versions of such exposure models which only separate indoor and outdoor exposures might be adequate. Considerable data are now available on indoor levels of pollutants, but they by no means provide systematic or representative coverage of all indoor environments. For outdoor-generated pollutants, a single value for the ratio of indoor to outdoor levels by building type may be adequate (e.g., WHO,

TABLE 6-3 Microenvironments Used in SHAPE Exposure Model

Indoors	Home
Indoors	Store/restaurant
Indoors	Recreation
Indoors	Parking garage
In-vehicle	Auto
In-vehicle	Bus
In-vehicle	School bus
In-vehicle	Truck
In-vehicle	Rail
Outdoors	Center city sidewalk
Outdoors	Residential sidewalk
Outdoors	Park, open area ($>$100 m from streets)
Outdoors	Bicycle

Source: From Ott, 1981.

1982; Yocom, 1982), but for pollutants that are wholly or partially generated indoors, estimates of concentrations in different rooms may be necessary. Multicompartment models to estimate indoor levels in different
rooms of various kinds of buildings are described in NAS (1981), but most
models in use for exposure assessment are of a one-compartment type. A
newly available multicompartment model is described by Sparks (1989).
A number of factors involved in indoor exposure modeling, along with
comparisons of model predictions for radon and indoor measurements in
controlled experiments and in actual houses is given by Knutson (1988).

The risk of an exposure is dependent not only on the concentration
of pollutants in the air, but also on conditions which determine how much
of the pollutant actually is retained in the body. These are characteristics
of the pollutant itself and of the exposed individual. The respiratory
system has numerous self-protective systems built-in. The laws of physics
also affect what fraction of the pollutant inhaled is retained and where in
the system it is retained. Most of the air that is inhaled is immediately
exhaled, along with many of the pollutants it contained. Reactive gases
such as ozone or sulfur dioxide are more likely to be retained than inert
gases. The more reactive they are, the higher up in the respiratory system
they are likely to be trapped. Particles are more complex. In addition to
diffusion to the sides of the respiratory tract, they are removed by impaction at bifurcations. Impaction depends on particle size and mass (combined into aerodynamic diameter, a measure of effective particle size).
The respirability of particles is thus a function of particle size. To make
matters more complex, hydroscopic particles (those which absorb water
from the air) quickly grow as they enter the respiratory tract which is at
close to 100% relative humidity.

Finally, pollutant intake is influenced by the breathing rate. The "standard man" inhales 20 m^3/d (ICRP, 1975; Poston, 1982). He might breathe
at half that rate while at rest and 50% higher while engaged in hard
physical activity. This difference in breathing rate should be accounted
for in microenvironment-based models so that the unit time weighting for
exposures while sleeping or relaxing should be proportionally less than
for exposure while engaged in strenuous work or sports. In addition,
everyone is not the "standard man." Since activity patterns of men,
women and children may differ, it should be recognized that women on
average have lower breathing rates because of their smaller size. Children
are more complicated. Their lungs are, of course, smaller, but young
children (preteen) have a faster breathing rate. Their overall amount
breathed is not greater than "standard man" but it is sometimes of importance to remember that the amount of air children breath per unit body
weight is greater than in adults.

A few cross-media exposures are important to consider in estimating inhalation exposure. Volatile carcinogens contained in water can be released into the air during cooking and bathing.

Ingestion

Water

"Standard man" consumes water at a rate of two liters/day (ICRP, 1975). Like breathing, this also varies with a person's constitution and other factors such as climate. In general, however, no attempts are made to modify this factor on such grounds. When calculating exposures, it is important to recognize that the average person does not drink eight glasses of water each day. The two liters includes water contained in milk, soft drinks, coffee, tea, soups, and other foods. It is often assumed that the entire population of a community, whose water supply comes from a polluted source, each drinks 2 liters/day of water containing the same concentration of pollutant as the environmental transport model predicted to be in the river at the point of the intake to the water treatment plant. This is a worst-case assumption. First, some of the two liters comes from bottled beer, soft drinks and even spring water for which the water generally comes from a more remote source not subject to the same contamination. Second, the water coming out of the tap at home is quite different from the water drawn from the river or other raw water source. Often, data are available on removal rates at water treatment plants and interactions of the chemicals of concern with chemicals added to water supplies such as chlorine. Third, many carcinogens are volatile and are released during cooking so that their concentration in water served in foods may be reduced. These volatiles then enter the air in the kitchen resulting in potential inhalation exposures.

Another air exposure of volatiles in water is from showering. Andelman et al. (1986) demonstrated that important inhalation exposures to organic water contaminants such as trichloroethylene can stem from showering and bathing.

Preliminary risk assessments may assume the entire population along a river, for example, obtains its drinking water from that source. This can be grossly mistaken. Groundwater sources may be used or water drawn from more remote locations. New York City is on the Hudson River but obtains its water from upstate reservoirs. A complete exposure assessment must determine the water supply source. In an assessment of health effects of toxic emissions from a coal-fired power plant, for example, Bolten et al. (1987) compiled data on each water company or authority drawing water from the Susquehanna River, the point of intake, the treatment processes used, the size of the population served (disaggregated by adults, teenagers, children, and infants), and the percentage of the total water supply coming from the river. Information on water source, system type, treatment processes used, and average daily population served in each of the over 200,000 public water supplies in the United States is available in the EPA Federal Reporting Data System maintained under the Safe Drinking Water Act (Wentworth et al., 1986).

Food

Food chain models estimate the concentration of pollutants in various foods produced at different distances from the source. These models generally end with the food product at the farm; effects of later processing are not included and may be difficult to determine. Even foods consumed raw are washed which may remove some forms of pollution. Cooking may drive off volatiles. A comparison of six internationally recognized models for transfer of radionuclides through food chains found that only one included removal during processing and preparation; in that model, however, the effect was highly significant: 90% of the radioactivity was removed in green vegetables and 85% in cereals (Hoffman et al., 1984). Pollutants may concentrate in parts of the food not eaten such as the skin of fruits and vegetables or the kidneys of animals. A literature review on the particular chemical of concern or chemically similar substances may reveal information which could be incorporated into an exposure assessment.

Given pollutant concentrations in food, there are different approaches to assessing exposure. Information is available on the amounts of different foods eaten by "standard man" (ICRP, 1975). When exposure assessments are made on the basis of standard dietary intake, it should be disaggregated by specific food groups. If in a simple assessment total food consumption is used, care should be taken to avoid double counting with drink. Freeman et al. (1986) gives food consumption alone as 1.5 kg/day with a ±40% error. For preliminary exposure estimates it is often assumed that *all* food requirements are met by locally grown food (without regard to actual local food production). This maximizes the contribution of a source being assessed but is seldom realistic. Information is readily available on the amount of food produced in a region from the Census of Agriculture, published by the Department of Commerce, and various data sources published by the Department of Agriculture; these data are often included in food chain models. A common assumption is that all food produced locally is also consumed locally, and additional requirements met with foods imported from outside the region. This is the assumption made by Bolton et al. (1987). Peculiarities of local diet among subgroups of the population should be investigated. These might stem from regional customs, ethnic or religious background, poverty, or locally available supplies. Fish or game are common example, of the latter; subgroups of the population may eat considerably more than the national average of these in areas where fishing and hunting are common. Reliable data on dietary habits, however, are difficult to obtain. Risk assessments usually have to rely on "standard man" or national average data (NCHS, 1979) which may be of variable reliability (Jensen et al., 1984; Block, 1982). Potential high-exposure groups are usually assessed based on assumptions and sensitivity analysis.

These approaches all focus on the local population. Sometimes it is the national impact of a source of pollution which is of concern. This is especially true when the area involved is an agricultural production center supplying a wide food market. The approach taken for exposure assessment depends on the dose–response model to be used. If a linear model is assumed, then each increment of exposure adds a proportional increment of cancer risk regardless of the total exposure. One can simply estimate the total mass of the pollutant contained in the agricultural products and assume that it is all eaten by someone. In one study, a total of 5.2 g/y of polycyclic aromatic organic material was estimated to be added to leafy vegetables, produce, grain for human consumption, milk, and beef in the area impacted by a hypothetical synthetic fuels plant (Morris et al., 1984). Considering that this food might be distributed anywhere, cancers resulting from this exposure were estimated without regard to where they might occur or even how many people were exposed. The amount of food involved was known, and using the "standard man" estimates of dietary intake of different foods, a "full-time equivalent" exposed population size was calculated as the minimum size of the exposed population. This is the population that, for a given food group, could have its complete dietary requirement met. This provides a means of estimating the maximum individual risk as well as the total societal risk. Since the food from this area would be mixed with foods from other areas, the actual population exposed would be much larger and the true individual risk much smaller. Under the linear hypothesis, however, the total number of cancers produced would be the same.

Further adjustments made at this stage of the analysis might also take into account particular features of local agricultural products. For example, food chain models typically model "meat" as beef. The predominant meat production in an area, however, might be sheep or other animals. Adjustments could be made to account for differences in uptake of pollutants or distribution of pollutants within the animal.

One area of ingestion not generally included in food-chain models is

TABLE 6-4 Average Soil Ingestion Rates (mg/d) by
Age Group

Age (years)	LaGoy (1987)	Hawley (1985)
0–1	50	—
1–6	100	150[a]
6–11	50	23[b]
Over 11	50[c]	60[d]

[a]2.5-year old.
[b]6-year old.
[c]25 mg/day more appropriate for nonsmoking adults who do
not engage in outdoor activities.
[d]Adult.

direct ingestion of soil. Children, in particular, are prone to ingest soil
either through normal "mouthing" of fingers or nonfood items or through
pica, an abnormal tendency to ingest nonfood materials. Pica has received
considerable attention in connection with children eating flakes of lead-
based paint. Estimating the amount of soil ingested is difficult. Results of
two recent detailed studies are given in Table 6-4. Household dust contains
a substantial amount of soil and is a source of exposure, but most of the
exposure results from direct contact outdoors. The values in any case,
therefore, will depend on the activity patterns of the population.

Environmental Contamination

Although damage to the environment per se is an important concern, it
is, in general, not part of cancer risk assessment which focuses entirely on
human exposures. Information on environmental contamination is often
available as a byproduct when the movement of pollutants through environmental pathways is estimated. One instance when cancer risk assessments may include environmental contamination as an endpoint is when
carcinogens are trapped or stored for long periods in environmental media.
This generally applies to soil or groundwater. A discharge of a carcinogen
to groundwater poses a potential threat for the future even if no one
currently draws on that aquifer or if the nearest well is at such a distance
that decades or more would be estimated to intervene before anyone is
exposed. For example, The Nuclear Waste Policy Act of 1982 required
demonstration that any release to groundwater would take over 1000 years
to reach a well supplying drinking water. Yet, this was clearly based on
providing assurance of containment or provision of a safety factor for
clean-up since, based on other laws [e.g., CERCLA (The Comprehensive
Environmental Response, Compensation, and Liability Act of 1980),
amended by SARA (the Superfund Amendments and Reauthorization
Act of 1986)], such a contaminated plume would not be tolerated. It is

clear that exposure assessment conducted as part of QCRA must report the extent of estimated soil and groundwater contamination even if no current or projected exposures are quantified.

SUMMARY

Exposure assessment focuses on exposures to people. It begins with estimation of source terms or the development of emissions scenarios. Releases to the environment are then tracked through various environmental pathways using a variety of models which generally have their basis in environmental research or regulatory applications and thus may not be well suited to exposure modeling for cancer risk assessment. Parallel to environmental modeling, data on the exposed population must be developed. These two efforts are then brought together by additional models, calculations and assumptions necessary to estimate population exposure.

REFERENCES

Akan, A.O. 1987. Pollutant washoff by overland flow. *ASCE J. Environ. Eng.* 113:811-823.

Ambrose, R.B., S.I. Hill, and L.A. Mulkey. 1983. User's manual for the chemical transport and fate model TOXIWASP (EPA-600/3-83-005). U.S. Environmental Protection Agency, Athens, GA.

Ambrose, R.B. 1986. Modeling volatile organics in the Delaware estuary. *ASCE J. Environ. Eng.* 113:703-721.

Andelman, J.B., A. Couch, and W.W. Thurston. 1986. Inhalation exposures in indoor air to trichloroethylene from shower air. In F.C. Kopfler (ed.), *Environmental Epidemiology: The Importance of Exposure Assessment* (EPA/600/9-86-030). U.S. Environmental Protection Agency, Research Triangle Park, NC, pp. 193-205.

Baes, C.F., C.L. Begovich, W.M. Culkowski, K.R. Dixon, D.E. Fields, J.t. Holdeman, D.D. Huff, D.R. Jackson, N. M. Larson, R.J. Luxmore, J.K. Munro, M.R. Patterson, R.J. Raridon, M. Reeves, O.C. Stein, J.L. Stolzy, and T.C. Tucker. 1975. The unified transport model. Oak Ridge National Laboratory, Oak Ridge, TN.

Block, G. 1982. A review of validations of dietary assessment methods. *Am J. of Epidemiol.* 115:492-505.

Bolten, J.G., P.F. Morrison, S.A. Resetar, and K.A. Wolf. 1987. Health risks of toxic emissions from a coal-fired power plant (R-3507-EPRI). The RAND Corporation, Santa Monica, California.

Borneff, J. 1977. Fate of carcinogens in aquatic environments. In I.H. Suffet (ed.), *Fate of Pollutants in the Air and Water Environments* (part 2). John Wiley & Sons, New York, pp.393-408.

Brown, L.C. and T.O. Barnwell, Jr. 1985. Computer program documentation for the enhanced stream water quality model QUAL2E (EPA/600/3-85/065). U.S. Environmental Protection Agency, Athens, GA.

Burns, L., R. Lassiter, and D. Cline. 1982. Documentation for the Exposure assessment modeling system (EXAMS) (EPA 600/3-82-023). U.S. Environmental Protection Agency Environmental Research Laboratory, Athens, GA.

Burns, L.A., D.M. Cline, and R.R. Lassiter. 1985. Exposure analysis modeling system: reference manual for EXAMS II (EPA-600/3-85-038). U.S. Environmental Protection Agency, Athens, GA.

Burt, E.W. 1977. Valley model user's guide (EPA 450/2-77-018). U.S. Environmental Protection Agency, Research Triangle Park, N.C.

Chapin, F.S., Jr. 1974. *Human Activity Patterns in the City.* J. Wiley and Sons, New York.

Codell, R.B., K.T. Key, and G. Whelan. 1982. A collection of mathematical models for dispersion in surface water and groundwater (NUREG-0868). U.S. Nuclear Regulatory Commission, Washington, D.C.

Conway, R.A., F.C. Whitmore, and W.J. Hansen. 1982. Entry of chemicals into the environment. In *Environmental Risk Analysis for Chemicals.* Van Nostrand Reinhold Co., New York, pp. 61-84.

Crowther, M.A., H.C. Thode, Jr., and S.C. Morris. 1980. Modules for estimating solid waste from fossil fuel technologies (BNL 51474). Brookhaven National Laboratory, Upton, NY.

Dass, P., G.R. Tamie, and C.M. Stoffel. 1977. Leachate production at sanitary landfills. *ASCE J. Environ. Eng.* 103:981-988.

Donigian, A.S., Jr. and S.M. Brown. 1983. A workshop on water modeling needs and available techniques for synfuels risk assessment. Georgia Institute of Technology, Atlanta, GA.

Duan, N. 1980. Mircoenvironment types: a model for human exposure to air pollution. SIMS Technical Report, Department of Statistics, Stanford University, Stanford, CA.

Eadie, W.J. and W.E. Davis. 1979. The development of a national interregional transport matrix for respirable particles (PNL-RAP-37). Pacific Northwest Laboratory, Richland, WA.

EPA. 1977. Compilation of Air Pollutant Emission Factors, 3d edition and supplements (AP-42), Office of Air and Waste Management. U.S. Environmental Protection Agency, Research Triangle Park, NC.

EPA. 1986a. Guidelines for estimating exposures. *Fed. Reg.* 51:34042-34054 1986a.

EPA. 1986b. CDM-2.0-Climatological Dispersion Model User's Guide (EPA/600/8-85/029) U.S. Environmental Protection Agency, Research Triangle Park, N.C.

EPA. 1988. Superfund exposure assessment manual (EPA/540/1-88/001), U.S. Environmental Protection Agency, Washington, D.C.

Fay, J.A. and J.J. Rosenweig. 1979. Analytical diffusion model for long distance transport of air pollutants (EPA-600/4-79-037). U.S. Environmental Protection Agency, Research Triangle Park, N.C.

Freeman, T., T. Eger, I. Harding-Barlow, J. Lautzenheiser, and S. Brown. 1986. Techniques and models to estimate the health benefits of controlling toxic substances emitted from coal-fired power plants (EA-4490). Electric Power Research Institute, Palo Alto, CA.

Freni, S.C. and D.L. Phillips. 1987. Estimation of the time component in the movement of chemicals in contaminated groundwater. *Environ. Health Perspec.* 74:211-221.

Fugas, M. 1975. Assessment of total exposure to an air pollutant. In Proceedings of the International Conference on Environmental Sensing and Assessment (IEEE 75-CH-1004-1). Las Vegas, Nevada.

Hanna, S.R., G.A. Briggs, and R.P. Hosker, Jr. 1982. *Handbook on Atmospheric Diffusion* (DOE/TIC-11223). Technical Information Center, U.S. Department of Energy, Oak Ridge, TN.

Hawley, J.K. 1985. Assessment of health risk from exposure to contaminated soil. *Risk Analysis* 5:289-302.

Heffter, J.L. A.D. Taylor, and G.J. Ferber. 1975. A regional continental scale transport diffusion and disposition model (NOAA-TM-ERL-ARL 50). U.S. Department of Commerce, National Oceanic and Atmospheric Administration, Washington, D.C.

Hoffman, F.O., U. Bergstrom, C. Gyllander, and A.-B. Wilkens. 1984. Comparisons of predictions from internationally recognized assessment models for the transfer of selected radionuclides through terrestrial food chains. *Nuclear Safety* 25:533-546.

Horie, Y. and A.S. Chaplin. 1977. Population exposure to oxidants and nitrogen dioxide in Los Angeles (EPA-450/3-77-004). U.S. Environmental Protection Agency, Research Triangle Park, NC.

Hosker, R.P., Jr. 1980. Practical application of air pollutant deposition models — current status, data requirements, and research needs. In S.V. Krupa and A.H. Legge (eds.), *Air Pollutants and Their Effects on the Terrestrial Ecosystem*, Wiley-Interscience, New York, pp. 505-567.

Huyakorn, P.S. and G.F. Pinder. 1983. *Computational Methods in Subsurface Flow*. Academic Press, New York.

ICRP. 1975. *Report of the Task Group on Reference Man* (ICRP 23). International Commission on Radiological Protection. Pergamon Press, New York.

ICRP. 1979. Radionuclide Release Into the Environment: Assessment of Doses to Man (ICRP 29). International Commission on Radiological Protection. Pergamon Press, New York.

Jaffe, P.R. and F.L. Parker. 1984. Uncertainty analysis of first order decay model. *ASCE J. Environ. Eng.* 110:131-140.

Jensen, O.M., J. Wahrendorf, A. Rosenqvist, and A. Geser. 1984. The reliability of questionnaire-derived historical dietary information and temporal stability of food habits in individuals. *Am. J. of Epidemiol.* 120:281-290.

Jirka, G.H., A.N. Findikakis, Y. Onishi, and P.J. Ryan. 1982. Transport of Radionuclides in surface waters. In J.E. Till and H.R. Meyer (eds.), *Radiological Assessment* (NUREG/CR-3332). U.S. Nuclear Regulatory Commission, Washington, D.C., pp. 3-1 to 3-58.

Kaye, S.V., F.O. Hoffman, L.M. McDowell-Boyer, and C.F. Baes. 1984. Development and application of terrestrial food chain models to assess health risks to man from releases of pollutants to the environment. In *Health Impacts of Different Sources of Energy*. International Atomic Energy Agency, Geneva, pp. 271-298.

Kayes, P.J. (ed.). 1985. *Manual of Industrial Hazard Assessment Techniques*. Office of Environmental and Scientific Affairs, World Bank, Washington, D.C.

Knutson, E.O. 1988. Modeling indoor concentrations of radon's decay products. In W.W. Nazaroff and A.V. Nero, Jr. (eds.), *Radon and Its Decay Products in Indoor Air*. John Wiley & Sons, New York, pp. 161-202.

LaGoy, P.K. 1987. Estimated soil ingestion rates for use in risk assessment. *Risk Analysis* 7:355-359.

Lange, R. 1973. ADPIC: a three-dimensional computer code for the study of pollutant dispersal and deposition under complex conditions (UCRL-51462). Lawrence Livermore National Laboratory, Livermore, CA.

Lee, S.S. 1982. Mathematical modeling for prediction of chemical fate. In R.A. Conway (ed.), *Environmental Risk Analysis for Chemicals*. Van Nostrand Reinhold Company, New York, pp. 241-256.

Linsley, R.K. and J.B. Franzini. 1979. *Water-Resources Engineering*. McGraw Hill, New York.

Mashburn, R.G., R.C. Durfee, and R.G. Edwards. 1976. REGRID, a generalized grid-to-grid transformation procedure (ORNL/RUS-18). Oak Ridge National Laboratory, Oak Ridge, TN.

Mercer, J.W., L.R. Silka, and C.R. Faust. 1983. Modeling ground-water flow at Love Canal. *ASCE J. Environ. Eng.* 109:924-942.

Meyers, R.E., R.T. Cederwall, and W.D. Ohmstede. 1979. Modeling regional atmospheric transport and diffusion: some environmental applications. In J.R. Pfallin and E.N. Ziegler (eds), *Advances in Environmental Science and Engineering*. Gordon and Breach, New York, pp. 118-184.

Morgan, M.G. and S.C. Morris. 1977a. Individual air pollution monitors, 2: examination of some non-occupational research and regulatory uses and needs (BNL 50637). Brookhaven National Laboratory, Upton, NY.

Morgan, M.G. and S.C. Morris. 1977b. Needed: a national R&D effort to develop individual air pollution monitor instrumentation. *J. Air Pollution Control Assoc.* 27:670-673.

Morris, S.C., K.M. Novak, and L.D. Hamilton. 1979. Use of county level data in health, energy, demographic, environmental, and economic analysis (BNL 51041). Brookhaven National Laboratory, Upton, NY.

Morris, S.C., J.I. Barancik, H. Fischer, L.D. Hamilton, S. Jones, P.D. Moskowitz, J.Nagy, S. Rabinowitz, and H.C. Thode, Jr. 1984. Extrapolation to health risk: use of comparative approaches. In K.E. Cowser (ed.), *Synthetic Fossil Fuel Technologies, Results of health and Environmental Studies*. Butterworth Publishers, Boston, pp. 323-340.

Morris, S.C., C. Grimshaw, P.D. Kalb, W.H. Medeiros, C.G. Miles, J. Nagy, K.M. Novak, B. Royce., V.M. Fthenakis, E. Kaplan, A.F. Meinhold, P.D. Moskowitz, and L.D. Hamilton. 1986. Evaluations of models to assess health impacts of possible radiation releases from an operating geologic repository (BNL 39210). Brookhaven National Laboratory, Upton, NY.

Moskowitz, P.D., S.C. Morris, H. Fischer, H.C. Thode, Jr., and L.D. Hamilton. 1985. Synthetic-fuel plants: potential tumor risks to public health. *Risk Analysis* 5:181-194.

Mountain West Research, Inc. 1981. Bureau of Reclamation economic assessment model (BREAM) technical description and users guide. U.S. Bureau of Reclamation, Denver, CO.

NAS. 1981. *Indoor Pollutants.* Committee on Indoor Pollutants, National Research Council, National Academy Press, Washington, D.C.

NCHS. 1979. Dietary intake source data, United States, 1971-74 (DHEW PHS 79-1221). National Center for Health Statistics, Hyattsville, MD.

NRC. 1977. Calculation of annual doses to man from routine releases of reactor effluents for the purpose of evaluating compliance with 10CFR Part 50, Appendix I, Revision 1 (Regulatory Guide 1.109). U.S. Nuclear Regulatory Commission, Washington, D.C.

OECD. 1984. Emission standards for major air pollutants from energy facilities in OECD member countries (ISBN 92-64-12574-5). Organization for Economic Cooperation and Development, Paris.

Oster, C.A. 1982. Review of ground-water flow and transport models in the unsaturated zone (NUREG/CR-2917). Battelle Pacific Northwest Laboratories, Richland, WA.

Ott, W.R. and D.T. Mage. 1975. A method of simulating the true human exposure of critical population groups to air pollutants. In *Recent Advances in the Assessment of the Health Effects of Environmental Pollution* (EUR 5360). Commission of the European Communities, Luxembourg, pp. 2097-2107.

Ott, W.R. 1980. Models of human exposure to air pollution (SIMS Technical Report no. 32). Department of Statistics. Stanford University, Stanford, CA.

Ott, W.R. 1981. Exposure estimates based on computer generated activity patterns. Presented at the 74th Annual Meeting of the Air Pollution Control Association, Philadelphia, Pennsylvania.

Ott, W.R. 1985. Total human exposure. *Environ. Sci. and Technol.* 19:880-886.

Pinder, G.F. and W.G. Gray. 1977. *Finite Element Simulation in Surface and Subsurface Hydrology.* Academic Press, New York

Poston, J.W. 1982. Reference man: a system for internal dose calculations. In J.E. Till and H.R. Meyer (eds.), *Radiological Assessment* (NUREG/CR-3332). U.S. Nuclear Regulatory Commission, Washington, D.C., pp. 6-1–6-31.

Rowe, M.D. 1980. Human exposure to sulfates from coal-fired power plants. *J. Air Pollution Control Assoc.* 30:682-684.

Rowe, M.D. 1981. Human exposure to particulate emissions from power plants (BNL 31305). Brookhaven National Laboratory, Upton, NY.

Seiler, F.A. 1987. A methodology for the selection of environmental dispersion models in health risk assessments. *Environ. Int.* 13:351-357.

Shor, R.W., C.F. Baes, III, and R.D. Sharp. 1982. Agricultural production in the United States by county: A compilation of information from the 1974 Census of Agriculture for use in terrestrial food chain transport and assessment models (ORNL-5768). Oak Ridge National Laboratory, Oak Ridge, TN.

Slade, D.H. (ed.). 1968. *Meteorology and Atomic Energy* (TID-24190). U.S. Atomic Energy Commission, Oak Ridge, TN.

Southworth, G.R., B.R. Parkhurst, S.E. Herbes, and S.C. Tsai. 1982. The risk of chemicals to aquatic environment. In R.A. Conway (ed.), *Environmental Risk Analysis for Chemicals*. Van Nostrand Reinhold Company, New York, pp. 85-153.

Sparks, L.E. 1989. Indoor Air Quality Model Version 1.0 (EPA/600/8-88/097) U.S. Environmental Protection Agency, Research Triangle Park, N.C.

Stenehjem, E.J. 1978. Summary description of SEAM: the social and economic assessment model (ANL/IAPE/TM/78-9). Argonne National Laboratory, Argonne, IL.

Szalai, A. (ed.). 1972. *The Use of Time, Daily Activities of Urban and Suburban Populations in Twelve Countries*. Mouton, The Hague.

Till, J.E. and H.R. Meyer. 1982. *Radiological Assessment, A Textbook on Environmental Dose Analysis* (NUREG/CR-3332). U.S. Nuclear Regulatory Commission, Washington, D.C.

Travis, C.C., C.F. Baes, III, L.W. Barnthouse, E.L. Etnier, G.A. Holton, B.D. Murphy, G.P. Thompson, G.W. Suter II, and A.P. Watson. 1983. Exposure assessment methodology and reference environments for synfuel risk analysis (ORNL/TM-8672). Oak Ridge National Laboratory, Oak Ridge, TN.

Travis, C.C., G.A. Holton, E.L. Etnier, C.Cook, F.R. O'Donnell, D.M. Hetrick, and E.Dixon. 1986. Assessment of inhalation and ingestion population exposures from incinerated hazardous wastes. *Environ. Int.* 12:533-540.

Turner, D.B. 1970. Workbook of atmospheric dispersion estimates (AP-26). U.S. Environmental Protection Agency, Research Triangle Park, NC.

Van Genuchten, M.Th. and W.J. Alves. 1982. Analytical solutions of the one-dimensional convective-dispersion solute transport equation (Technical Bulletin 1661). U.S. Department of Agriculture, Washington, D.C.

Vaughn, B.E. 1984. State of research: environmental pathways and food chain transfer. *Environ. Health Perspec.* 54:353-371.

Wentworth, N.W., K.K. Wang, and J.L. Westrick. 1986. Drinking water quality data bases. In F.C. Kopfler (ed.), *Environmental Epidemiology: The Importance of Exposure Assessment* (EPA/600/9-86-030). U.S. Environmental Protection Agency, Research Triangle Park, NC, pp, 127-135.

Wenzel, W.J. and A.F. Gallegos. 1985. EFFECTS: documentation and verification for a BEIR III cancer risk model based on age, sex, and population dynamics for BIOTRAN (LA-10371-MS). Los Alamos National Laboratory, Los Alamos, NM.

Yocke, M.A., G.E. Anderson, S.M. Greenfield, T.W. Tesche, G.Z. Whitten, and D.A. Stewart. 1984. Final report of second workshop on air dispersion modeling for risk analysis (SYSAPP-83/237). Systems Applications, Inc., San Rafael, CA.

Yocke, M.A., B.R. Weir, and S.M. Greenfield. 1985. Workshop on atmospheric dispersion modeling III: toxic organic compounds (SYSAPP-85-094). Systems Applications, Inc., San Rafael, CA.

Yocom, J.E. 1982. Indoor-outdoor air quality relationships, a critical review. *J. Air Pollution Control Assoc*. 32:500-520.

Warwick, J.J. and W.G. Cale. 1986. Effects of parameter uncertainty in stream modeling. *J. of Environmental Engineering* 112:479-489.

WHO. 1982. Estimating human exposure to air pollutants (Publ. no. 69). World Health Organization, Geneva.

WHO. 1983. Compendium of Environmental Guidelines and Standards for Industrial discharges (EFP/83.49). World Health Organization, Geneva.

7

Pharmacokinetics

Up to this point, measurements and models for exposure assessment have focused on exposure or what toxicologists call "administered dose." Until the mid-1970s, risk analysts, epidemiologists, and even toxicologists were content with that for most purposes. There was an implicit assumption that what might be called the "biologically effective dose" was proportional to exposure. One exception was the concern of those assessing risks of internal radiation exposure who found it necessary to know the distribution and residence times of inhaled or ingested radionuclides in the body so that doses to individual organs or tissues could be calculated.

As interest in quantitative cancer risk assessment grew throughout the 1970s and 1980s, several models were proposed to express the cancer dose–response relationship (see Chap. 9). For many people, the essence of QCRA became the fitting of animal bioassay data with a dose–response model, and the shape of the model had as much influence as the data in determining the result. The dose–response model related "biologically effective dose" with cancers produced, only the dose data put into the model was not the biologically effective dose but the administered dose. An important example through which this problem received attention was the case of vinyl chloride. The active carcinogen is a metabolite of vinyl chloride (O'Flaherty, 1985). Although the linear dose–response model was generally accepted for regulatory purposes, results of long-term animal studies with vinyl chloride showed a distinctly nonlinear dose–response function. Gehring and co-workers (1977; 1978; 1979) showed that the rate of metabolism of vinyl chloride in rats was a function of dose, and much of the nonlinearity in the dose–response could be attributed to the nonlinear relationship between administered dose and biologically effective dose.

The distribution of a pollutant chemical and its metabolites from the point of entry to the different organs and tissues of the body is the role of pharmacokinetics. This is a highly developed science, but there remains a long way to go in developing a full understanding and an ability to predict how chemicals are distributed. As the name indicates, pharmacokinetics developed principally to study the action of drugs in the body and its application to environmental pollutants is a relatively minor speciality. The fields covered by pharmacokinetics include: (1) factors that determine the rate and extent of absorption of a substance from the point of entry; (2) factors that govern the distribution and elimination of the substance, and the formation, distribution, and elimination of biologically active metabolites, if any; and (3) factors that affect the rate or extent of reaction of the substance with target substances such as DNA and enzymes.

Pharmacokinetics has four important roles in risk assessment (Clewell and Anderson, 1987). *First*, pharmacokinetic models allow the biologically effective dose to be predicted from exposures or administered doses. A nonlinear relationship between exposure or administered dose and the biologically effective dose is a crucial factor in extrapolating from the high doses of occupational exposure or animal studies to the low doses of public exposure. The linkage of pharmacokinetics with high-dose to low-dose extrapolation models was proposed by Hoel et al. (1983) and furthered by Lutz and Dedrick (1987). *Second*, pharmacokinetics allow extrapolation of the dose–response function from one route of entry to another because in each case, the biologically effective dose in the organ of interest can be calculated. The dose to an organ such as the liver will differ for the same amount of substance administered through ingestion or inhalation. Yet, while inhalation is often the important exposure route in people, ingestion is by far the more common experimental method in the laboratory. *Third*, pharmacokinetics is also important in extrapolating results found in laboratory animals to humans, since pharmacokinetic factors differ among species. *Fourth*, pharmacokinetics helps in translating the well-controlled, easily characterized exposures in the laboratory or the specialized character of occupational exposure to the discontinuous, variable environmental exposures human populations face. This includes prediction of temporal variations in tissue concentration that might occur after exposures with different time sequences than used in bioassay studies. Here the emphasis is on providing a basic understanding and appreciation of these roles. An extensive review of the application of pharmacokinetics in risk assessment can be found in the recent report of that title by a committee of the National Research Council (NAS, 1987).

ALLOMETRY

Allometry describes the disporportionate relationship of the size or function of isolated features in animals with body size or mass (Lindstedt,

TABLE 7-1 Power Relationship of Named Items with Total Body Mass

Lung capacity	1.0
Heart volume	1.0
Skeletal mass	1.1
Metabolic rate	0.75
Heart and respiratory rate	−0.25
Physiological time	0.25

Source: Data from Lindstedt, 1987.

1987). Although all mammals share much in common in bodily structure and function, larger animals are not proportionally scaled to smaller animals. In larger animals, for example, the skeleton comprises a greater proportion of the total mass than in small animals while smaller animals have a higher metabolism rate per unit mass. This relationship is generally described as a power function:

$$Y = aM^b$$

where

Y is the specific structural of functional feature
M is the body mass, and
a and b are derived empirically.

Example values of the coefficient b are given in Table 7-1. A common allometric scaling factor is $b = 2/3$, the ratio of body surface area to mass. Another important source of scaling is physiological time.

Physiological Time

There is apparently a common body-sized dependent clock among all mammals, to which physiological events are timed. Thus, although all animals must contend with identical lengths of days and seasons, these span disproportionately longer physiological periods in small animals than in large animals (Lindstedt, 1987). Pharmacokinetic effects occur in physiological time; when viewed in physiological time, species variability in pharmacokinetic variables may disappear. Blood circulation rate, respiratory cycle, and growth times all appear to be tuned to a constant physiological time with a body mass exponent of about 0.24. An animal with twice the mass of another might be expected to have $2^{-0.24}$ times the blood circulation rate. Lindstedt points out that since volumes and capacities are linear with mass while times go as the 1/4 power of mass, then clearance rates (volume/time) must vary as the 3/4 power of mass, and that the ratios of various rates must be uniform among species.

The concept of physiological time provides the basic premise for extrapolation of cancer incidence from laboratory animals to people at all. In humans, a 10- to 20- year latent period intervenes between exposure and the first appearance of most forms of cancer, and it takes a further 40-50 years for the full effect of a carcinogen exposure to be expressed in a human population. Effects in small animals with 2-year lifespans can be extrapolated to humans because these events are not functions of chronological time, but of physiological time. The latent period and the period of expression of cancer is attuned to the lifespan, not the absolute chronological time intervals. In terms of scaling as a function of mass, however, it has been suggested that the human lifespan is disproportionately long relative to the expectation for a 70-kg animal (Hill et al., 1986).

Limitations of Allometry

There are, of course, differences among species which go beyond scaling. Larger species are more complex than smaller ones. Some species have enzyme systems and even organs which others lack. Marked differences in tissue to blood partition ratios exist. In some specific cases, these differences may be important. In general, however, allometric scaling is a useful first-level analysis. It is in the special situations where there are greater differences among species than can be handled by simple scaling that more complex pharmacokinetic models are necessary.

METABOLISM

The greatest difference among species in the pharmacokinetic handling of chemical pollutants is due to differences in routes, mechanisms, and rates of metabolism (Withey, 1985). The metabolic process is designed to eliminate nonnutritious substances from the body. It tends to break down large, complex molecules into smaller ones with lower molecular weight and to convert substances insoluble in water into soluble conjugates. These metabolites may be further metabolized, bound in tissue, or excreted. Breaking down molecules and converting them to soluble forms both increase the ability of the substance to diffuse through tissue and membrane barriers and the tendency, therefore, is to facilite excretion. Metabolic processes were not designed to deactivate carcinogens. They may either detoxify or activate a substance. For many "carcinogenic" substances, it is their metabolites which are the true carcinogens.

Metabolic processes generally involve enzymes. Such enzymatic processes have saturation limits which vary among species. In the simplest case of a single saturable pathway, the rate of change of concentration with time (i.e., the speed with which the substance is metabolized) is described by the Michaelis-Menten equation (e.g., see Gehring et al., 1976; O'Flaherty, 1985):

$$\frac{dC(t)}{dt} = \frac{V_m C(t)}{K_m + C(t)}$$

where

$C(t)$ is the concentration at time t;
V_m is the maximum rate of elimination, achieved when all elimination sites are occupied;
K_m is the Michaelis constant, equal to the concentration of the substance when the rate is $V_m/2$.

When the concentration is large relative to K_m, the metabolic rate of the substance approaches its maximum, V_m. When the concentration is small relative to K_m, the metabolic rate of the substance is proportional to its concentration, with a proportionality factor of (V_m/K_m). This shows that when the exposure to the pollutant is sufficient to saturate the capacity of the enzymatic process, the whole nature of the system changes. New processes may come into play and new metabolic products or marked changes in the mixture of metabolic products may appear.

This equation is one of the foundations of pharmacokinetics. Metabolism is, of course, much more complex than depicted by the Michaelis-Menten equation. Seldom is only one enzyme involved; metabolism of pollutant compounds may involve combinations of several types of reactions (e.g., oxidation, dehydrogenation, hydrolysis, sulfation, glucuronidation, and glutathionyl conjugation reactions), each catalyzed by several different enzymes. Knowledge of the Michaelis-Menten parameters of a single enzyme alone is seldom sufficient to predict either the concentration of the parent substance or any of its metabolites. In addition, other substances within cells may limit metabolic rates. The validity of the simple form of the Michaelis-Menten equation in these cases depends on the kinetics of the mechanisms govening the concentration of these other substances. With the focus on the Michaelis-Menten equation, the importance of other methods of elimination which affect the concentration of the parent compound may be overlooked (Gillette, 1987). The ability to observe and measure the effects of metabolism varies with the kind of metabolite. Table 7-2 lists functional classes of metabolites based on their

TABLE 7-2 Functional Classes of Metabolites

1. Ultrashortlived metabolites. Metabolites never leave the enzyme (suicie enzyme inhibitors).
2. Shortlived metabolites. Metabolites never leave the cell.
3. Intermediately lived metabolites. Metabolities never enter aortic blood.
4. Longlived metabolites. Negligible amounts of metabolites excreted into air, bile, and urine.
5. Ultralonglived metabolites. Metabolites extensively excreted into air, bile, or urine.

Source: From Gillette, 1987.

persistence. Obviously the shorter the life of a metabolite, the more difficult to find it experimentally. Finally, significant quantitative and even qualitative differences in metabolism of pollutant substances exist among individuals. This interindividual variability adds to the overall uncertainty of predictions of biologically effective dose and response.

PHARMACOKINETIC MODELS

As with other models, pharmacokinetic models simplify reality. It is not necessary to understand and incorporate every step in a model, but the overall scheme and the limiting steps must be recognized (Blancato, 1986). The models provide the framework which provides insight into the mechanism that control the time history of contaminants in the body (Lutz and Dedrick, 1987).

In addition to anatomical and metabolic factors discussed above, pharmacokinetic models may include parameters representing physiological, clearance, thermodynamic, and transport processes in the body. Physiological parameters include blood flow rate. Clearance mechanisms include urinary and fecal elimination processes which involve the kidney and liver. Thermodynamic parameters include protein binding and tissue partitioning which depend on physical interactions between the contaminant and biological tissues. Many thermodynamic parameters can be evaluated in vitro. Transport is generally via blood, but in some cases may be limited by the rate of transport across cell membranes. The latter may be by passive diffusion or the contaminant may first bind to a carrier protein on the cell membrane surface and then the whole complex transported through the membrane (Lutz and Dedrick, 1987).

There are basically two approaches to pharmacokinetic modeling. The classic approach is empirical and focuses on data fitting; the newer approach, physiologically based pharmacokinetic modeling (PB-PK), is predictive. O'Flaherty (1987) describes the role of each class of model and how the need for interspecies conversion of animal data led to the development of PB-PK models.

Classical Models

The bases, formulations, and applications of these models are described by Gehring et al. (1976). The complexity of the body is reduced in the model to a small number of separate compartments. Each compartment represents those organs, tissues, and cells with similar uptake and subsequent clearance of a chemical substance. The pharmacokinetics of most substances are studied in one- to three-compartment models (Fig. 7-1). In a three compartment model, one compartment may be thought of as the vascular system into which the substance has been introduced. The second compartment represents those organs with an abundant blood supply, which quickly equilibrate with the vascular system. The third compartment represents tissues such as bone and fat which are slower to equilibrate. If the second compartment were to equilibrate extremely fast, it would be indistinguishable from the vascular system and the two might be combined into a single compartment. This would leave a two-compartment model. If, then, the third compartment equilibrated so slowly that it could be ignored in the analysis, one would be left with a one-compartment model. The parameters of the models are the concentrations (or amounts) of the substance in each compartment, the rates of adsorption and elimination, and the rates of transfer between the central vascular compartment and any other compartments. The models are driven by measurements of concentrations or amounts.

Once the model and its rate parameters are defined, numerical integration techniques can be used to estimate the total quantity of contaminant adsorbed in the body in a given period given estimates of the exposure

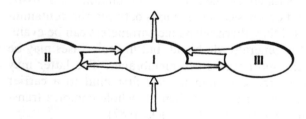

Figure 7-1 Schematic diagram of a three compartment model (after Gehring et al., 1976).

rate; conversely, the exposure rate could be estimated using measurements of the amount excreted in urine (Ramsey and Gehring, 1981).

Although they represent mixes of organs and other tissues, the compartments usually have no anatomic or physiologic reality; a compartment is simply a fluid volume that is kinetically homogeneous. They are sufficient, however, to estimate the quantitative parameters describing the fate of chemicals in the body. Concepts of biological half-life, clearance, integrated total exposure, and steady state following a chronic exposure were derived from such models. Moreover, because their compartments are not constrained to physiological reality, the widest latitude is available to statistical fitting of the data and to comparison of results among different experimental conditions, doses, or chemicals.

Physiologically Based Pharmacokinetic Models

The strength of the classical models is also their weakness. Since they have no specific physiological or biochemical basis, they cannot form a reliable basis for extrapolation of results from one species to another. This need was a principal reason for the development of PB-PK models. In these, the compartments represent actual organs and tissues with known blood flows, enzyme activities, etc. They are more simulation models than models designed for reduction of experimental data and testing of hypotheses. The history and scientific bases of PB-PK models is given by Bischoff (1987) while risk assessment applications are discussed by Clewell and Andersen (1987).

Each organ in the body need not be represented individually. Bischoff (1987) notes that the main features needed to describe the distribution of a foreign substance in the body can be had in models containing little detail. Body parts with a definite anatomic and physiologic basis that can be described by a single concentration level are lumped together into compartments, which Bischoff refers to as "regions" to avoid confusion with the more abstract "compartments" of classical pharmacokinetic models. Figure 7-2 shows a general schematic. The pharmacokineticist's judgment is needed to decide how many regions must be included to model a particular substance. For example, if a substance is not lipid soluble, the fatty tissues may not be represented in detail. Figure 7-3 shows a schematic formulation from an actual case.

Once the basic structure of the model is established, the model is quantified using known physiological and biochemical parameters such as organ volumes, blood flow rates to each region, partition coefficients of the relative solubility of the substance in blood and tissue, and physical

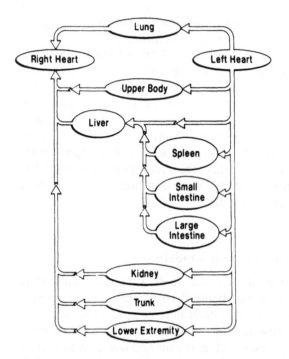

FIGURE 7-2 Schematic diagram of general mammalian flow diagram for pharmacokinetic modeling (after Bischoff, 1987).

and biochemical constants of the modeled substance. Mass balance equations are written, accounting explictly for free and bound forms of the substance modeled. The model *predicts* the time course of the substance in the body rather than merely fitting the data as in a classical model. Incorporating more physiological factors increases accuracy. This results, however, in increased complexity, the need for greater numbers of physiological and biochemical parameters, and added demands on computer capacity (Standaert, 1986; Clewell and Andersen, 1987). These problems are not insurmountable. Much precompiled physiological data are available; a set of reference physiological parameters for pharmacokinetic modeling is being developed at Oak Ridge National Laboratory under EPA sponsorship. Membrane transport parameters are, perhaps, the least available, and because of their absence, modeling often follows the expedient course of assuming membrane resistances are not rate controlling.

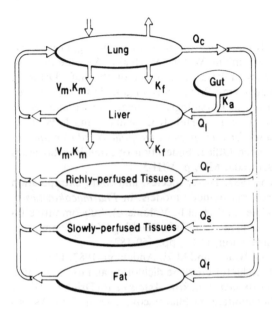

FIGURE 7-3 Schematic diagram of an example pharmacokinetic model (after ethylene dichloride model of D'Souza et al., 1987). The only important metabolism in this case was assumed to occur in the lung and liver where V_m and K_m refer to a saturable (Michaelis-Menten) metabolic pathway and K_f a linear pathway.

SUMMARY

Pharmacokinetics makes four important contributions to risk assessment: (1) It provides the means to translate exposure or administered dose to the dose at the site of biological importance. This is especially important in separating nonlinearities in exposure to dose from those in dose–response. (2) It allows an exposure-response relationship derived from one route of exposure (e.g., ingestion) to be used in an assessment of the risk from another route of exposure (e.g., inhalation) because in each case the dose at the target tissue can be calculated. (3) It allows improved extrapolation of results in laboratory animals to humans. (4) It helps in translating well-controlled, easily characterized exposures in the laboratory to the variable environmental exposures human populations face. In particular, PB-PK models have great promise in improving cancer risk assessment.

164   CHAPTER 7

REFERENCES

Bischoff, K.B. 1987. Physiologically based pharmacokinetic modeling, in *Pharmacokinetics in Risk Assessment* (Drinking Water and Health, Volume 8), Subcommittee on Pharmacokinetics in Risk Assessment of the Safe Drinking Water Committee. National Academy Press, Washington, D.C., pp. 36-61.
Blancato, J.N. 1986. Design and use of physiologic pharmacokinetic models for use in risk assessment (abstract), in T.A. Hill, R.C. Wands, and R.W. Leukroth, Jr. (eds), *Biological Bases for Interspecies Extrapolation of Carcinogenicity Data*, Life Sciences Research Office, Federation of American Societies for Experimental Biology, Bethesda, MD, p. VIII-5.
Clewell, H.J. and M.E. Andersen. 1987. Dose, species, and route extrapolation using physiologically based pharmacokinetic models, in *Pharmacokinetics in Risk Assessment* (Drinking Water and Health, Volume 8), Subcommittee on Pharmacokinetics in Risk Assessment of the Safe Drinking Water Committee. National Academy Press, Washington, D.C., pp. 159-182.
D'Souza, R.W., W.R. Francis, R.D. Bruce, and M.E. Anderson. 1987. Physiologically based pharmacokinetic model for ethylene dichloride and its application in risk assessment, in *Pharmacokinetics in Risk Assessment* (Drinking Water and Health, Volume 8), Subcommittee on Pharmacokinetics in Risk Assessment of the Safe Drinking Water Committee. National Academy Press, Washington, D.C., pp. 286-301.
Gehring, P.J. and G.E. Blau. 1977. Mechanisms of carcinogenesis: dose response. *J. Environmental Pathol. Toxicol.* 1:163-179.
Gehring, P.J., P.G. Watanabe, and G.E. Blau. 1976. Pharmacokinetic studies in evaluation of the toxicological and environmental hazard of chemicals. In M.A. Mehlman, R.E. Shapiro, and H. Blumenthal (eds.), *New Concepts in Safety Evaluation*. Wiley and Sons, New York, pp. 195-270.
Gehring, P.J., P.G. Watanabe, and C.N. Park. 1978. Resolution of dose–response toxicity data for chemicals requiring metabolic activation: example—vinyl chloride. *Toxicol. Appl. Pharmacol.* 44:581-591.
Gehring, P.J., P.G. Watanabe, and C.N. Park. 1979. Risk of angiosarcoma in workers exposed to vinyl chloride as predicted from studies in rats. *Toxicol. Appl. Pharmacol.* 49:15-21.
Gillette, J.R. 1987. Dose, species, and rout extrapolation: general aspects, in *Pharmacokinetics in Risk Assessment* (Drinking Water and Health, Volume 8), Subcommittee on Pharmacokinetics in Risk Assessment of the Safe Drinking Water Committee. National Academy Press, Washington, D.C., pp. 96-158.
Hill, T.A., R.C. Wands, and R.W. Leukroth, Jr. 1986. Biological bases for interspecies extrapolation of carcinogenicity data, prepared for the Food and Drug Administration by Life Sciences Research Office, Federation of American Societies for Experimental Biology, Bethesda, MD.
Hoel, D.G., N.L. Kaplan, and M.W. Anderson. 1983. Implications of nonlinear kinetics on risk estimation in carcinogenesis. *Science* 219:1032-1037.

Lindstedt, S.L. 1987. Allometry: body size constraints in animal size, in *Pharmacokinetics in Risk Assessment* (Drinking Water and Health, Volume 8), Subcommittee on Pharmacokinetics in Risk Assessment of the Safe Drinking Water Committee. National Academy Press, Washington, D.C., pp. 65-79.

Lutz, R.J. and R.L. Dedrick. 1987. Implications of pharmacokinetic modeling in risk assessment analysis. *Environ. Health Perspec.* 76:97-106.

NAS. 1987. *Pharmacokinetics in Risk Assessment* (Drinking Water and Health, Volume 8), Subcommittee on Pharmacokinetics in Risk Assessment of the Safe Drinking Water Committee. National Academy Press, Washington, D.C.

O'Flaherty, E.J. 1985. Differences in metabolism at different dose levels, Chapter 3 in D.B. Clayson, D. Krewski, and I. Munro (eds.), *Toxicological Risk Assessment, Volume I, Biological and Statistical Criteria.* CRC Press, Boca Raton, FL, pp. 53-90.

O'Flaherty, E.J. 1987. Modeling: an introduction, in *Pharmacokinetics in Risk Assessment* (Drinking Water and Health, Volume 8), Subcommittee on Pharmacokinetics in Risk Assessment of the Safe Drinking Water Committee. National Academy Press, Washington, D.C., pp. 27-35.

Ramsey, J.C. and P.J. Gehring. 1981. The integration and application of pharmacokinetic principles in realistic estimates of risk, in C.R. Richmond, P.J. Walsh, and E.D. Copenhaver (eds), *Health Risk Analysis.* The Franklin Institute Press, Philadelphia, pp. 213-223.

Standaert, F.G. 1986. Absorption and distribution of xenobiotics, in T.A. Hill, R.C. Wands, and R.W. Leukroth, Jr. (eds), *Biological Bases for Interspecies Extrapolation of Carcinogenicity Data.* Life Sciences Research Office, Federation of American Societies for Experimental Biology, Bethesda, MD, pp. III-1–III-29.

Withey, J.R. 1985. Pharmacokinetic differences between species, in D.B. Clayson, D. Krewski, and I. Munro, *Toxicological Risk Assessment, Volume I, Biological and Statistical Criteria*, CRC Press, Boca Raton, FL.

PART III

DOSE–RESPONSE ASSESSMENT

The ability to demonstrate a gradient of response to increasing dose levels has long been a criterion in biomedical studies for deciding if a relationship was causal. The need to quantify dose–response curves is more recent and is tied directly to quantitative risk assessment. Dose–response assessment is the evaluation and quantitative characterization of the relationship between level of exposure and health related response. It differs from other parts of risk assessment in that it is often developed independently of the application on which the risk assessment focuses, using data from other sources, and is equally applicable to many risk assessment applications.

The term dose–response function most commonly means exposure-response function. Exposure is the concentration (or amount) of a pollutant one is exposed to in the environment, e.g., 25 $\mu g/m^3$ in the air breathed. Dose is the physiologically significant amount reaching the target tissue. The dose of concern may not even be the same material as the exposure, but a chemically altered metabolite. The exposure-response function includes metabolic, pharmacokinetic, and other processes which intervene between the initial point of exposure and the tissue of interest, which can be highly dependent on how the person was exposed, and which may vary considerably within a population. The true dose–response function may be difficult to determine since the actual dose to the target tissue is difficult to measure.

The risk analyst must be familiar with the methods and literature of several biomedical sciences which provide the information upon which dose–response assessments are based. This section begins with a chapter on toxicology which focuses on long-term animal bioassays. This comes first, not because it is most important, but because it is the most all encompassing and provides a good base for examining other approaches. Since it is people we are interested in rather than animals, the following chapter considers extrapolation from animals to people. This is followed by a chapter dealing with short-term approaches including models which relate chemical structure to biological activity and in vitro bioassays such as the Ames test. Next is a chapter on epidemiology, the science which examines the relationship between exposures and cancer in human populations directly. The final chapter illustrates how this information is put together to make a dose–response assessment.

8

Toxicology

INTRODUCTION

Toxicology is the study of the harmful actions of chemicals on biologic tissue (Loomis, 1974). This includes an understanding of pharmacokinetics and metabolism included in the previous chapter because, for the present purpose, they fit more closely under exposure and dose assessment. Experiments to develop dose–response data must, of course, also include measurement or calculation of exposure and dose. This chapter focuses on experiments to determine carcinogenic dose–response directly in mammals. It provides some basic understanding of the methods by which dose–response information is developed in controlled experimental approaches. Application of this information to risk assessment is covered in the following chapter. Presenting animal studies first does not mean they are superior to epidemiological studies or cellular level bioassays. Animal studies simply seem to be the simplest and most straightforward way to present concepts which form a basis from which to expand the discussion to other approaches. Toxicology also includes studies using other species of animals and plants as well as bacteria and cells in culture; some of these are covered in Chapter 10. Modern toxicology began in the early 1800s. Since that time, a number of general principles have become apparent (Table 8-1).

Although generally well accepted, there remains controversy over application of some of these principles. The general usefulness of quantitative extrapolation from animals compared to direct use of human observation is still debated by some (e.g., see Gori, 1980) and the concept of a threshold of effect is in general rejected in the case of cancer. Controversy over thresholds is based more on a philosophy of how to deal with uncertainty than it is on the science of the matter since it is essentially impossible to distinguish between a threshold, i.e., a dose below which

TABLE 8-1   General Principles of Toxicology

1. In order for a chemical agent to produce a biologic effect, it must come into immediate contact with the biological cells under consideration
2. There will be some quantity of each chemical below which there will be no detectable effect on biologic systems, and there will be some greater amount of each chemical at which a significant effect will be present on essentially all biologic systems. Between that amount of each chemical which produces no effect and that amount which produces a significant effect, there will be a range of amounts of the chemical that will produce significant effects on some types of biological systems
3. Cells having similar functions and similar metabolic pathways in various species in biology generally will be similarly affected by a given chemical entity
4. Small changes in the structure of a chemical agent may greatly influence the biological action of that agent

Source: From Loomis, 1974.

there is no response, and a progressively decreasing response which in any experiment reaches a point below which the effect can no longer be detected.

The acceptance of animal models by the risk assessment community is exemplified by a set of principles (Table 8-2) established for EPA by the National Research Council Committee on Drinking Water and Health (NAS, 1977; 1986). The last principle is of especial interest here, since it advocates quantitative risk assessment, rather than qualitative determination of a "safe" or "not safe" level. EPA's Gene-Tox Carcinogen Data Base provides a means to evaluate the ability of various bioassays to predict carcinogenicity of chemicals (Nesnow et al., 1986).

TABLE 8-2   Principles for Assessment of Effects of Long-Term Exposure to Carcinogens

1. Effects in animals, properly qualified, are applicable to humans
2. Methods do not now exist to establish a threshold for long-term effects of toxic agents
3. The exposure of experimental animals to toxic agents in high doses is a necessary and valid method of discovering possible carcinogenic hazards in humans
4. Agents should be assessed in terms of human risk, rather than as "safe" or "unsafe"

Source: From NAS, 1977, 1986.

EXPERIMENTAL DESIGN

Toxicology is an experimental science. To understand, interpret, and use the results of toxicological experiments, the risk analyst must have an understanding of what is involved in those experiments that can shape the results. A number of issues affecting experimental design are discussed below. This discussion draws heavily on two authoritative reviews of issues involved in animal carcinogen testing (OSTP, 1984; NTP, 1984). Most carcinogen testing is done with standard designs in a routine manner. Since each chemical's toxic properties are different, however, each test

TABLE 8-3 Standard Carcinogen Animal Bioassay Designs

	NCI	FIFRA	TSCA
Species	Rats & mice	Rats & mice	Rats & mice
No. animals (M/F) at each dose	50/50	50/50	50/50
Dosages	2: MTD, MTD/2 or MTD/4 No dose control	3: MTD MTD/2 or MTD/4 MTD/4 or MTD/8 no dose control	3: HDL HDL/2 or HDL/4 HDL/4 or HDL/10 no dose control
Dosing regimen			
Start	6 weeks	In utero or 6 weeks	6 weeks
End	24 months	Mice: 18-24 months Rats: 24-30 months	24-30 months
Observation period:	3–6 months after end of dosing	NS	NS
Organs and tissues to be examined	All animals: external and histopathologic exam (ca. 30 organs and tissues)	All animals: external exam; some animals pathological exam of 30 organs and tissues, other animals: fewer organs and tissues	All animals: external and histopatho-logic exam of (ca. 30 organs and tissues)

Abbreviations: NCI, National Cancer Institute;
FIFRA, Federal Insecticide, Fungicide and Rodenticide Act;
TSCA, Toxic Substances Control Act;
MTD, Maximum tolerated dose, causes minor acute toxicity;
HDL, high dose level, causes some acute toxicity;
NS, not specified.
Source: From OTA, 1981.

can involve its individual set of judgments associated with its design, performance, and interpretation. Table 8-3 compares some features of standard designs Although different regulatory agencies set their own design criteria, the leading U.S. organization in animal carcinogen testing is the National Toxicology Program (NTP). The NTP was established in 1978 to bring together the relevant programs, staff, and resources of the National Cancer Institute, National Institute of Environmental Health Sciences, National Center for Toxicological Research, and the National Institute for Occupational Health and Safety. Detailed reports of all NTP carcinogenesis bioassays are publicly available.

Objective

The design of an experiment is obviously influenced by the kind of information sought. The basis of current design stems from experiments looking for both carcinogenic potential and mechanism. In the 1960s, this developed into 'a more or less standard bioassay system for testing carcinogenicity which had as its emphasis the qualitative question, is the material a carcinogen or not. This resulted in what Gori (1980) calls an "understandable preoccupation with increasing the odds of inducing cancer" and a lack of interest in negative studies. The design basically compared an exposed group to a nonexposed group, attempting to maximize the chances of detecting a difference in tumor production between them to increase the sensitivity of the test, with a lesser regard for avoiding false positives. With a shift in emphasis toward QCRA, there were some modifications in the design. These primarily involved increasing the number of dose levels included in the experiment from two doses plus a control to three doses plus a control (Table 8-3). In general, the attempt has been to combine both qualitative and quantitative objectives in one bioassay design, although a design which is optimal for one may be inefficient for the other (Portier, 1985). The emphasis in both qualitative and quantitative analysis was on the fraction of animals to develop tumors. An emphasis in quantifying the time to tumor development would require different consideration in experimental design requiring more animals and more interim sacrifice of animals. McKnight and Crowley (1984) discuss the importance of interim sacrifice for obtaining quantitative tumor incidence rates from a statistical perspective.

Species and Strain

Of all the animal species, which should be used for a bioassay? Some criteria are given in Table 8-4. Only three species meet these criteria: the mouse, the rat, and the hamster. Of course, other species may be ideally suited for specific carcinogens, examination of effects on specific tumor

TABLE 8-4   Criteria for Selection of Test Species

Availability
Economy
Life span of reasonable length, long enough to allow time for tumors to develop
   and short enough to allow bioassays to be conducted relatively quickly (i.e.,
   2–3 years)
Small size, easy to handle, and live and breed well in captivity
Extensive knowledge available on the biology of the species
Similarity to humans in metabolism and pathologic responses
Strains used should be likely to be susceptible to cancer from the chemical being
   analyzed, yet not hypersensitive

sites, or certain research questions. It is important for research that a wide variety of species and strains be available for use so that the most appropriate can be selected for each experiment. We are not discussing cancer research here, however, but general bioassays which must produce comparable results for different chemicals. For this purpose, a high degree of standardization is appropriate. While these two or three species are the only ones currently to meet the requirement for standardization, there remains some feeling that insufficient attention has gone into selection of test species and a need exists to build a greater body of information on a variety of species and to stimulate comparative biology in order to improve our ability to predict human response from animals (NAS, 1985a).

There is some controversy over the use of inbred strains of these species rather than genetically heterogeneous animals. Inbred rodent species are often regarded as the biologist's equivalent to pure chemicals for the chemist. That is, inbred strains provide the uniform experimental material that results in more precise and stable results. Further, by focusing on a few particular strains, much greater understanding can be developed about pharmacokinetics and metabolism of various kinds of chemicals, increasing the ability to design better experiments and to better interpret results. A drawback is that, by relying on a body of information developed on a particular strain and on the relative precision of the results, the genetic integrity of that strain becomes vitally important. Impurities accidentally and unknowingly introduced into the strain or genetic shifts over time could cause devastating results. This requires constant checking and verification, adding to the expense of maintaining pure strains of animals. More heterogeneous animal populations are hardier, less expensive to breed and maintain, and less prone to high spontaneous cancer rates. In addition, a heterogeneous animal population is said to more closely reflect the human population, which is of course genetically heterogeneous. Although the heterogeneity of the human population is something to be considered in extrapolating results of animal studies, this is an insufficient argument for using an animal population of unknown heterogeneity in a bioassay. A switch to a heterogeneous research animal population would introduce greater variability in the results, possibly necessitating more animals per dose level. Use of a controlled group of multiple strains would be prohibitively expensive. The selection of a test animal is always something of a compromise, and these are factors which must be considered in such a compromise.

An issue meriting discussion here is the use of animal strains with high spontaneous tumor rate, illustrated particularly by the B6C3F1 hybrid mouse, the standard mouse used in the NTP bioassay (Reynolds et al., 1987). The male of this strain has a high spontaneous liver tumor rate and frequently shows increases in liver tumors upon exposure to chemicals which yield no other increase in tumors and no increase in liver tumors in female mice or in rats. This follows the objective of increasing the sensitivity of the test; a test system which demonstrates tumors at lower doses or with fewer animals has greater sensitivity. The question of whether this is sensitivity to the desired outcome or not is addressed below in the discussion of interpretation of animal studies. In terms of species and strain selection, there are two points to be made from this example. First, selection of a test species is not made lightly, and the longer a test species is used, the more of a body of knowledge is built upon that particular species and strain. For this reason, there has been a reluctance to change to another strain which may not seem to have such a problem, but of which less is known. Beyond this is the need to decide how to settle such problems of interpretation. The problem is not "solved" simply by making it go away by switching to a different strain which does not exhibit the problem. The situation is further complicated by differences of opinion over whether the particular liver lesions should, in fact, be interpreted as cancers. Moreover, decisions of this kind are made in a political fishbowl. Switching to a different strain might well result in some chemicals which would be labeled carcinogens in the present bioassay being labeled noncarcinogens. Changes with such ramifications must have strong scientific justification. The second point is that the male B6C3F1 mouse not only exhibits this propensity for liver tumors, but also seems to exhibit a wide variation in spontaneous liver lesions among laboratories. This may argue for a lack of genetic integrity among the population of B6C3F1 mice. Along similar lines, there seems to be a recurring phenomenon in chemical-induced tumors in Fischer 344 rats, in which increased incidence of liver tumors is associated with decreased incidence of leukemia or lymphoma in exposed animals (Haseman 1985).

This association does not occur in control animals. It has been hypothesized that chemicals initiate a tumor in the liver which, in turn, influences the leukemia response, but neither the reason nor the biological significance is actually known.

Dose

In animal toxicology, "dose" usually means the amount of the test chemical administered to the animal rather than the amount reaching the target tissue, although the latter meaning is sometimes used also. The first consideration for dose is to assure that the right chemical is being administered. That may sound obvious, but with testing often being carried out on esoteric industrial chemicals, care must be taken. NTP (1984) gives an illustration of bioassays of nitrosodiphenylamine in two different laboratories. The report from one laboratory described the chemical as dark brown, whereas the other laboratory reported it to be colorless. This raises the question of whether the same substance was tested in both laboratories. The obvious parallel question for risk assessment is whether the substance being tested in the bioassay is the same as the one to which the population at risk is exposed. This is particularly important in cases where the dose–response information is being taken from the literature. Impurities in a chemical may themselves be carcinogens, resulting in false positive results. This is even more important in extrapolating results of an earlier study reported in the literature to a human exposure which may be a different variant of the chemical. The impurities may also be part of the human exposure, but for estimating risk and for devising control strategies, it is important to know whether the chemical itself or impurities associated with it are the harmful agent.

Of obvious importance in experimental design is the route of administration. Different routes result in differences in absorption, distribution, and metabolism of the chemical. The route should be relevant to existing or anticipated human exposure when possible, but consideration must also be given to the relevance of the route to the test species and other experimental conditions. A rodent spreads its feeding over a much longer period than a human, for example, and thus an equivalent dose on a daily basis may produce a different absorption, blood level, and elimination profile in the two species. For some substances oral gavage in the rodent may more closely mimic the human exposure situation.

Inhalation is usually an important route for environmental and occupational pollutants, yet inhalation exposures are the most complex and expensive in toxicology. This is particularly true for exposures that include a particulate phase. Particles deposit on the hair of rodents and then are ingested during grooming, complicating the dose. Reactive gases and aerosols will plateout on the walls of the chamber or react with ammonia and other gases associated with wastes making the actual exposure different than what would otherwise have been calculated. It is thus important to measure the key constituents of the air the rodents are actually breathing in a test chamber and not to rely on a measured amount being piped in. Complications associated with complex mixtures are dealt with separately below, but it should be mentioned here that some air pollutant mixtures are difficult to duplicate. Sometimes great efforts must be undertaken to produce the desired exposure. Auto exhausts, for example, have been duplicated by running actual auto engines, diluting and cooling the exhaust and then directing it into a test chamber. The actual exposures must then be measured in the chambers. Even this, however, does not reproduce the photochemical smog produced by aged exhaust exposed to sunlight and mixed with pollutants from other sources.

Sometimes actual environmental samples are taken on filters or on charcoal or other absorbent. These are then extracted with a solvent in the laboratory for administration to the animal. Such environmental samples are often used for skin painting. Some of the solvents may themselves be carcinogenic or may affect the experiment by drying the skin. Vegetable oils are frequently used as a vehicle to administer chemicals that are not water soluble in feeding or gavage studies. They are also used for chemicals which are volatile, irritating, or which have a taste or odor objectionable to the rodent. These vegetable oils may affect the dietary balance of the animal, increasing intake of dietary fat and thus affecting the tumor rate. To account for this in the analysis, a separate control group given only the vehicle is often used (see below).

Finally, the most obvious consideration of dose in experimental design is the number and selection of dose levels to be administered. Most standard study designs call for the highest dose to be the maximum tolerated dose (MTD) predicted from preliminary, subchronic data. This is varyingly defined as "the highest dose that can be given that would not alter the animals' normal lifespan from effects other than cancer" (OTA, 1981) or the dose that will produce no more than a 10-12% depression in body weight if administered over a lifetime (but estimated in a 90-day study). More recent suggested refinements call for selection of the MTD on the basis of other signs of toxicity including gross and microscopic pathology, alterations in enzyme levels or other biochemical or pharmacological indices of abnormality. For a qualitative measure of carcinogenicity, the optimal design is to divide the available animals into two groups, one receiving the MTD and the other an unexposed control. This maximizes the chances of detecting a difference in tumor rates. The standard NCI protocol (Table 8-3) calls for an intermediate dose of one-half the

MTD. This provides additional information, but its primary purpose is to provide a substitute dosed group so the experiment would not be lost in case the MTD was wrongly estimated and acute toxic effects appear in the high dose group. The common method of determining lower dose rates remains simple fractions of the MTD (e.g., 1/2, 1/4, 1/10). Pharmacokinetic and metabolic information on possible dose-dependent and time-dependent processes affecting disposition of the test substance and its metabolites throughout the body should also be used to determine dose selection (including the MTD). Kociba (1987) discusses issues in MTD selection, although focussing on qualitative results. To aid in later quantitative extrapolation, preliminary modeling can be used to help select dose levels which will maximize the usefulness of the results in developing quantitative dose–response functions (see Chap. 9).

Number and Selection of Test Animals and Control Groups

Standard bioassay designs generally call for 50 animals in each experimental group with four groups (male and female rats and male and female mice) at each dose level. Thus, a bioassay with two dose levels and one zero-dose control would involve a total of 600 animals. Adding an additional dose level adds 200 additional animals. Although an equal number of animals in each dose group is the standard approach, there are several recommendations for using different numbers of animals at different dose levels. As lower doses are included in the design, more animals are required to maintain reasonable uncertainty bands on the tumor estimates, although Gaylor et al. (1985) argue this gains no advantage.

Several kinds of control groups are used. The purpose of the control group is to provide the baseline comparison against which tumor development in the other groups can be measured, or, in the case of quantitative dose–response function development, to provide a zero dose point on the dose–response curve. The standard control group is composed of animals which are not dosed, but which otherwise receive concurrent treatment identical to the experimental groups. Sometimes vehicle controls are used, as mentioned above. These are treated only with the vehicle that the dose is delivered in, and as the plain control group, are treated otherwise identical to the experimental groups. Sometimes a shelf control is used, particularly when animals are housed or handled in an unusual manner. This is a concurrent, undosed control group which is housed in a conventional manner and does not undergo all the other handling and treatment that the experimental animals undergo. Another kind of control is the positive control. The positive control is a group which is administered a known carcinogen, but otherwise treated as the experimental groups. The expected tumor rate in this group is known, and any significant deviation from that rate will indicate abnormal conditions in the experiment. If genetic drift in the animal population or experimental difficulty is suspected, or if a new aspect is being added to the experimental protocol, positive controls may be useful. The use of positive controls is controversial. Some investigators believe they have great value, others believe they have no value and can even be misleading. It is difficult to see how they cannot add additional information and verification to the experiment, so long as the standard control group is also used.

Vehicle, shelf, and positive controls are additions to the standard controls; they do not substitute for them. All must also be contemporaneous with the experimental group. That is, their selection, treatment, and sacrifice must coincide in time with the experimental groups. They are designed to provide a base of comparison which reflects all aspects of the experimental animals' life except for the administered dose. This must include the laboratory conditions *at the time of the experiment*. A testing laboratory which does repeated standard bioassays develops an extensive record of the spontaneous tumor rate in the control groups. While recognizing that these data are subject to additional sources of variation which does not exist in the contemporaneous controls and which must be taken into account in the analysis, these historical controls can add substantial increases in precision in certain circumstances, provide helpful information on the assessment of rare tumors, and help in the evaluation of a marginally significant result relative to concurrent controls (Krewski et al., 1985). In using historical control data, it is important to keep in mind that the thoroughness of pathological diagnosis may have evolved and nomenclature changed over time. NTP has identified substantial variability over time and among different laboratories in historical controls (Haseman, 1984). Continuing review of historical controls is useful in uncovering such variations. Sometimes such sources of variability may be corrected. It is important that analysis relying on historical controls be clearly indicated in any reports so as not to mislead the reader.

Duration

Cancer latent periods, the delay between exposure and manifestation of a clinically diagnosed cancer, range in humans from 10 to 40 years or more, a significant portion of the human lifespan. Fortunately for the sake of animal experimentation, latent period appears to be associated with lifespan than the absolute number of years. That is, a cancer which might take decades to appear in a human appears in a rat within 20 months. The lifespan of a mouse is about 30 months and for a rat 36 months. To assure that these latent cancers are captured, the general policy is that the experiment should last for the majority of the normal life of the animal. Unless the number of survivors in the low dose or control groups drops to 20-25% earlier, studies are usually terminated at the end of 120 weeks for mice and 130 for rats. It has been shown that if the period of observation were reduced to 12 months, a significant number of otherwise positive assays would have appeared negative. In terminating the study before all animals have died one must be sure that negative results will be valid. Existing data suggest, however, that most of the common neoplasms in a commonly used laboratory animal, the Fischer 344 rat, could be found upon pathological examination before 100 weeks of age. This may well vary by chemical, however. On the other hand, it is not advisable to continue the study until all animals live out their lifespans. Like people, spontaneous tumors increase with age and high background rates in the last weeks of life may increase the variability in the results and could increase false positives. There are also practical reasons. Animals dying natural deaths may be lost to cannibalism or decay. There are thus no rigid rules for determining the end of the experiment. A fully informed decision would require knowledge of incidence and growth rate of both spontaneous and exposure-induced tumors at each organ site. This information is, at best, not available until after the experiment is over. The typical bioassay itself may be insufficient to provide this information. The decision falls back on the general knowledge and judgment of the toxicologist, subject to some validation after the data are analyzed.

Because of the latent period, dosing of the animals could well be stopped weeks before the experiment was terminated. Since it is not known how early this can be done, however, and since continued dosing may have some influence on the continued progression of tumors, dosing is usually continued until the end unless the presence of residual chemical in the animal may pose a hazard to those processing the rodent tissues.

Husbandry

Valid and consistent experimental results are dependent upon good facilities, personnel, and management. The key animal environmental factors important to a long-term study are: filters, bedding, temperature, humidity, air quality, light, noise, sanitizing agents, vaccines, feed, water, and caging (NTP, 1984).

Data Collection

Standard practice is that animals be checked carefully at least twice each day. Body weight and food intake should be determined for each animal weekly for the first 13 weeks and monthly after that. Any clinical signs should of course be recorded, particularly any visible tumor development. The principal data source, however, is the detailed pathological examination.

Tumor incidence is ordinarily calculated as the number of tumor-bearing animals having tumors at a specific organ site divided by the total number of animals that survived long enough to have been at risk for that specific type of tumor (OSTP, 1984). Separate reporting and interpretation of benign and malignant tumors and life-shortening and nonlife shortening tumors are discussed below as well as the usefulness of the overall net tumor rate for risk assessment.

While microscopic examination of all tissues is desirable, practical limitations force a selective approach. It should go without saying that the experimental groups and control groups must be treated exactly alike.

INTERPRETATION OF ANIMAL STUDIES

Interpreting the results of a long-term animal bioassay is not a straightforward task in which the data can simply be dumped into a statistical package. There are a number of subjective issues involved in deciding what the data collected mean. In some of these areas, rules or guidelines have been developed either on a scientific or policy basis. In other cases, much is left to the judgment of the investigator. The "rules" of science require any such judgments to be explicitly reported as part of the report of the investigation, but frequently the risk assessor, in searching the literature for animal data appropriate to the problem, finds reports lacking in this regard. In some cases, even key experimental features are omitted. This is not the case with NTP reports which are complete and highly detailed. The results of animal studies are an important source of dose–response information for risk assessment and lack of sufficient information to interpret the results can exclude potentially important data from the assessment. It is the policy based on the assessment and eventually someone's health that suffers the loss.

The original investigator has the right and obligation to interpret the results. The risk assessor must review and often reinterpret the results, however, for several reasons. The purpose of the risk assessment is often different than the purpose of the original investigator and the data must be reinterpreted (and sometimes reanalyzed) in light of a new objective. For example, the original study may have been done to investigate mechanisms while the assessment requires a quantitative dose–response function. New information from other studies may have become available since the report of the original investigation, and the results must be reinterpreted in light of these additional data. Finally, the original investigator may have focused on a particular interpretation, while the risk assessor must examine the degree to which the data support or refute several alternative approaches or hypotheses. The risk assessor may not be personally qualified to make some of the necessary judgments and will rely on experts in the field. It is important, however, that the risk analyst understand the kinds of uncertainties requiring judgments and the kinds of questions that must be asked. The following paragraphs discuss some of the factors involved in interpretation of different aspects of animal studies.

Subjective Diagnosis of Tumors

The diagnosis of tumors is subjective and, although there may be guidelines established, pathologists may disagree on diagnoses. This is particularly true in cases that are not clear-cut. Frequently, the difficulty is in classifying the lesion as benign or malignant. OSTP (1984), for example, indicates that distinguishing between an adenoma and an adenocarcinoma in a number of organs is so difficult that the two should be lumped into one category for statistical purposes. Galli (1984) points out that, while lesions are often "classified on the basis of cytologic or histologic features generally associated with malignancy, such as hypercellularity, hyperchromatism, increased mitotic activity, and apparent local invasion . . . , the predictive value of these criteria can vary markedly depending on tumor type, organ, and species." In a reply, Konstantinidis et al. (1984) support the subjectiveness of the criteria saying, "the 'state of the art' in this context is that honest disagreements are not infrequent in judging whether histologic features represent actual or potential threats . . . ." Compounding this subjectivity, most pathologists do not review microslides "blind" (OSTP, 1984). That is, they know when reading them which slides are from treated animals and which from controls. Doing analysis "blind" is an important scientific principal to eliminate subjective bias and can be especially important in histologic examination which is rather subjective. Claimed disadvantages of blind pathology include (Haseman, 1984):

1. Control animals must be examined first to determine the natural incidence and severity of neoplastic and nonneoplastic lesions;
2. Blind pathology requires increased time;
3. Blind pathology leads to increases in coding errors;
4. An experienced pathologist can generally distinguish which tissues are from the control animals and which from the dosed animals anyway.

Speaking more from the statistical than the pathological point of view, none of these arguments seem compelling. The last, however, raises a consideration that, were the evaluations done apparently blind, if the pathologist could tell which were the controls, they would not actually be blind. It would seem preferable to do the work blind and keep this caveat in mind, rather than give up entirely to subjectivity. NTP uses a compromise solution: the original pathology is done nonblind. If a dose effect is seen, those tissues are reviewed blindly to determine if the results can be verified under a more rigorous protocol (Haseman, 1984). Since the most likely effect of nonblind evaluation would be an increase in false positives, this seems to be a reasonable procedure.

In addition to interpretation in reading slides, selection of tissues for examination and the methods used for their preparation introduce subjectivity. Finally, in dealing with studies from the literature, it is important to recognize that both the "rules" and practices for selecting and preparing tissue and reading slides change over time as new information and techniques develop. This possibility must be investigated when explaining differences (or similarities) among studies from different times or different countries.

Malignant versus Benign Tumors: Which to Count

There are many different types of tumors and many sites at which they occur. How should they be counted and reported? This has been the subject of considerable debate. Those favoring a risk-adverse cancer policy generally support including benign tumors since it leads to more chemicals being named as possible carcinogens (Rushefsky, 1986). Most published guidelines deal with this qualitative question rather than quantifying dose–response curves. Many of the same scientific arguments apply to both. NTP (1984) lists reasons for and against combining benign and malignant tumors (Table 8-5).

Based on an evaluation of these arguments, NTP (1984) developed extensive guidelines by organ system of which tumor types at which organ sites should be combined and which should not. Because it complicates statistical analysis (see below), OSTP (1984) also argues that "life shortening tumors should not be combined with nonlife shortening tumors." EPA, noting that chemicals which cause benign tumors frequently also induce malignant tumors, stated as a policy that benign and malignant tumors will be combined unless the specific benign tumors are not considered to have the potential to progress (EPA, 1986).

TABLE 8-5   Reasons for Combining Benign and Malignant Tumors

Advantages:
1. The terms benign and malignant are convenient for classification and, at times, clinical prognosis, yet their use may be an artificial division/separation of neoplastic development and progression.
2. For some neoplasms there is substantial evidence for progression from benign to malignant. In such cases evaluating benign and malignant tumors in isolation of each other may mask a true effect.
3. The morphologic criteria for differentiating benign and malignant tumors is often subjective and sometimes arbitrary. In fact, for certain lesions it is difficult to differentiate hyperplasia from neoplasia.
4. The categorization of a neoplasm as benign or malignant may bear little relevance to its adverse biologic potential. Some benign tumors are as life-threatening as their malignant counterparts.
5. In carcinogenesis studies time and resources do not allow for stepsectioning (multiple sections) of a given lesion diagnosed as benign to determine if malignant areas are present. Also the use of interim sacrifices to determine the progression from nonneoplastic lesions through the neoplastic stage is not always feasible.

Disadvantages:
1. Differentiating benign and malignant neoplasms provides at least circumstantial evidence for the aggressiveness of a particular type of tumor, thereby providing a better data base for interpretation of carcinogenicity and hazard assessment.
2. In some tissues the difference between benign and malignant neoplasms is clear. In organs where differentiation is less clear and possibly arbitrary it is still useful to differentiate between low and highly aggressive neoplasms. Malignant tumors may also appear to arise de novo.
3. The knowledge that for a given compound the treated animals had a higher incidence of malignant (or benign) neoplasms than the controls is valuable even though the total incidence of neoplasms (benign and malignant) may be comparable. Malignancy implies more extensive damage to the host and by definition irreversibility.
4. Some benign neoplasms have the ability to regress to nonneoplastic lesions.
5. Neoplasia is a complex disease involving many mechanisms. To diagnose a lesion merely as neoplastic or nonneoplastic would ignore this complexity and would not communicate to other scientists the type of information needed for decisionmaking.

Source: From NTP, 1984.

Tumor Induction or Promotion?

There is considerable debate over whether agents that initiate tumors by inducing mutations in DNA should be classed separately from agents which promote the growth of tumors that have already been initiated. One difficulty is in identifying which is which. If, in order to increase the sensitivity of the bioassay, animals are used which have a high background tumor rate (and thus a presumed greater sensitivity to tumor induction), than an increase in observed tumors may be additional tumors induced by the exposure or simply an increase in spontaneous tumors which have been "promoted" to appear earlier. Implications for human cancer risk are particularly important if the promotion is an effect of the high dose used in the bioassay and does not happen at the lower doses to which human populations are exposed. The mutagenic capacity of an agent may be measured in short-term in vitro tests (Chap. 10), but these usually depend on specific genetic effects and an agent might act to initiate a tumor in a different way from that measured in the in vitro test.

An example introduced earlier is the B6C3F1 hybrid mouse, the standard mouse used in the NTP bioassay. This mouse has a high spontaneous liver tumor rate. The question has been raised of whether such an increase in liver tumors has any implication for human carcinogenicity. As of June, 1984, 50% of all agents found to be carcinogenic on NTP and NCI bioassays gave positive responses in the mouse liver (Maronpot, in press). More than 28 compounds have been identified for which the mouse liver was the only site with increased incidence of tumors. Epidemiological evidence strongly suggests that at least one of these agents (phenobarbital), is not a human carcinogen Clayson (1987).

A new capability of examining the mechanism of tumor formation at the molecular level by investigating the pattern of oncogene activation directly in the mouse liver holds promise as a method of resolving the question of the B6C3F1 mouse liver tumors (Reynolds et al., 1987). The first reported results suggest that, in the case of two agents, the increased incidence of mouse liver tumors was caused at least in part by induction of weakly activating point mutations.

Net Tumor Rate

OSTP (1984) indicates that "most experts agree that the incidence of total tumors at all organ sites is not a very useful expression of cancer incidence, nor in the calculation of the incidence of total benign or total malignant tumors. Most useful appears to be the number of histologically unique tumors at specific organ sites." Clearly, to provide the fullest understanding of the carcinogenic effect of the agent, identification and reporting by specific organ site and histological type is important. It is also recognized that the amount of "digging" for information in the available tissue involves some degree of economic trade-off. All reasonable detail should be reported to assist in the interpretation of the experiment. It should also be recognized that, although sophisticated computer models may be used in extrapolating human risks from animal bioassay data (see Chap. 9), the data actually drawn from the bioassays is extremely simple, often basically the number of animals and number of animals with particular tumors in each group. Most of the detailed information supports the qualitative decision. Contrary to "most experts," the net increase in tumors, perhaps weighted by their degree of threat to life (although this is not done), would seem to be more useful for quantitative risk estimates. Often, risk extrapolations are based on data from only one organ site. Yet, it is well known that a carcinogen may affect different organs in different species. Does it make sense then to extrapolate the quantitative cancer rate in, say, a rat liver to predict a quantitative estimate of increase in liver cancer in humans when the agent may express its carcinogenic effect in a totally different organ in people? If quantitative extrapolation at the individual organ level were accepted, why extrapolate only from the organ with the greatest increase in tumors? Why not extrapolate the risk for all organs and produce a combined net cancer rate? A related problem that arises from the latter question is the problem of what have been termed "ambiguous carcinogens" by Weinberg and Storer (1985). These are carcinogens which increase the incidence of tumors at some sites, but at the same time *decrease* the tumor incidence at other sites. The suggestion that the net effect on the total incidence of all tumors be used in determining carcinogenicity produced considerable controversy (Cumming, 1985; Haseman, 1985; Albert, 1985; Storer and Weinberg, 1985). The question of quantitative extrapolation gets lost in the more immediately political issue of defining a substance as a carcinogen. Weinberg and Storer argue that for the purpose of the Delaney Amendment and other regulatory rulings, a substance should not be considered a carcinogen unless it produces a net increase in the total incidence of all cancers. Opponents argue that the definition of a carcinogen is well established as an agent which increases the incidence of cancers at any site. This argument is primarily one of policy and those who take a risk-adverse approach will argue for the decision of carcinogenesis to be made based on a tumor increase at any site while those who take a more liberal approach to risk will argue for the more stringent criteria of a net increase (Rushefsky, 1986).

The rules for quantitative assessment are not as institutionalized as *those for qualitative* assessment, and those with opposing views are not forced into such rigid positions. Other factors also come into play; background rates are an example. A large relative risk for a site which has a low background rate in humans may produce a lower quantitative estimate of risk than a lower relative risk for a site with a larger background rate. For example, a 10% increase in lung cancer would have a much greater effect than a 50% increase in liver cancer. Using tumor incidence at only one site, albeit the site of greatest increase in risk in the test species, could overestimate the net risk if other tumors decreased and underestimate the net risk if other tumors increased.

Statistical Considerations

Many statistical issues arise in the evaluation of results of long-term animal bioassays. Traditionally, qualitative determination of carcinogenesis in bioassays has been made on the basis of comparing an exposed group with a control group. Recently, the trend has been to have two or more exposed groups, dosed at different levels and a control group. Under these circumstances a test for an existence of a dose–response relationship, a trend defined as "progressiveness of response with increasing dose," may be the most important statistical test even for qualitative decisions on carcinogenicity (Ciminera, 1985). A dose–response relationship is a stronger indicator of an effect than one group having a higher rate than another.

　　Haseman (1984) notes that the sensitivity of trend tests discouraged their use by some investigators because of a fear of false positives, but that their use will increase as:

1.　Standard designs begin including more dose groups
2.　The likelihood of false positives becomes more understood
3.　More is learned about patterns of chemically induced dose–response trends

　　Despite the use of a dose–response relationship as a criteria of causation, the standard analysis of NTP studies aims at the qualitative question of carcinogenesis. Results are classified into one of five categories based on the strength of experimental evidence without regard to potency or mechanism (these were described in Chap. 3).

　　If it has not already come up in the design stage, it is at the point of statistical analysis that the decision must be made of what exactly is it that we measure to determine if a chemical is a carcinogen. The basic comparison, particularly in the past, was the proportion of tumor-bearing animals in the dosed group versus the proportion in the control group. That sounds simple enough; if the dosed group has a higher proportion of animals with tumors, and the difference is statistically significant, then the chemical is a carcinogen. Unfortunately the world is not so simple. Suppose several animals in the dosed group died during the course of the experiment from causes unrelated to carcinogenesis. There may then be a lower proportion of tumors in the dosed group since some of the animals that may have gotten tumors have died. Should we ignore non-tumor-bearing animals that die early and count only the proportion of tumors in the remaining animals? This approach has been used, but it is more rigorous, and less wasteful of the animals, to include the total experience of the experiment in the analysis, correcting for what is called intercurrent mortality. The tumor incidence rate then becomes the important parameter, rather than the final proportion. Carcinogenesis is presumably a process that exists from initiation to the final manifestation of the tumor, the point at which it can be clinically detected and identified. In animals, this usually means identified at autopsy. To determine the rate, the experiment becomes more complicated. Instead of killing all the animals at the end of the study, smaller groups are killed and autopsied at different intervals throughout the study and the proportion of animals with tumors determined within each of these groups. There are still some troublesome animals that die on their own at the wrong time. If they have tumors, it may have been that the tumor caused their death and the incidence of the tumor was near the time of death. But the tumor may have been incidental, death being due to a completely independent cause. In that case the "incidence" of a tumor would otherwise have been counted at the animals scheduled death rather than at this early, unscheduled time. The chance event of the animal dying early could thus distort the experimental results. Although the question of whether a tumor is lethal is of secondary interest to whether the chemical increases the production of tumors (McKnight and Crowley, 1984), it is an important distinction for the purposes of the analysis (Haseman, 1984). Several methods have been explored to deal with this problem statistically, including logistic regression which has the advantage that additional factors such as cage location and litter effects can be examined. There is also discussion among pathologists as to the reliability of classifications of "fatal" or "incidental" (Haseman, 1984). The main problem is not with the statistics or the pathology, however, but with the nature of the experiment. If the tumor is "occult," i.e., cannot be identified without cutting open the animal, one never knows when the tumor would be clinically identifiable, only that it was at some time before the animal was cut open to look. Largely because the degree to which the tumor contributes to the death cannot always be determined with confidence, the standard analyses used in the NTP include three statistical methods: (1) a life-table method which assumes tumors in animals dying before the end of the study were "fatal"; (2) an analysis which estimates incidence rate but assumes all such tumors were "incidental" rather than "fatal"; and (3) an unadjusted analysis which does not adjust for survival differences. When the three give similar answers, there is no problem. When they differ, interpretation depends on the extent to which the tumor under consideration is regarded as the cause of death (NTP, various).

Animals are given large doses to assure that a carcinogenic effect will be seen in the relatively small number that it is feasible to use in toxicology studies. But what is the chance of a false negative? If 100 animals are given the chemical in a dosage of 1% of their diet and none develop a tumor, then, using the binomial upper limit, there is only a 2.5% chance the true underlying incidence is greater than 3.6%, the actual result of zero being due to random variability. If we are concerned with the risk to people at, say, 1000 times less or 10 parts per million in their diet, and if everything scaled linearly (which may well not be the case), then the same upper bound would be 3.6×10^{-5}. As pointed out by Maugh (1978) this is a small risk, but if 200 million people were exposed, this upper bound would be nearly 10,000 tumors. This is one reason for concern about the implications of using animal studies. The implications of this more properly belong under a discussion of risk management.

Time to Tumor

Some design and analysis considerations of time to tumor were discussed above. It is difficult to collect appropriate data to evaluate time to tumor. In addition, there are likely mechanistic differences between agents which produce additional tumors and agents which decrease the latent period of tumors which would otherwise have appeared naturally, only later. Many strong carcinogens have both effects, but chemicals which only produce the latter effect require careful interpretation. Decreased latency period can result from nonspecific effects such as high doses leading to excessive cell proliferation, changed food intake, and other experimental artifacts (Interdisciplinary Panel, 1984).

Dose-Rate Effects and Age at Exposure

Animal studies with ionizing radiation and with chemical carcinogens have shown that protraction of dose over time leads to lower tumor rates than the same dose given over a shorter time period (NRC, 1975; NAS, 1986). This indicates some nonlinear mechanisms, perhaps repair of the genetic damage. For at least some materials, dose-rate may be more important than total dose, although most risk assessment models rely solely on the total cumulative dose.

Because the background cancer incidence increases rapidly with age, it seems likely that environmental induction of cancer has something to do with age. The important parameter may be age at exposure or age at the expression of the cancer, although the former is usually the focus of attention when age effects are considered. There seems to be growing evidence of such an age effect in human populations, although discussion of this will be deferred to Chap. 11. Animal data appear mixed (BEIR, 1980). It may be that the latent period begins to extend beyond the animals' lifespan for exposures begun in later life. This may be one instance where the longer human lifespan may make a difference. There are clearly additional unexplained factors involved, however. There may be especially sensitive periods in life. The fetus and the young are especially sensitive to certain radiation-induced cancers.

Multiple Comparisons and False Positives

Separate statistical analyses are carried out routinely for approximately 30 different tumor types or combinations for two sexes and two species in each bioassay (NTP, 1984). That is a total of 120 separate pairwise comparisons. All other things being equal, one would expect to obtain by pure chance, a finding of a difference which is statistically significant at the 5% level in one out of every 20 analyses made. Under such circumstances one might expect a totally benign agent to yield statistically significant results in 6 of these 120 comparisons—more than sufficient to brand it as a carcinogen. Moreover, since each paired comparison is subjected to three separate statistical analyses and three p values calculated, plus p values for a dose–response trend, the possibility of a chance result could be even higher. It has been calculated that if the decision was made solely on the basis of a p value less than 0.05 in any single paired comparison, the false positive rate would be as high as 20-50%. Haseman (1984) discusses this problem. False positives are largely a concern with common tumors, since it would be difficult to have sufficient numbers of rare tumors to achieve statistical significance. The answer to the simple statistical calculation above is that the decision on carcinogenesis is not made mechanically from the statistical results. The p values are mathematical results, but must be interpreted using biological judgment. There are statistical methods available to calculate appropriate "critical values" for multiple comparisons, against which to compare p values. These require smaller and smaller values of p to achieve statistical significance as the number of comparisons increase (e.g., see Snedecor and Cochran, 1967). The general practice, however, has been to rely more on subjective judgment of the toxicologist.

One way to evaluate "biological judgment" in this area is to define a statistical rule which produces the same results as are achieved in practice. One examination of 25 NTP feeding studies developed the following rule which mimicked the actual judgments made:

> Regard as carcinogenic any chemical that produces a high-dose increase in a common tumor that is statistically significant at the 0.01 level or a high-dose increase in an uncommon tumor that is statistically significant at the 0.05 level (Haseman, 1983).

The false-positive rate associated with this rule is 7 to 8%. Thus, in actual practice, the rate of such false positive results is substantially less then expected from "naive calculations" (NTP, 1984). Greater reliance on dose–response trends, multiple logistic regression, and other methods which look more at the data as a whole rather than as multiple separate comparisons and which lead more directly to quantitative dose–response may eventually simplify this problem. Moreover, as noted above, using the net tumor rate for quantitative extrapolation will also help to reduce the multiple comparison problem.

Statistical Analysis not Enough

The quantitative analyst may tend to rely on the results of statistical analysis in the interpretation of animal studies even more than others. It

TABLE 8-6 Factors Considered in Biological Meaningfulness

---

1. Was the effect dose-related?
2. Was the effect supported by related nonneoplastic changes?
3. Was similar evidence seen in other sex-species groups?
4. Did the effect occur in a "target organ," one which pharmacokinetics would suggest is dosed?
5. Were there other forms of toxicity present in the target organs?
6. Could the effect have been influenced by the relative survival rate of dosed and control animals?
7. How does the effect compare with the historical rate of the particular tumor?
8. Were tumors observed in the dosed group of a type that are rarely seen in controls?
9. Was there a decrease in latency period time to tumor as well as an increase in proportion of animals with tumors?
10. Were there time- and dose-related changes in the incidence of preneoplastic lesions?

Sources: Haseman, 1984; Interdisciplinary Panel, 1984; EPA, 1986.

should be clear by now, however, that statistical analysis is not enough. Decisions on carcinogenesis, and even decisions on the means of extrapolating the carcinogenic risk to lower doses and to other species, must consider the biology of the situation as well as the statistics themselves.

Even the most sophisticated statistical analysis cannot replace the biology. The qualitative judgments of the toxicologist and pathologist add information that cannot be reduced to statistics. Table 8-6 lists example factors considered in determining biological meaningfulness. On the other hand, such judgment must not blindly overrule the statistical analysis. The latter must be consistent with the biology. If the results are inconsistent or counterintuitive, then the biology must be re-examined for a rationale which might justify the results. The statistical results must then be interpreted with regard to the current understanding of the validity of the underlying biological rationale. If no underlying biological rationale can be found, then the results must be regarded with suspicion and interpreted with great caution.

Synergisms, Antagonisms, and Complex Mixtures

Complex mixtures are a recurrent theme in this volume because they plague every aspect of risk assessment of chemical carcinogens. The use of indices to measure complex mixtures and their constantly changing characteristics were discussed in Chap. 4. Their implications for dose–response are introduced here with animal toxicology but the discussion continues on in the following chapters.

The combined effect of a combination of pollutants may be markedly different than the sum of the effects of its components individually. For toxicologic effects, these interactions appear to take two forms. The presence (or past presence) of one or more chemicals either (1) changes the availability of other chemicals for target-site interaction or (2) alters the reactivity of the target macromolecule for these other chemicals (NAS, 1980). These effects have been described more specifically as including (1) chemical and physical interactions in the mixture; (2) effects on the timing, route and conditions of exposure; (3) physiological factors influencing absorption; (4) mutual influences of absorbed materials and metabolites on metabolism, pharmacokinetics, and target organ dose; (5) relative affinities at the target site for toxicity; and (6) various relationships among the pollutants in their toxicologic action including independent actions, additive effects, antagonism, potentiation, and synergism (Ballantyne, 1985).

Synergism is an often misused and misunderstood term. Most people think that if the effect of exposure to two agents is the sum of what the effect of the individual exposures would have been separately, the effect is "additive"; if the combined effect is greater than that, particularly if it is more like the product of the two separate effects, it is synergistic. Consider, however, an agent which has a nonlinear effect. Exposure to one unit produces an effect of level A. Exposure to two units produces an effect greater than $2 \times A$ because of the nonlinear dose–response curve. Is the agent synergistic with itself? Of course not, and two different agents with the same mechanism of effect may act in the same way and produce what may at first appear to be a synergistic effect.

Seiler (1987a) and Seiler and Scott (1987b) provide a clear framework for the mathematical understanding of interactions of two agents. For simplicity, we assume a dose–response relationship in which the effect is proportional to a power of the dose,

$$r_i = a_i \cdot D_i^m$$

Then we must realize that there is a "natural" background cancer rate in the population, and exposure to even a single agent may interact with the mechanisms which produce that background rate. In evaluating the results of an experiment, any such interactions will will automatically be included in the excess risk assigned to the single agent. The combined risk of two agents in the presence of a background risk r_0 is

$$R = r_0 + r_1 + r_2 + r_{(1)(2)} - \{Q\}$$

where r_1 and r_2 are the separate excess risks for agents 1 and 2, $r_{(1)(2)}$ is the excess risk due to their interaction, and Q, the overlap if the risks are independent, contains higher order terms, and can generally be neglected for low-dose, low-risk situations. The combined risk in terms of dose is

$$R = a_0 + a_1 D_1^m + a_2 D_2^m + a_{(1)(2)} D_1^p D_2^q$$

The four parameters, a_i and a_{ij}, must be determined from the experimental data. If it is assumed that factors such as age, sex, and lifestyle are the same for all parameters and that exposure is the only significant factor, than one can divide through by background risk, r_0, and express the equation as a relative risk model in which the combined risk is proportional to the background risk. The combined risk is then given as

$$R/r_0 = [1 + f_1 + f_2 + f_{(1)(2)}]$$

where f_i and f_{ij} are the fractional excess risks for the two agents and their interaction. Expressing this in terms of dose gives

$$R/a_0 = [1 + b_1 D_1^m + b_2 D_2^m + b_{(1)(2)} D_1^p D_2^q]$$

and only three parameters, b_i and b_{ij} need be determined from the experimental data.

In cases of two or three pollutants, these interactions can be explored experimentally, although the experiments can be quite complex and expensive. With more than three pollutants, there is no possibility of exploring all possible interactions among each of the individual pollutants in the mixture. The mixture is then termed a complex mixture. Animal inhalation studies have been done with complex mixtures, but the generation of the mixture is difficult and the interpretation of the results may also present a problem. For example, an extensive set of toxicological studies was done to assess the effect of exposure to diesel engine exhaust. Actual diesel engines were run to generate the exhaust which was then mixed in a manifold to cool it and to obtain the desired concentrations (Mokler et al., 1984). The difficulties of maintaining a uniform mixture over the time of a long-term animal exposure are obvious. The mixture to which the animals were exposed, however, was only one of an infinite number of potential mixtures which might exist in urban air as the diesel exhaust ages, is exposed to sunlight, and mixes with other pollutants in the air. Each change in the mix potentially changes the balance of synergisms and antagonisms among the constituents. The results are thus a single snapshot in time with no way to extrapolate the effects of any changes.

It is clear that, from a dose–response standpoint, the prospect of being able to predict carcinogenic effects of complex mixtures is not bright. Coupled with a reminder that complex mixtures are the only kind of real world exposures that exist, the situation appears grim. In fact, the problem is a long way from an ideal solution. But, animal toxicology is the most difficult medium in which to address the question of complex mixtures. The situation will improve in the following chapters on short-term tests and epidemiology. We should not expect too much, but we can move ahead.

POTENCY

Examining results of animal bioassays for many chemicals, it becomes clear that all carcinogens are not equal. Some have a much more "potent" effect than others. This is the first step toward quantification. Even reports which term quantitative extrapolation from animals to man as "a leap of faith" concede that, "one can make statements about the magnitude of dose required to produce a particular tumor incidence in a given test system for one chemical as compared to another" (OSTP, 1979). This report goes on to say that "few would argue that a chemical which requires *several grams* to produce cancer in a given test animal must be viewed with as much concern as another chemical requiring only a few micrograms to produce a similar type and frequency of cancer in the same animal."

The principle of potency seems well agreed upon. Now, how to measure it? Since the ultimate goal is generally extrapolation to estimate human cancer risk at low doses, EPA measured potency as the slope of the animal dose–response curve at its low-dose end (Albert, 1984). The method has ranged from simply drawing a straight line from the origin to the lowest significant data point to the fitting of stochastic models such as the one-hit or the multistage models. In the latter case, the slope of the linear (or essentially linear) component at low dose, or the slope of an upper bounding estimate was taken as the potency. Appropriate modification factors could then be applied to convert the animal potency estimate into a "unit risk" (CAG, 1980).

A problem in this approach, which will be addressed in more detail in the next chapter, is that extrapolation to low dose introduces additional uncertainty into the potency estimate. If one is willing, for the moment, to turn from the direct goal of estimating human risk and address the simpler question of the carcinogenic potency of the agent in the test animal itself, this additional uncertainty can be avoided. Why be concerned about potency in the animal itself? Because it can define the relative carcinogenic potency of different chemicals, allowing a new chemical to be evaluated quantitatively against a well-known carcinogen, for example. While such a relative ranking cannot directly lead to an estimate of the absolute cancer risk for a given exposure in humans, it can be useful in making quantitative decisions on a relative basis. Moreover, as will be seen in Chap. 12, potency can be used to modify epidemiologically based risk estimates in related chemicals to estimate absolute risks in humans for chemicals for which there is no human data. Further, potency levels of the same chemical in different test species for the same route of exposure, or in the same species for different routes of exposure or other experimental differences, can help to understand interspecies differences and the implications for cancer risk of factors such as route of exposure.

A National Research Council committee recommended that potency factors, called "Carcinogenic Activity Indicators" (CAI), be calculated for each data point on a dose–response curve by dividing the excess percentage of tumor-bearing animals in the exposed population by the normalized administered dose, expressed as the number of molecules ingested divided by the animal's body weight (OTA, 1981). The committee did not recommend these potency factors be used for extrapolating human risks, however. This approach to estimating potency has not gained any widespread use.

A standardized approach to potency estimation without low-dose extrapolation that has drawn more support was suggested later (Sawyer, et al., 1984; Peto, et al., 1984). This approach was modeled on the LD_{50}, the dose at which half of the animals die, a time-tested parameter which has proved useful for evaluating acute toxins. Called the TD_{50}, this potency measure is the chronic dose rate expressed in mg/kg body weight/ day which halves the actuarially adjusted percentage of tumor-free animals at the end of a standard lifespan experiment. An extensive data base of TD_{50} potency factors has been compiled (Gold et al., 1984; 1986; 1987). This work is a monumental effort, and has already demonstrated its usefulness in several studies based on the data base (e.g., Gaylor and Chen, 1986). Of course, since no two experiments are exactly alike, potency factors may differ among experimental results due to differences among the experiments. Differences in experimental protocol, specific strain within the species and time to tumor differences are not considered in the data base. The question of benign or malignant tumors does not go away either, but potency factors can be calculated for each end-point. Sometimes the definition of benign or malignant may vary in different reports. As put by Jones (1984) in response to a question at a conference, "If the investigator in the original publication of the animal study called the response a tumor, then I called it a tumor. If he called it a cancer, then I called it a cancer." This philosophy carries into the TD_{50} database the experimentalist's analysis of results on an organ and histological type specific base. Nonetheless, the database appears quite robust. In general, a TD_{50} is available for a specific tumor type and site, not the overall probability of an animal developing a tumor.

Because it is associated with an extensive published database which continues to be maintained and updated, the TD_{50} will probably continue to be a standard measure of potency. An interesting and appealing variation has been proposed, however, that converts the TD_{50} into what may be a more suitable metric similar to the chemical measure of pH (Clayson, 1987). Clayson suggests defining potency as:

$$potency = 7 - \log_{10}(TD_{50})$$

although he calls the TD_{50} the ED_{50} and measures it in micromoles/kg body weight/week instead of mg/kg/day. The 7 is an arbitrary constant to keep all the values of potency positive. Use of a logarithmic scale removes small variations from notice, a reasonable attribute since the uncertainty in the estimates probably makes them of no significance anyway. The result is that one can easier focus on the big differences among potencies. Clayson reminds us that "the potency value is no more than a number that integrates and reflects the outcome of a particular bioassay." Thus the log transformation does not destroy any inherent sacred quality of the TD_{50}.

SUMMARY

Animal experiments offer many advantages over attempts to derive cancer dose–response functions directly from human data. Experiments can be much better controlled, higher doses given, lifetime studies carried out more easily and quickly, and invasive techniques used. Although there are differences among species, all mammals, including humans, share many biological features. Use of animal bioassay data is based upon the commonly accepted premise that effects in lower mammals, properly qualified, are applicable to humans (OTA, 1981). Although the degree of this applicability is often argued, the cancer process is similar in humans and lower mammals. Differences in susceptibility do exist, but virtually every form of human cancer has an animal counterpart. On the other hand, it must be remembered that mice and rats are not little people. They have physical and metabolic characteristics and sensitivities different than humans. Further, experimental exposures and conditions are quite different from those under which human populations are exposed. The risk analyst must be fully aware of these differences in when using animal data.

REFERENCES

Albert, R. 1984. A comparative potency approach for estimating the carcinogenic response of various agents In O. White (ed.), *Workshop on Problem Areas Associated with Developing Carcinogen Guidelines* (BNL 51779). Brookhaven National Laboratory, Upton, NY, pp. II-23–29.

Albert, R.E. 1985. The practical importance of anti-tumor bioassay responses in carcinogen risk assessment. *Risk Assessment* 5:165.

Ballantyne, B. 1985. Evaluation of hazards from mixtures of chemicals in the occupational environment. *J. Occup. Med.* 27:85–94.

BEIR. 1980. *The Effects on Populations of Exposure to Low Levels of Ionizing Radiation*. Committee on the Biological Effects of Ionizing Radiation, National Academy of Sciences, Washington D.C.

CAG. 1980. Method for determining the unit risk estimate for air pollutants. Carcinogenic Assessment Group, Environmental Protection Agency, Washington, D.C.

Ciminera, J.L. 1985. Some issues in the design, evaluation, and interpretation of tumorigenicity studies in animals. In *Proceedings of the Symposium on Long-Term Animal Carcinogenicity Studies: A Statistical Perspective*. American Statistical Association, Washington, D.C.

Clayson, D.B. 1987. The need for biological risk assessment in reaching decisions about carcinogens. *Mutat. Res.* 185:243–269.

Cumming, R.B. 1985. "Ambiguous carcinogens"—another look. *Risk Assessment* 5:157–159.

EPA. 1986. Guidelines for carcinogenic risk assessment. U.S. Environmental Protection Agency. *Fed. Reg.* 51:33992–34003.51: 33992–34003.

Galli, S.J. 1984. Uncertainty of histologic classification of experimental tumors (letter). *Science* 226:352–353.

Gaylor, D.W., J.J. Chen, and R.L. Kodell. 1985. Experimental design of bioassays for screening and low dose extrapolation. *Risk Analysis* 5:9–16.

Gold, L.S., C.B. Sawyer, R. McGaw, G.M. Buckman, M. deVecidna, R. Levinson, N.K. Hooper, W.R. Havender, L. Bernstein, R.Peto, M.C. Pike, and B.N. Ames. 1984. A carcinogenic potency database of the standardized results of animal bioassays, *Environ. Health Perspec.* 58:9–319.

Gold, L.S., M. de Veciana, G.M. Backman, R. McGaw, P. Lopipero, M. Smith, M. Blumenthal, R. Levinson, L. Bernstein, and B.N. Ames. 1986. Chronological supplement to the carcinogenic potency database: Standardized results of animal bioassays published through December 1982. *Environ. Health Perspect.* 67:161–200.

Gold, L.S., T.H. Slone, G.M. Backman, R. McGaw, M. DaCosta, P. Lopipero, M. Blumenthal and B.N. Ames. 1987. Second chronological supplement to the carcinogenic database: Standardized results of animal bioassays published through December 1984 and by The National Toxicology Program through 1986. *Environ. Health Perspect.* 74:237–329.

Gori, G.B. 1980. The regulation of carcinogenic hazards. *Science* 208:256–261.

Haseman, J.K. 1983. A re-examination of false-positive rates for carcinogenicity bioassays. *Fund. Appl. Toxicol* 3:334–339 (as cited in Haseman, 1984).

Haseman, J.K. 1984. Statistical issues in the design, analysis and interpretation of animal carcinogenicity studies. *Environ. Health Perspec.* 58:385–392.

Haseman, J.K. 1985. Evaluating the carcinogenic potential of a chemical that appears to both increase and decrease tumor incidence. *Risk Analysis* 5:161-1–64.

Interdisciplinary Panel. 1984. Criteria for evidence of chemical carcinogenicity. *Science* 225:682–687.

Jones, T. 1984. A dose–response model that provides an estimate of potency factors for neoplastic potentiation. In O. White (ed.), *Workshop on Problem Areas Associated with Developing Carcinogen Guidelines* (BNL 51779). Brookhaven National Laboratory, Upton, NY, pp. II-8-22.

Kociba, R.J. 1987. Issues in biochemical applications to risk assessment: How should the MTD be selected for chronic bioassays? *Environ. Health Perspec.* 76:169–174.

Konstantinidis, A., J.B. Smulow and C. Sonnenschein. 1984. (letter). *Science* 226: 353.

Krewski, D., R.T. Smyth, and R.T. Burnett. 1985. The use of historical control information in testing for trend in quantal response carcinogenicity data. In *Proceedings, Symposium on Long-term Animal Carcinogenicity Studies: A Statistical Perspective*. American Statistical Association, Washington, D.C., pp. 56–62.

Loomis, T.A. 1974. *Essentials of Toxicology*, 2d ed. Lea & Febiger, Philadelphia.

McKnight, B. and J. Crowley. 1984. Tests for differences in tumor incidence based on animal carcinogenesis experiments. *J. Am. Statis. Assoc.* 79:639–648.

McKnight, B. and J. Crowley. 1984. Tests for differences in tumor incidence based on animal carcinogenesis experiments. *J. American Statistical Assoc.* 79:639–648.

Maronpot, R.R. In press. as cited by Reynolds et al., 1987.

Maugh, T.H. 1978. Chemical carcinogens: how dangerous are low doses? (research news). *Science* 202:37–41.

Mokler, B.V., F.A. Archibeque, R.L. Beethe, C.P.J. Kelly, J.A. Lopez, J.L. Mauderly, and D.L. Stafford. 1984. Diesel exhaust exposure system for animal studies. *Fund. Appl. Toxicol.* 4:270–277.

NAS. 1977. *Drinking Water and Health*. National Academy of Sciences, Washington, D.C.

NAS. 1980. Principles of toxicological interactions associated with multiple chemical exposures, report of the National Research council Panel on Evaluation of Hazards Associated with Maritime Personnel Exposed to Multiple Cargo Vapors. National Academy Press, Washington, D.C.

NAS. 1985a. Models for Biomedical Research: A New Perspective. National Academy Press, Washington, D.C.

NAS. 1986. *Drinking Water and Health*, Vol. 6. National Academy Press, Washington, D.C.

Nesnow, S., M. Argus, H. Bergman, K. Chu, C. Frith, T. Helmes, R. McGaughy, V. Ray, T.J. Slagu, R. Tennant and E. Weisburger. 1986. Chemical carcinogens, a review and analysis of the literature of selected chemicals and the establishment of the Gene–Tox Carcinogen Data Base, a report of the U.S. Environmental Protection Agency Gene–Tox Program. *Mutation Research* 185:1–195.

NTP. Various. Statistical Methods in National Toxicology Program Technical Report Series. National Toxicology Program, Research Triangle Park, NC.

NTP. 1984. Report of the NTP Ad Hoc Panel on Chemical Carcinogenesis Testing and Evaluation. Board of Scientific Counselors, National Toxicology Program, U.S. Department of Health and Human Services.

OSTP. 1979. Identification, characterization, and control of potential human carcinogens: a framework for federal decision-making. Office of Science and Technology Policy, Executive Office of the President, Washington, D.C.

OSTP. 1984. Chemical carcinogens; notice of review of the science and its associated principles. Office of Science and Technology Policy. *Fed. Reg.* 49:21594–21661 (May 22).

OTA. 1981. Assessment of Technologies for Determining Cancer Risks from the Environment. Office of Technology Assessment, Washington, D.C.

Peto, R., M.C. Pike, L. Bernstein, L.S. Gold, and B.N. Ames. 1984. The TD_{50}: A proposed general convention for the numerical description of the carcinogenic potency of chemicals in chronic-exposure animal experiments. *Environ. Health Perspec.* 58:1–8.

Portier, C.J. 1985. Design of animal carcinogenicity experiments: dose allocation, animal allocation, and sacrifice times. In *Proceedings, Symposium on*

Long-Term Animal Carcinogenicity Studies: A Statistical Perspective. American Statistical Association, Washington, D.C., pp. 42–50.

Reynolds, S.H., S.J. Stowers, R.M. Patterson, R.R. Maronpot, S.A. Aaronson, and M.W. Anderson. 1987. Activated oncogenes in B6C3F1 mouse liver tumors: implications for risk assessment. *Science* 237:1309–1316.

Rushefsky, M.E. 1986. *Making Cancer Policy.* State University of New York Press, Albany.

Sawyer, C., R. Peto, L. Bernstein, and M.C. Pike. 1984. Calculation of carcinogenic potency from long-term animal carcinogenesis experiments. *Biometrics* 40:27–40.

Seiler, F.A. 1987a. Mixtures of toxic agents and the risk of health effects, in R.H. Gray, E.K. Chess, P.J. Hellinger, R.G. Riley, and D.L. Springer (eds.), *Health & Environmental Research on Complex Mixtures* (CONF-851027) Pacific Northwest Laboratory, Richland, Washington, pp. 725–735.

Seiler, F.A. and B.R. Scott. 1987b. Mixtures of toxic agents and attributable risk calculations. *Risk Analysis* 7:81–90.

Snedecor, G.W. and W.G. Cochran. 1967. *Statistical Methods*, 6th ed. The Iowa State University Press, Ames.

Storer, J.B. and A.M. Weinberg. 1985. "Ambiguous carcinogens"—the main point. *Risk Assessment* 5:167.

Weinberg, A.M. and J.B. Storer. 1985. Ambiguous carcinogens and their regulation. *Risk Assessment* 5:151–156.

9

Mouse to Man: Extrapolation from Animals

INTRODUCTION

If sufficient epidemiological data were available, much of the difficulty and controversy in cancer risk assessment would not arise. For most carcinogens and potential carcinogens, however, little or no adequate human data are available. Without human data, the next best source of information is from other mammals. For current purposes, animal studies fall into two classes: (1) research studies designed to learn something about the mechanisms producing cancer and (2) bioassays, studies using standard protocols designed to determine whether a substance meets certain criteria to be considered a carcinogen and providing a standard data set for generation of a dose–response function. This chapter is primarily concerned with the analysis of data from bioassays. The standard long-term cancer bioassay design was discussed in the previous chapter, along with a number of considerations for the interpretation of the results. In this chapter, the more quantitative aspects of the analysis of these experiments to estimate cancer dose–response functions is presented. Although human and cellular level studies are important, in most cases animal experiments are the dose–response basis of quantitative cancer risk assessment.

The problem of deriving a dose–response function has many facets. Animal experiments must use high doses to get results with a reasonable number of animals. A dose level producing a risk of 1 in 100 would be expected to result in less than one extra tumor in a group of 50 animals; no effect could be demonstrated at all, aside from generating data for a dose–response curve. High doses are therefore the rule. The first problem, then, is the need to extrapolate the dose–response function from high to low dose. Even in this high-dose range, only a limited number of groups with different exposure levels can be used. The standard bioassay design provides only three data points. It should not be surprising that the results of these bioassays are inadequate to shed much light on the question of the *shape* of the dose–response function even in the moderate- to high-dose region, and can have nothing to contribute to its shape in the low-dose region. In fact, using the data from standard bioassays, one is unable to reject any of several common model shapes even in the high-dose region (Food Safety Council, 1980). The functional form of the dose–response curve embodies the knowledge or assumption about the mechanism underlying the process. Since the data are insufficient to determine this empirically, it must be derived from a theory of carcinogenesis. We will examine several different popular functions, each based on a different theory. Unfortunately, while current understanding of mechanisms is sufficient to suggest some likely forms, it is inadequate to justify any particular equation over another (Anderson et al., 1983). Since the various equations in common use often diverge sharply at low doses, this is an important contribution to overall uncertainty in cancer risk estimates. The shape of the dose–response function (i.e., the form of the equation) must be assumed; the extrapolation analysis only quantifies the parameters. The quantitative estimate of risk often depends more on the shape of the dose–response function used than on the data.

It is easy to fall into the trap of assuming that developing a dose–response function is simply an exercise in curve fitting. For too long, cancer risk assessment did not go much beyond that, but it is certainly a gross oversimplification. Every beginning student of regression analysis is warned to beware when extrapolating the regression line beyond the data, particularly when the mechanisms at work are not well understood. Yet, in cancer risk assessment the dose–response function is routinely extrapolated orders of magnitude below the lowest dose level in an animal experiment. There is, of course, a data point at zero dose from the control group. This places some limitation on the curve, but the shape or slope of the curve near zero cannot be determined from bioassay data.

Not surprisingly, the theories of cancer development on which early models were based were simple; this followed a rule of parsimony: if you do not understand a process, there is no sense in using a complicated model to analyze it. Moreover, these theories focused primarily on cancer initiation. The result was an attempt to explain all of the complicated processes going on between administering a dose to an animal and production of a cancer through a single equation based on a theory of cancer initiation. The better understanding of pharmacokinetics and of the other stages of carcinogenesis and the ability to measure intermediate events, such as the formation of DNA adducts, all gained through decades of *basic and applied biomedical* research, is finally beginning to seep into extrapolation models. There is still a long way to go; eventually high-dose to low-dose extrapolation may be incorporated into a chain of models, each depicting a stage in the dose and carcinogenic process.

High- to low-dose extrapolation is only one part of the "mouse to man" extrapolation. Neither the low-dose nor the high-dose risk in mice is the same as in man. A variety of scaling factors are generally used before and after the low-dose extrapolation. The more widespread understanding and use of pharmacokinetics is changing this aspect of extrapolation from simple scaling coefficients to more realistic, biologically based models.

HIGH- TO LOW-DOSE EXTRAPOLATION MODELS*

This section introduces the traditional quantal response models that formed the core of quantitative cancer risk analysis during its formative period from the 1960s into the 1980s and are still the basis of many dose–response coefficients in current use and much cancer risk regulation. These models are based on experiments in which animals are exposed in groups; one unexposed control group and two or more groups at various exposure levels. The animals are followed for some specific period (usually a substantial fraction of their lifetime) and the number of animals in each group that develop tumors or cancers are counted. This is the experimental design in the standard animal carcinogenesis bioassay of the National Toxicology Program. An animal either does or does not develop a tumor during the course of the bioassay. The analysis may also be specific as to organ or histologic type, e.g., an animal either does or does not develop a liver tumor of a specific histologic type. The general form of the models used to extrapolate these experimental results is that the probability of a single animal developing a tumor is a function of dose, $P = F(d)$. This function is in the form of a cumulative probability density function (CDF) such that the probability, P, lies between 0 and 1, and the probability associated with one dose level is greater than that associated with another only if the first dose level is greater than the second. The specific form taken by the function $F(d)$ is, in effect, the mathematical expression of a biological "model" of carcinogenesis, and the models can be categorized by the biological concepts on which they rest.

Statistical Models

The first group of models are tolerance-distribution models; these are sometimes called statistical models. They are based on a standard tenet

---

*Parts of this section draw on Morris et al., 1982.

of classical toxicology, that each individual has a tolerance level to an environmental agent, below which it is not affected and above which, in this case, a cancer develops. The distribution of tolerance levels in the population is the tolerance distribution. Probit, logit, and Weibull distributions are frequently used to characterize the tolerance distribution. Other than the fact that these models generate a sigmoid or S-shaped cumulative dose–response curve, commonly observed throughout the field of toxicology, there is little biological basis for using any particular statistical model for the tolerance distribution. In particular, there is no biological evidence to justify extending any shape curve into the low-dose region. Since all of these models produce curves that pass through the origin, some fraction of the population will be predicted to develop cancer at any dose level.

Probit

The probit is a lognormal tolerance model that has long been used in toxicology. Bliss (1934) noted that the distribution of critical dose for several different forms of drug applications could be represented by the lognormal distribution. The probit model can be pictured on linear graph paper by transforming the dose into its logarithm and expressing response in probits. This is a linearizing transformation effectively corresponding to the use of log-probability graph paper. The model, without the probit transformation, is given by

$$P(d) = (2\pi)^{1/2} \int_{-\infty}^{\alpha + \beta \log d} \exp(-\mu^2/2) \, d\mu \tag{1}$$

where α and β are the parameters to be estimated. The model can be run using standard computer routines by taking the probit of the data and regressing it on the logarithm of the dose (Food Safety Council, 1980):

$$\text{probit } P(d) = a + b \log(d) \tag{2}$$

Its use in analysis of animal carcinogen experiments was introduced by Bryan and Shimkin (1943). Mantel and Bryan (1961) suggested a modified version of the probit model in their landmark paper for low-dose extrapolation. Instead of estimating the probability of an animal developing a tumor at a given dose, the modified model estimated a "virtually safe dose," that is, the dose associated with a conservatively low level of risk. The method consisted of setting β to a conservative value (usually 1), and fixing the probability of a tumor at a predetermined "acceptable risk" of one in a million (10^{-6}). This was an early approach to the problem faced by regulatory agencies to set a standard that incorporates a "margin of safety." An "improved" version of the Mantel–Bryan procedure was introduced a decade later (Mantel et al., 1975). The

Mantel–Bryan procedure was thought to be an advance over the earlier "safety factor" approach in which the "safe" dose was defined as 1/100th of the lowest dose at which no tumors were seen in experimental animals, without regard to the design of the experiment. It permitted higher "safe" doses to be deduced from large experiments in which few positive responses were observed than from small experiments with the same response frequencies (Mantel and Schneiderman, 1975). Despite its built-in conservatisms, the increased risk over background in the Mantel–Bryan procedure approaches zero rapidly and will generally give a lower estimate of risk in the low-dose region than any of the other quantal models (Krewski and Van Ryzin, 1981). Crump et al. (1976) argued that using the probit model for extrapolation was incompatible with low-dose linearity that stemmed from assumptions of single-cell cancer induction and additivity of background, and is appropriate only for what are sometimes called epigenetic carcinogens. Cornfield (1977), however, pointed out that while biological data frequently appear to be normal or lognormally distributed, they often deviate from these distributions in the tails. He judged that the probit model would overestimate the probability of cancer response at low dose.

Logit
The logit model is similar to the probit, but characterizes the tolerance distribution with the logistic function rather than the normal distribution.

$$P(d) = (1 + \exp(-a + b \log(d)))^{-1} \tag{3}$$

where a and b are the parameters to be estimated. Unless the sample size is large, it is difficult to distinguish between the probit and logit models (Prentice, 1976). The logit curve approaches zero response more slowly, however, and thus in the low-dose region the probit generally gives a lower estimate of risk at a given dose (Krewski and Van Ryzin, 1981).

Weibull
The Weibull model characterizes the tolerance distribution as a power transformation of the exponential model. It has been closely associated with time-to-failure models of electronic systems, but has no compelling explicit theoretical basis as a cancer tolerance distribution, although it is a generalization of the stochastic hit model in a statistical form. The Weibull model is given by:

$$P(d) = 1 - \exp(-bd^m) \tag{4}$$

where b and m are the parameters to be estimated.

The Weibull model has greater flexibility in fitting model curvature than the probit or logit, allowing more accuracy in the fit of the model to the data. Since it is not clear what the best way to estimate effect in the low dose region is by detailed extrapolation of the shape suggested by a small number of data points at much higher doses, the flexibility is not necessarily an advantage. Even perfect agreement between observation at high doses and a given distribution offers no assurance that extrapolation to the far tail of the distribution is valid. Murdoch et al. (1987) note that if one changes the focus of a hit model (see below) from a single cell to a tissue, and considers many different cell lines in a tissue competing to produce tumors, the resulting model is a Weibull distribution. They conclude the Weibull thus has a stronger rationale than the multihit.

Stochastic Models

Stochastic models are based on a different biological hypothesis. Rather than a tolerance distribution, they assume everyone in the population is equally susceptible to cancer, but that a cancer is initiated only as a result of one or more independent, stochastic—or randomly occurring—events.

One-Hit

The simplest stochastic model is the 1-hit model, first introduced to describe the mechanism of radiation-induced cell killing and later carcinogenesis. Imagine that a cell contains a critical target; if this target is "hit" by a gamma ray, a process begins that leads inevitably to a cancer. If one is exposed to gamma radiation, it is only a matter of chance whether the critical target in a cell is "hit." The chance is a function of dose; the more radiation one is expose to, the greater the probability of a "hit." A lucky person might be exposed to high doses and never receive an effective "hit." Even at the lowest dose, however, there is still some probability of a "hit," so "hit" models are nonthreshold; they will estimate some cancer risk in a population at any dose above zero. In a more sophisticated sense, the critical target is usually thought of as the DNA in the cell nucleus and the "hit" the production of a somatic mutation that is assumed to be the initiating event for a cancer. While the word "hit" may seem appropriate in the radiation example, in the case of chemical carcinogens a variety of possible biochemical events may constitute a "hit;" one is a somatic mutation resulting from the formation of a DNA adduct. The mathematical form of the 1-hit model is

$$P(d) = 1 - \exp(-bd) \qquad (5)$$

where b is the expected rate of hits per unit dose and is the parameter to be estimated. Although the equation is exponential, the 1-hit model is sometimes referred to a the linear model because in the low-dose region d is small and the equation is approximated by the linear form

$$P(d) = a + bd \tag{6}$$

The model is simple and the low-dose linearity introduces many further simplifications in later stages of the analysis. The cumulative population dose can be estimated as the mean dose in the population multiplied by the number of people in the population. A 1 rad dose to each of 10 people (10 person-rad) produces the same risk in the population as an 0.1 rad dose to each of 100 people (also 10 person-rad). The 1-hit also meets the axiom that in the face of uncertainty about which model to use, the simplest model should be the choice. It has been asserted both that the linear model accurately represents what is happening on the molecular level and that it provides an upper bound of possible effects, providing the "margin of safety" desired by regulators. It was an attractive model for regulatory purposes and was used extensively in radiation and environmental chemical carcinogen risk management. In comparisons with other models, the 1-hit predicts the highest effect and produces the greatest slope at low dose (Scientific Committee, 1980). From the perspective of "safe" dose estimation, estimates of "safe" doses obtained using the one-hit model are usually much lower than those obtained from the same experimental data using the Mantel–Bryan probit procedure (Guess and Crump, 1977). Stating this the other way around, the one-hit model usually yields higher estimates of risk at low doses than the probit.

Multi-hit

Since the process of cancer development is clearly more complex than the activation of a single target, the 1-hit model was expanded into a more general form of the multihit model. The expanded theory is that, of a number, M, critical targets available, m must be altered to induce a response (where m is a number smaller than M), and producing each alteration requires k "hits." In general, it was assumed that each target required the same number of hits (Danzer, 1934). The order of the hits is not important. Table 9-1 is a modified listing of Danzer's postulates describing a general hit theory. A virtually infinite number of possible multihit models can be constructed on the basis of this general theory. If the probability of k or more hits, given a specific dose d, is governed by a Poisson process where b is the expected rate of hits per unit dose, the probability of a tumor is (Krewski and Van Ryzin, 1981):

$$P(d) = 1 - \sum_{j=0}^{k-1} \exp(-\lambda d) \frac{(\lambda d)^j}{j!} \tag{7}$$

The 1-hit model is a special case in which k = 1. Two other special cases are the two-hit model and the two-target model. The parameters in a multihit model are generally estimated in a way that lets the data determine the number of hits (within often tight restrictions on model fit). Because they have one (or more) additional parameters, multi-hit models in general provide a closer fit to the data than the 1-hit model

In multihit theory, the exact biological definition of a "hit" is no longer as clear as it was in the 1-hit model, but it still can be thought of as a unique event that either happens or does not happen. If we can no longer picture exactly what a "hit" is, the next logical step is to hypothesize that the "hit" does not necessarily have to be a unique event, but can represent part of a continuous process. Then the number of "hits" can be chosen from a continuous scale and 1.32 "hits" would be perfectly acceptable. Rai and Van Ryzin (1979) developed such a model, known as the generalized k-hit dose–response model. It is also sometimes called the gamma multihit model, although it is quite far removed from the original concept of "hit" models and, in fact, can be interpreted as a statistical tolerance model based on a gamma density function with scale parameter 1/b and shape parameter k:

$$P(d) = \int_0^d (\beta t)^{kc}(-\beta t)/t\Gamma(k)\, dt \tag{8}$$

where

$$\Gamma(k) = \int_0^\infty t^{k-1}e^{-t}\, dt$$

Because $P(d)/d^k$ is constant at low doses, $P(d)$ is linear for $k = 1$ (one-hit), concave upward for $k < 1$, and convex upward for $k > 1$, in the low-dose region.

Multistage

An analogy to a multihit model requiring one hit on each of two targets would be flipping two coins where "heads" constitute a "hit." Each of the coins would be flipped a given number of times depending on the dose. Success in producing a cancer would require only that both coins come up "heads" at least once during the course of the flipping. The probability of heads for each coin is the same (Postulate 6 in Table 9-1). If the model required two hits on each of two targets, each coin would have to come up "heads" at least twice; the probability of a "head" on each flip is the same (Postulate 4). If the targets are distinguishable (*eliminate Postulate 6*), or if successive hits have different rate constants

TABLE 9-1   Postulates Describing General Hit Models

---

1. A subject has M critical targets
2. The subject produces a response if m < M or more of the critical targets are altered
3. A critical target is altered if it is hit k or more times
4. For a given dose, the probability of a hit is the same for all targets
5. The probability of a target being hit is independent of any other target being hit; similarly, all hits on a specific target are independent of each other
6. The probability of exactly n hits occurring to a single target at a given dose d is defined by a Poisson process with the average probability rate βd, the expected number of hits that occur at dose d, where β > 0 is the same at all dose level. This implies that the probability of a hit increases as the dose increases.

Source: From Turner, 1975.

from preceding hits (eliminate Postulate 4), than a whole new class of models is created. This class of models might be called "multievent." An analogy of one type would be throwing a die and flipping a coin where a "one" and a "heads" constitute success. If the order of the die-throw and the coin flip is inconsequential, the model is an unordered multievent. In a biological system, one can easily envision situations in which the first event must succeed to enable a second event. In the analogy, "heads" obtained in the coin flipping do not count until after a "one" has been thrown on the die. These ordered multievent models are called multistage models.

The multistage model was first proposed as a description of cancer development by Armitage and Doll (1954) based on observations of human cancer rate patterns with age. It incorporates more of a biological basis into cancer models. Peto (1977) describes the underlying biological hypothesis as follows: "a few distinct changes (each heritable when cells carrying them divide) are necessary to alter a normal cell into a malignant cell . . . human cancer usually arises from the proliferation of a clone derived from a single cell that has suffered all the necessary changes and then started to proliferate malignantly." The general mathematical requirements can be stated more simply. In the multistage process, "k [distinct] initiating events must occur in some particular time sequence" (Crump et al., 1976). While there are any number of models that might be constructed to fit this criterion, only one is currently in common use (Guess and Crump, 1976, 1978; Crump et al., 1976, 1977). This assumes the transition rate of a cell through each stage is linearly related to the dose rate and, consequently, the residence time of a cell at each stage has an exponential distribution (Crump and Howe, 1984). The resulting form of the model is given in Eq (9), where d is the dose and k the number of stages. The coefficients, q_i, must be nonnegative, i being an integer from 1 to k.

$$P(d) = 1 - \exp[-(q_1 d + q_2 d^2 + \cdots + q_k d^k)] \tag{9}$$

This model is capable of reflecting both linear and nonlinear dose–response relations. It is thus more flexible in shape than either the 1-hit or the probit models and estimates of "safe" doses may range widely, depending on the experimental data. Its confidence limits should include some factors previously expressible only qualitatively as "model-dependent" uncertainties rather than quantitatively as uncertainty in the numerical value of model parameters (Guess and Crump, 1977). Whittemore (1979) notes, however, that using this model in a mode to produce "safe" doses guarantees nonthreshold linearity at low dose rates, making the procedure so insensitive to response at experimental dosages that it is unable to distinguish between low levels of potent carcinogens and noncarcinogenic substances.

This model has been used widely in federal carcinogen regulation by EPA, OSHA, and the Consumer Product Safety Commission. The usual justification is that it is believed to have a greater biological basis than the previous models, although this justification is often stated together with the caveat that there is actually little justification to choose one model over another. Most biologists readily agree that cancer is a multistage process and, providing they accept the concept of low-dose extrapolation at all, that a multistage model is the most suitable for low-dose extrapolation. Few biologists have examined the biological meaning of the specific mathematical formula used to compare it with their concept of the multistage cancer process.

In using the multistage model, however, regulatory agencies do not use the best fit of the model (the maximum likelihood estimate, MLE), but an 95% confidence limit (the upper confidence limit on risk or conversely, the lower confidence limit on the virtually safe dose) that is linear in dose. Crump and Howe (1985) describe approaches for setting confidence limits and give examples using the multistage and other models. There are four reasons for reliance on the 95% upper bound:

1. Regulatory agencies exhibit a natural conservatism, feeling obligated to err on the side of protecting public health; in the presence of uncertainty they are inclined to opt for a conservative bounding estimate.
2. Although it is usually assumed in extrapolation modeling that the

agent of concern acts independent of the background risk, it is recognized that, in reality, this is probably not the case. Even a small amount of interaction with background would be expected to lead to low-dose linearity (Crump et al., 1976; Hoel, 1980). Therefore, it is felt desirable that the extrapolation become linear with dose at low doses. This has been shown to be the case for most of the extrapolation models discussed above. The multistage model is nonlinear, and, at least with some data sets, is nonlinear throughout the entire dose–response range. An upper confidence limit may be generated, however, that is linear at low doses.

3. When the trend does not have a definite linear component, only the upper confidence limit will be stable (Guess et al., 1977). It has been shown that slight, biologically insignificant changes in the data can lead to large changes in the MLE of the multistage model, while the confidence limit remains robust. It hardly seems logical to accept a "best" estimate that might vary by orders of magnitude if in one experimental dose-level group of the bioassay 1 instead of zero animals out of 150 had developed a tumor.

4. Although different model forms may produce radically different MLE and lower confidence limits, the upper confidence limits are usually similar and highly linear as long as the model does not rule out low-dose linearity by assumption (Guess et al., 1977).

All these points have merit, but they also require a closer look. They violate a tenet of risk analysis that, if possible, risks should be expressed as a best estimate with confidence bounds, not as upper bounds alone. This allows the level of confidence (or margin of safety) to be established by the policy maker, or vice-versa, the safety factor associated with a decision made on other bases to be calculated. This will be discussed further in Chap. 16, along with the question of the regulatory agencies' need for conservatism. Of more technical importance, the risk estimate from the multistage model extrapolation is not the final risk estimate. This number is usually one of a series of estimates (e.g., emissions, transport rates, population size) multiplied together to estimate the population risk. Use of an upper-bound estimate prevents the correct approach to propagation of uncertainty through this calculation. Often the final risk estimate presented to decision makers and the public is the product of several upper-bound estimates, a number likely to be far out on the tail of the distribution. Perhaps more importantly, such estimates contain an unknown degree of conservatism that probably varies among pollutants.

One way of thinking about the inexorability of linearity at low doses is to recognize that, if an equation that fits the bioassay data in the experimental range has even a small linear component, that linear component will come to dominate the risk estimate as the dose approaches zero and the higher order terms approach zero faster than the linear. Even if the equation of best fit to the experimental data does not include a linear term, adding a small linear term would not affect the fit enough to reject the addition, and, as before, would dominate at low dose (Guess et al., 1977). That shows that linearity at low dose could occur, and even that it may be likely, but does not prove it exists. Crump et al. (1976) demonstrate low-dose linearity in a multievent model such as the multihit or multistage under assumptions of additivity. Additivity suggests that causes of cancer other than the agent of interest act in a similar, additive, manner. These might be other chemicals or spontaneous events. Thus, the incidence rate at zero dose of the agent of interest can be thought of as a risk imposed by these other causative factors whose cumulative exposure might be expressed as an effect dose of the agent of interest. Hoel (1980) further demonstrates that if even a small fraction of the background incidence is attributable to additive effects low-dose linearity applies. The effect applies only to carcinogens that act on a single cell. Crump et al.'s proof of low-dose linearity does not apply to nongenotoxic carcinogens or carcinogens with a threshold effect. Moreover, although Crump et al. (1976) show that approximate linearity holds over a fairly long range, this range can be considerably reduced if the underlying effect, as exhibited in the experimental data, is highly nonlinear. The scope of applicability of these assumptions should be reevaluated in light of the intervening decade of research on cancer mechanisms.

The statement that the MLE is mathematically unstable has more behind it than a problem with the MLE. The lack of stability is due to the requirement in the Crump model that the coefficients be nonnegative. When the data are such that the coefficients want to be negative, a discontinuity is formed in the risk surface. This could be interpreted not simply that the MLE is unstable but that this instability is an indication that the particular data set is unsuitable for analysis by the multistage model. In such a situation, does it make sense to use the upper bound of the multistage model? Or should one go back to the 1-hit or something else. This, again, is a question that deserves more exploration. Moreover, within the range where nonnegative coefficients provide the optimal fit, the opposite effect occurs. That is, the upper bound estimate is not sensitive to large changes in experimental data that suggest greatly different dose–response patterns while the MLE allows characterization of these changes (Sielken, 1987).

The Crump multistage model can be restricted or unlimited in the number of stages allowed. Following a general practice in regression analysis that the number of parameters to be fit should be fewer than the number of data points available, one approach is to run the model with the restriction that the number of stages be limited to 1 less than the number of dose levels in the experiment. While this seems a prudent restriction, it is severely limiting since the standard bioassay only has two dose levels plus a control group. Following the recommendations of a consensus workshop, the general practice has been to use the model in a generalized form with no restriction on the number of stages; this also increases the likelihood of a nonzero linear term (NAS, 1986).

Despite its presumed biological basis, the multistage model focuses on only one aspect of cancer development: initiation. It does not explicitly address promotion, suppression, progression, or other possible processes affecting cancer growth. Moreover, the dose of the model is the dose to the target tissue or even target cell, yet the dose used in applying the model is generally the dose administered to the animal or the environmental exposure to the population. It must be recognized that, given these circumstances, application of the multistage model is simply an exercise in curve-fitting no different than is the case with any of the other commonly used models. Hoel et al. (1983) suggested coupling the multistage model with a pharmacokinetic model so that the biological effective dose, represented as levels of specific carcinogen-DNA adducts, would be the dose term of the extrapolation model. A separate advance has been the gradual increase in interest in more biologically based cancer risk models discussed below.

MODELING EFFECTS OF TIME-VARYING DOSE

Low- to high-dose extrapolations commonly assume a uniform dose rate, often over the entire lifespan. Many different time patterns of dose can be envisioned, however: (a) a single, short exposure such as that received by the atomic bomb survivors; (b) rest periods between doses such as in occupational exposures and many animal experiments where the daily dose is constant for 5 days per week but there is no dose over the weekend; (c) highly variable dose rates such as a maintenance worker in a chemical plant might receive; (d) relatively constant dose over a fraction of lifetime, such as someone drinking water from a chemically contaminated well for a few years. Do these dosing patterns make a difference in extrapolation modeling? Hit models do not depend on time patterns of dose, and will give the same effect from different patterns as long as the total dose is the same (Morrison, 1987). Limited time-pattern dependency can be introduced using a hit model by applying it in a life-table analysis. Here, the cancer risk during each remaining year of life is calculated separately for the exposure during each year of life. Multi-stage models, however, are highly dependent on time-pattern of dose (Morrison, 1987).

EPA's generalized multistage model assumed a constant, uniform dose. While this assumption never truly holds for human exposure, it is generally adequate for risk assessment purposes. Situations arise, however, in which dose varies with time in animal experiments or marked changes occur in population exposure. A modified version of the model applicable to time-varying dose patterns has been developed (Crump and Howe, 1984). Kodell et al. (1987) investigated the implications of using average lifetime dose rate assumptions for intermittent exposures. They found that low-dose risk estimates based on average lifetime dose rate may overestimate the "true" risk as determined by a time-dependent dose multistage model by several orders of magnitude, although the degree of possible underestimation was limited. Implications of time-dependent exposures were further explored by Murdoch and Krewski (1988), who compared the effect in the multistage model and the Moolgavkar-Venzon-Kundson model (see below), and Chen et al. (1988), who examined the time-pattern implications of three types of carcinogens, initiators, completers, and promoters, in the MVK model.

BIOLOGICAL MODELS AND MATHEMATICAL MODELS

For too long, risk assessors focused on the cancer-initiating event. This is like looking for the lost keys under the light pole, where you can see, rather than in the dark, where you dropped them. To the biomedical cancer researcher, cancer development is an extremely complex, virtually unfathomable process. To the risk assessor, it has too often been a simple and direct function of dose. The one-hit model, the earliest and still one of the most popular of many risk assessment models, assumes that one "hit" on the DNA of a single cell inevitably leads to development of a cancer, and that "hit" is a simple function of dose.

The multistage model is widely used because biomedical researchers believe cancer is a multistage process, but to what extent does the mathematical model most generally used actually represent the multistage process the researchers are talking about? Perhaps first we should ask, do the biomedical researchers know what they are talking about? Armitage and Doll's (1954) advancement of a multistage process was based on mathematical analysis of observed patterns of cancer with age, not on molecular biology. Moolgavkar and Knudson (1981) claim that "when kinetics are taken into account, two stages are sufficient to generate the whole spectrum of cancer incidence curves observed in human populations . . ." and, moreover, "no more than two distinct stages [initiation and promotion] have been experimental demonstrated." Indeed, there are no established explanations of what the five or six stages often predicted by the model actually represent in biological terms. Nonetheless, something must be going on between that hypothetical cancer-initiating event and manifestation of the cancer some 20 or more years later. Even dividing this period up into ill-defined stages, however, it seems to be stretching the imagination to expect that every stage is a function of the dose of the initiating agent. In the well-known two-stage process, demonstrated in mouse skin painting tests, initiation is dependent on the dose of one substance, while promotion is dependent on application of a different agent.

There would seem to be room for improved models that would be better aligned with biomedical knowledge. Stochastic and statistical models are each based on a single concept of carcinogenesis; both have independent merit. It is possible that both mechanisms simultaneously play a role. Statistical models assume people vary in tolerance or susceptibility while stochastic models assume that a dose is effective when one or more probabilistic interactions between a cell and a carcinogen occur. Joint formulations could include, for example, a statistical range of tolerance to stochastic processes. The same event might score a successful "hit" on one person, but not on another depending on their tolerance level. Or, given a successful initiating event, the rate constants of later stages might depend on individual susceptibility (say a distribution in the activity of repair processes) instead of or in conjunction with dose. More complex models will generally require larger bioassays to supply the data. It does no good to have a model with four or five parameters if you only have two data points. The problem goes further, though. If the "carcinogenic potency" of the substance is only one factor in the equation, than the data needs cannot be supplied by a bioassay on one substance. It may be necessary to know more about the make-up of the complex mix of exposures in the population and about the distribution of genetic susceptibility in the exposed population. All the information needed may not be available now, but more research in developing the list of what is needed is the beginning. Once that list is available, the information may not be as difficult to get as might seem at first. The techniques for genetic screening of populations are available, and the database is actually growing. For some time, medical researchers have been interested in the tolerance distribution for cancer, not to support better quantitative risk assessment, but to identify people who might be particularly susceptible so they can be warned to avoid exposures.

BIOLOGICALLY BASED CANCER RISK MODELS

The multistage model, presumably the most well-based biologically of any model used in regulatory practice, is grounded in the biological understanding of the 1950s. It provides for multiple stages in the development of a tumor, but these stages do not represent specific, known, biological mechanisms. The parameters for each stage must be determined simultaneously from dose and tumor production data, one cannot physically measure each parameter specifically. While a complete understanding of the carcinogenic process remains elusive, biomedical science has advanced considerably in this area since the 1950s. A better appreciation of the many different mechanisms involved in tumor initiation and development has been gained (Chap. 2). Quantitative research models have been developed for many of these precesses (see, e.g., Thompson and Brown, 1987). In addition, the ability to measure quantities previously unheard of has advanced rapidly; this ability allows quantification and verification of mechanistic models. As was the case for pharmacokinetics (Chap. 7), cancer risk modeling is also moving to more biologically based models. The call for such change was made strongly by Wilson (1986) in an editorial in *Risk Analysis*.

A biologically based cancer risk model that provides a framework for incorporating new biomedical information was developed by Moolgavkar and co-workers (Moolgavkar and Venzon, 1979; Moolgavkar and Knudson, 1981; Moolgavkar, 1983; Thorslund et al., 1987; Moolgavkar et al., 1988). This will be referred to as the MVK model. The structure of the model is shown in Figure 9-1. It is a two-stage model that explicitly incorporates the kinetics of tissue growth and development. The basic assumptions of the model are (1) tumors develop from a single progenitor cell; (2) two specific steps (or transformations) are required; (3) these

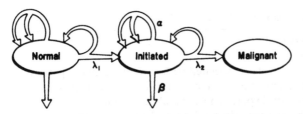

FIGURE 9-1 Schematic diagram of Moolgavkar–Verzon–Knudson (MVK) model. λ_1 is the rate at which normal cells are initiated by exposure to an initiator, λ_2 is the rate initiated cells undergo malignant transformation. α indicates the rate of cell birth through normal division while β is the rate of cell death. The difference, $(\alpha - \beta)$ is an indication of promotional activity in initiated cells (after Murdoch and Krewski, 1988).

transformations occur at cell division; (4) cells undergo these transformations independently of one another; (5) these transformations are irreversible. The model begins with a population of normal stem cells in a tissue. These normal cells may undergo three different kind of transformations: (1) divide into two normal daughter cells; (2) die or differentiate; (3) divide into one normal cell and one intermediate cell. The latter has undergone the first transformation, initiation, and is now a preneoplastic or initiated cell. Each of these processes occurs at a given rate that may be determined by fitting the model to data or actually measured experimentally (or in some cases inferred from a surrogate measure). Initiated cells accumulate in the model's second compartment where they are subject to a similar set of transformations: (1) they may divide into two daughter cells like themselves; (2) they may die or differentiate; or (3) they may divide into one cell like themselves and one tumor cell. The latter is assumed to result in the formation of a malignant tumor after a given time period, so its transformation rate must implicitly take into account defense mechanisms such as immune surveillance (Moolgavkar et al., 1988). As the ability to draw on direct measurements advances, there would seem to be no reason why the model could not be expanded to include these factors explicitly.

By assuming different tissue growth patterns, the model can fit the incidence curves of all human cancers (Moolgavkar and Knudson, 1981). Promotional activity is the difference of the cell birth and death rates among initiated cells. This model has the ability to explain many key phenomena (Table 9-2). It can accommodate time-dependent dose patterns (Moolgavkar et al., 1988; Murdoch and Krewski, 1988). The coupling of the MVK model with a pharmacokinetic model has also be demonstrated (Tan and Singh, 1987).

TABLE 9-2   Phenomena Explained by MVK Model

- Genetic predisposition to cancer
- Patterns in childhood cancer rates
- Changes in respiratory cancer rates associated with variable smoking patterns
- Observed increase of age-specific incidence rates for many human cancers
- Results of initiation-promotion experiments for multiple agents
- Lower tumor rates at very high experimental doses than at lower doses
- Additive, multiplicative, or antagonistic response to exposure to multiple carcinogens
- Regression and disappearance of some transformed cell masses after cessation of exposure

Source: From Thursland et al., 1987.

Sielken (1987) has adapted the MVK model to incorporate individual susceptibilities due to metabolic rates, tissue sensitivity, repair efficiency, and immune system characteristics. This model allows these susceptibilities to interact in the pharmacokinetic model used to provide the biologically effective dose term to the cancer risk model.

Which Comes First, The Model or the Data?

The current National Toxicology Program long-term animal cancer bioassay is designed to answer the qualitative question, "is the substance a carcinogen or not?". This can be expressed more specifically as, "do treated animals have a higher tumor rate than controls?". Yet, it is the data from these bioassays that are often the basis of extrapolation modeling for dose–response. That the goal of using the same bioassay to screen for carcinogenic activity and to explore the dose–response relationship leads to conflicting criteria for optimizing the experimental design was the subject of a National Toxicology Program panel (NTP, 1984). The panel recognized several recommendations for designs incorporating more dose levels and increasing numbers of animals at lower dose levels. It also considered a two-tiered test: a screening bioassay followed by later exploration of dose–response in chemicals that were positive on the screening. Depending on the fraction of substances tested that were positive on the screening test, this two-tiered process could be cost effective in testing. None of this takes into account cost-effectiveness in terms of legal costs or costs of bad decisions due to inadequate data. The panel rejected the two-tier design "on the grounds that a delay of several years between a positive finding of carcinogenicity and subsequent elaboration of dose-effect relationships could have intolerable consequences for the regulatory process" (NTP, 1984).

Gaylor et al. (1985) explored the selection of bioassay designs that would simultaneously detect carcinogens with relatively good power and supply enough data to drive low-dose extrapolation models. They thus implicitly reject the two-tier approach *a priori*. Their analysis is of interest because it uses an extrapolation model to help design the dose levels and number of animals in each dose group in an experiment. Since no model can be assumed to be the correct one, they further reject the notion of predicting best estimates of risk below the range of experimental data, instead focusing on predictions of upper bounds of risk by using a linear extrapolation below the experimental data range. To minimize effects introduced by a curve-fitting model, they take a straight line between zero and the upper confidence limit of the lowest experimental dose level as the upper bound of the dose–response curve. As an alternative that does not depend directly on a single data point, they suggest using a straight line between zero and the upper bound of the modeled risk estimate at a risk level of 1%, a risk sufficiently near the experimental data range to exclude large variations among models in its estimation.

Their criteria for the "best" design is the one that yields the lowest upper bound on risk at a given dose level for a wide variety of dose–response curves. Since the lower bound is, for practical purposes, zero, this is essentially a criteria of minimizing the uncertainty bounds on risk. It is not the only object one could imagine, but it is a good one. In their analysis, they generate simulated experimental data for 12 different designs using a Weibull model. These designs include different numbers of dose levels (2 to 4) at various fractions of the maximum tolerated dose (MTD), and with balanced and unbalanced numbers of animals per dose. Their conclusions were that, under the requirements they established, adding an additional dose level (at 1/4 the MTD) would provide a significant design advantage for low-dose extrapolation but there was no advantage demonstrated for deviating from the standard bioassay design with equal numbers of animals per dose group. Designs with uniform numbers of animals per dose group that incorporated lower experimental doses lead to a greater range of uncertainty on risk. This should not be surprising since risk at these lower doses would require a larger number of animals to achieve significant results.

The uncertainty of low-dose risk estimates depends on the bioassay design, including the number of experimental dose levels, their spacing, and the number of animals in each group; the extrapolation distance; and the uncertainty of not knowing which of several possible extrapolation models is appropriate, which can be restated as not knowing the true dose–response function (Wong, 1984). For a lengthy extrapolation, the latter is probably the limiting uncertainty. It is also one that is only slowly being reduced through biomedical research and its application in risk assessment. Some improvement might be made, however, by considering experimental designs for bioassays that produce data aimed specifically to drive an extrapolation model. The effectiveness of increasing the number of dose levels or the number of animals per dose level on reducing the uncertainty of the low-dose risk estimate can only be determined through the use of the extrapolation model and will vary with extrapolation distance. As often happens in statistical analysis, the proper design of the experiment cannot be determined until the results are known, a catch-22 that is resolved by doing a preliminary, pilot experiment to pre-estimate the necessary parameters to design the full experiment. This takes us back to something like the two-tier process rejected by the NTP panel (1984) above because of the delays it creates in the regulatory process.

Various aspects of this dilemma will be discussed in later chapters, but it should be clear that this is not a one-sided argument. Delays in the regulatory process are undesirable, especially after a preliminary study has suggested that a substance is a carcinogen. Some of the weight of this argument may be lifted by a reminder that the current regulatory process is not known for its speediness. Moreover, it is not unknown for regulations to be periodically revised in light of increasing knowledge. The key argument is that public policy and the regulatory process are presumably not enhanced by excessive uncertainty in the science on which regulations are based. There must be some room for trade-off between delay or the disruption caused by changing regulations and an improved knowledge base leading to better regulations.

MOUSE TO MAN

The dose–response assessment relationship developed from animal data applies to the experimental animal. Extrapolating to man is a further step. If the administered dose in the animal experiment is used as the "dose" for the dose–response extrapolation, some consideration must be given to physical, metabolic, and pharmacokinetic difference that may affect the biologically effective dose to the target cell or tissue. Experimental animals are not little people. Mice, rats, and other commonly used test species have physical and metabolic characteristics and sensitivities different from humans. Some have organs that humans do not have and lack organs humans do have (e.g., the rat lacks a gallbladder). While comparative anatomy is well understood, many of the differences between mouse and man, and especially the implications of these differences for extrapolation of mouse cancer rates to man, still retain considerable uncertainty. Not only may factors such as metabolism rates differ between species, but the way metabolism changes with different dose rates may differ between species. These differences were discussed in Chap. 7. Additional information can be found in a number of useful summaries and reviews (Hill et al., 1988; Crump, 1986; Lepkowski, 1978).

While use of pharmacokinetic models to estimate biologically effective dose is becoming more common, cancer dose–response functions in experimental animals have traditionally been converted for application in man by simplistic scaling factors. The most common is to express dose in terms of mg per m^2 body surface area, roughly proportional to body weight raised to the 2/3 power. Others conclude that scaling on a simple mg dose per kg body weight basis is best (Lepkowski, 1978, Dixon, 1976). More rarely, and particularly for agents taken by mouth, scaling is done on the basis of the fraction of agent weight to total diet, (mg/kg). The differences resulting from applying these different scaling factors when extrapolating from mice and rats to man are shown in Table 9-3. Because more than body weight or size is involved, however, simple scaling factors can never be right. Moreover, true interspecies differences will vary between different agents, since the metabolism, pharmacokinetics, promotion, type of damage to DNA, immunological reactions, and repair mechanisms all may differ for different agents. Thus, scaling factors may distort the ranking of chemicals by potency as well as introduce error in the absolute value of dose–response. Hoel (1979) suggests that greater errors are associated with use of scaling factors than with statistical extrapolation. Because of different kinds of uncertainties associated with epidemiological results in humans, it is difficult to test the variation resulting from scaling factors. Hoel (1979) describes the affect of different scaling factors in six chemicals that an earlier study (Meselson, 1975) had examined and concluded there were sufficient human data to develop dose–response estimates. Depending on "corrections" selected to account for deficiencies in the human results, either mg/kg or mg/kg$^{2/3}$ might be supported, but the quantitative error introduced by scale-up factors can be greater than that associated with the high- to low-dose extrapolation model. Additional information on scaling factors are reviewed by Travis and White (1988).

Even use of metabolic and pharmacokinetic models may not cover all bases for interspecies extrapolation, however. Clayson (1988) gives examples where differences in metabolism were thought to provide the reason for interspecies differences, but later other factors were shown to be responsible. These included detoxification; high background tumor rates in certain tissues for some laboratory test species, leading to increased tumor rates for agents that have primarily a promotional effect; and the effect of some agents on the endocrine system that may differ among species. The problem remains a difficult one, especially so because it is difficult to estimate the degree of error involved in assumptions that must be made. Greater application of biologically based cancer risk

TABLE 9-3 Differences in Human Risk by Scaling Technique

Experimental animal	Projected human risk for identical animal Dose (mg/kg) using indicated scaling method		
	mg/kg	mg/m^2 body wt	ppm in diet
Mouse	1	14	6
Rat	1	6	3

Source: From OTA, 1981.

models combined with the increasingly better data measuring interspecies differences are gradually reducing this problem.

In addition to extrapolating between species, variation within a species must be considered. Experimental animals are highly inbred to achieve homogeneity and reduce experimental error. The human population, however, is heterogeneous. This has the effect of a greater variation in susceptibility to cancer in the population than may appear random but is undoubtedly determined to some degree by genetic and other factors. These differences can be important when applying the results to different ethnic groups. These considerations are discussed further by Calabrese (1987).

SUMMARY

This chapter reviews methods to extrapolate animal bioassay data from high dose to low dose. It introduces commonly used models, discusses the multistage model in detail, and describes new, biologically based cancer risk models.

REFERENCES

Anderson, E.L. and the Carcinogen Assessment Group of the USEPA. 1983. Quantitative approaches in use to assess cancer risk. *Risk Analysis* 3:277-295.

Armitage, P. and R. Doll. 1954. The age distribution of cancer and a multistage theory of carcinogenesis, *Br. J. Cancer* 8:1-12.

Bliss, C.I. 1934. The method of probits. *Science* 79:38-39.

Bryan, W.R. and M.B. Shimkin. 1943. Quantitative analysis of dose–response data obtained with three carcinogenic hydrocarbons in strain C3H male mice. *J. Nat. Cancer Inst.* 3:503-531.

Calabrese, E.J. 1987. Animal extrapolation: a look inside the toxicologist's black box. *Environ. Sci. Technol.* 21:618-623.

Chen, J.J., R.L. Kodell, and D.W. Gaylor. 1988. Using the biological two-stage model to assess risk from short-term exposures. *Risk Analysis* 8:223-230.

Clayson, D.B. 1988. Needs for biological risk assessment in interspecies extrapolation. *Environ. Health Perspect.* 77:93-97.

Cornfield, J. 1977. Carcinogenic risk assessment. *Science* 198:693-699.

Crump, K.S. 1986. Methods for estimating human cancer risk from nonhuman data. In *Proceedings: New Directions on the Extrapolation of Health Risks from Animals to Man* (EPRI EA-447). Electric Power Research Institute, Palo Alto, CA, pp. 6-1–6-13.

Crump, K.S., D.G. Hoel, C.H. Langley, and R. Peto. 1976. Fundamental carcinogenic processes and their implications for low dose risk assessment. *Cancer Res.* 36:2973-2979.

Crump, K.S., H.A. Guess, and K.L. Deal. 1977. Confidence intervals and test of hypothesis concerning dose response relations inferred from animal carcinogenicity data. *Biometrics* 33:437-451.

Crump, K.S. and R.B. Howe. 1984. The multistage model with a time-dependent dose pattern: applications to carcinogenic risk assessment. *Risk Analysis* 4:163-176.

Crump, K.S. and R.B. Howe. 1985. A review of methods for calculating statistical confidence limits in low dose2 extrapolation. In D.B. Clayson, D. Krewski, and I. Munro (eds.), *Toxicological Risk Assessment*, Vol. I. CRC Press, Baco Raton, FL, pp. 187-203.

Danzer, H. 1934. Uber einige wirkungen von strahlen VII. *Physik* 89:421, as reported in Turner, 1975.

Dixon, R.L. 1976. Problems in extrapolating toxicity data for laboratory animals to man. *Environ. Health Perspect.* 13:43-50.

Food Safety Council. 1980. Quantitative risk assessment. *Food Cosmet. Toxicol.* 18:711-734.

Gaylor, D.W., J.J. Chen, and R.L. Kodell. 1985. Experimental design of bioassays for screening and low dose extrapolation. *Risk Analysis* 5:9-16.

Guess, H.A. and K.S. Crump. 1976. Low-dose extrapolation of data from animal carcinogenicity data. *Environ. Health Perspect.* 22:149-152.

Guess, H.A. and K.S. Crump. 1977. Can we use animal data to estimate "safe" doses for chemical carcinogens? In A. Whittemore (ed.), *Environmental Health Quantitative Methods*. SIAM Institute for Mathematics & Society, Philadelphia, pp. 13-28.

Guess, H., K. Crump, and R. Peto. 1977. Uncertainty estimates for low-dose-rate extrapolations of animal carcinogenicity data. Cancer Res. 37:3475-3483.

Guess, H.A. and K.S. Crump. 1978. Best-estimate low-dose extrapolation of carcinogenicity data. *Environ. Health Perspec.* 22:149–152.

Hill, T.A., R.C. Wands, and R.W. Leukroth, Jr. (eds.). 1988. Biological bases for interspecies extrapolation of carcinogenicity data, proceedings of a symposium, *Environ. Health Perspect.* 77:47-97.

Hoel, D. 1979. Low-dose and species-to-species extrapolation for chemically induced carcinogenesis. In V.K. McElheny and S. Abrahamson, (eds.), *Assessing Chemical Mutagens: the Risk to Humans*. Banbury Report No. 1, Cold Spring Harbor Laboratory, Cold Spring Harbor, NY.

Hoel, D.G. 1980. Incorporation of background in dose–response models. *Federation Proceedings* 39:73–75.

Hoel, D.G. N.L. Kaplan, and M.W. Anderson. 1983. Implication of nonlinear kinetics on risk estimation in carcinogenesis. *Science* 219:1032-1037.

Kodell, R.L., D.W. Gaylor, and J.J. Chen. 1987. Using average lifetime dose rate for intermittent exposures to carcinogens. *Risk Analysis* 7:339-345.

Krewski, D. and J. Van Ryzin. 1981. Dose response models for quantal response toxicity data. In M. Csorgo et al. (eds), *Statistics and Related Topics*. North-Holland Publishing Co., Amsterdam, pp. 201-232.

Lepkowski, W. 1978. Extrapolation of carcinogenesis data. *Environ. Health Perspect.* 22:173-181.

Mantel, N., N. Bohidar, C. Brown, J. Ciminera, and J. Tukey. 1975. An improved

Mantel–Bryan procedure for "safety" testing of carcinogens. *Cancer Res.* 35:865-872.

Mantel, N. and W.R. Bryan. 1961. Safety testing of carcinogenic agents. *J. Natl Cancer Inst.* 27:455-470.

Mantel, N. N.R. Bohidar, C.C. Brown, J.L. Ciminera, and J.W. Tukey. 1975. An improved Mantel–Bryan procedure for "safety" testing of carcinogens. *Cancer Res.* 35:865-872.

Mantel, N. and M. Schneiderman. 1975. Estimating "safe levels, a hazardous undertaking. *Cancer Res.* 35:1379-1386.

Meselson, M. (chairman). 1972. Report of the consultative panel on the health effects of chemical pesticides. National Academy of Sciences, Washington, D.C.

Moolgavkar, S.H. and D.J. Venzon. 1979. Two-event models for carcinogenesis: incidence curves for childhood and adult tumors. *Math. Biosci.* 47:55-77.

Moolgavkar, S.H. and A.G. Knudson, Jr. 1981. Mutation and cancer: a model for human carcinogenesis. *J. Natl Cancer. Inst.* 66:1037-1052.

Moolgavkar, S.H. 1983. Model for human carcinogenesis: action of environmental agents. *Environ. Health Perspect.* 50:285-291.

Moolgavkar, S.H., A. Dewanji, and D.J. Venzon. 1988. A stochastic two-stage model for cancer risk assessment. I. The hazard function and the probability of tumor. *Risk Analysis* 8:383-392.

Morris, S.C, H.C. Thode, Jr., J.I. Barancik, H. Fischer, P.D. Moskowitz, and J. Nagy. 1982. Methods for assessing cancer risks using animal and human data. Brookhaven National Laboratory, Upton, NY.

Morrison, P.F. 1987. Effects of time-variant exposure on toxic substance response. *Environ. Health Perspect.* 76:133-140.

Murdoch, D.J., D.R. Krewski, and K.S. Crump. 1987. Quantitative theories of carcinogenesis. In J.R. Thompson and B.W. Brown (eds.), *Cancer Modeling.* Marcel Dekker, Inc., New York, pp. 61-89.

Murdoch, D.J. and D. Krewski. 1988. Carcinogenic risk assessment with time-dependent exposure patterns. *Risk Analysis* 8:521-530.

NAS. 1986. Drinking Water and Health, Volume 6. Board on Toxicology and Environmental Health Hazards, National Research Council, R.D. Thomas (ed.). National Academy Press, Washington, D.C., pp. 254-255.

NTP. 1984. Report of the NTP ad hoc panel on chemical carcinogenesis testing and evaluation. Board of Scientific Counselors, National Toxicology Program, U.S. Public Health Service, Dept. of Health and Human Services.

Office of Technology Assessment. 1981. Assessment of technologies for determining cancer risks from the environment. U.S. Government Printing Office, Washington, D.C.

Peto, R. 1977. Epidemiology, multistage models, and short-term mutagenicity tests, in H.H. Hiatl, J.D. Watson and J.A. Winsten (eds.), *Origins of Human Cancer*, Cold Spring Harbor Laboratory, Cold Spring Harbor, N.Y. pp. 1403–1428.

Prentice, R.L. 19. A generalization of the probit and logit methods for dose response curves. *Biometrics* 32:761-768.

Rai, K. and J. Van Ryzin. 1979. Risk assessment of toxic environmental substances using a generalized multi-hit dose response model, in N.E. Breslow and A.S. Whittemore (eds.), *Energy and Health*, SIAM, Philadelphia, PA.

Scientific Committee of the Food Safety Council. 1980. *Food Cosmet. Toxicol.* 18:711-734.

Sielken, R.L., Jr. 1987. Cancer dose–response extrapolations. *Environ. Sci. Technol.* 21:1033-1039.

Tan, W.Y. and K.P. Singh. 1987. Assessing the effects of metabolism of environmental agents on cancer tumor development by a two-stage model of carcinogenesis. *Environ. Health Perspect.* 74:203-210.

Thompson, J.R. and B.W. Brown. 1987. *Cancer Modeling*. Marcel Dekker, Inc., New York.

Thorslund, T.W., C.C. Brown, and G. Charnley. 1987. Biologically motivated cancer risk models. *Risk Analysis* 7:109-119.

Travis, C.C. and R.K. White. 1988. Interspecific scaling of toxicity data. *Risk Analysis* 8:119-125.

Turner, M.E. 1975. Some classes of hit-theory models. *Math. Biosci.* 23:219-235.

Whittemore, A.S. 1979. Mathematical models of cancer and their use in risk assessment. SIMS Tech. Report. 27, Department of Statistics, Stanford University, Stanford, CA.

Wilson, J.D. 1986. Time for a change. *Risk Analysis* 6:111-112.

Wong, S.C.Y. 1984. Model uncertainty: Implications for animal low-dose cancer risk assessment experiments. Presented at·Society for Risk Analysis annual meeting, Knoxville, TN.

10

Quick Methods: Structure–Activity Relationships and Short-Term Bioassay

INTRODUCTION

Faced on one hand with thousands of potential chemical carcinogens in the environment and more being generated continuously as new chemical products or byproducts, and on the other with long-term animal testing requiring two years and half a million dollars just to get the beginnings of an answer on carcinogenicity on each chemical, regulators, policy makers, and scientists sought quicker answers. Organic chemists looked toward structure–activity relationships. What could be better than to be able to predict whether a compound was carcinogenic, and perhaps even its quantitative carcinogenic potency, simply from its molecular structure? The biologist looked to simpler lifeforms and biological indicators or precursors of tumors. With the development of the Ames test, which exposed a mutated bacterial culture to the chemical agent and measured revertants (back-mutation) as an index of the mutagenicity of the chemical, the biologists made a spectacular success. This test, and numerous others that followed, revolutionized our ability to test suspected carcinogenic agents. Compared to the half-million dollars or more for long-term animal tests, short-term bioassays can be conducted quickly for $1000 to $10,000 per chemical. In a period of about one decade, nearly 10,000 compounds have been tested in at least one short-term mutagenicity assay (Guidelines, 1986). While not as spectacular, the chemists made steady gains and structure-activity relationships have found an important niche in the process of identifying carcinogens.

While these quick methods have firmly established a role in the cancer assessment process, have become key techniques in the research area, and are undoubtedly the direction of the future, they are not yet sufficiently reliable to be the sole basis of regulatory action or quantitative cancer risk estimates.

225

STRUCTURE–ACTIVITY RELATIONSHIPS

The effect of a chemical pollutant on target tissues is believed to be a result of specific molecular interactions. Thus, the physiochemical properties associated with the molecular structure of the chemical pollutant determine the response of the biological system (McKinney, 1984). A thorough understanding of these structure-activity relationships (SAR) would make easy work of identifying carcinogens. A chemist could determine the molecular structure and know immediately if the compound could cause cancer. It is even possible to envision quantifying this relationship (QCRA) to predict the potency of carcinogens. This would eliminate the need for toxicology in QCRA. This ideal state has not yet arrived, but SAR does have something to offer now, particularly in the hazard assessment step of QCRA.

Early groundwork for subsequent work on SAR was laid in the 1870s (Kland, 1977). Since the 1930s, many useful drugs have been developed by applying knowledge of SAR (Craig and Enslein, 1981). The field has become very sophisticated and is an important method of developing new and more effective drugs today. Use of SAR in drug development, however, involves exploring modifications to chemicals for which much information is available concerning biological effect and the relationship between molecular structure and that effect.

By comparison, chemical carcinogens include a wide variety of structural types of compounds. Many have more than one functional group (e.g., the halogen or amino group) and, except for selected classes, there is no evidence that biological activity is determined by functional group (Rosenkranz et al., 1984). SAR is a potentially useful predictive tool for cancer risk assessment but, to date, has had limited impact. One reason is the lack of clear cancer dose–response information on which to base studies correlating molecular structure with carcinogenic activity. Understanding of SAR comes from analysis of a large number of compounds for which structure and biological response are known. To learn which chemical structures are predictive of carcinogenicity, one must know which compounds are carcinogenic and which are not. As we have seen earlier (Chap. 8), the latter is not always a clearcut decision.

Craig and Enslein (1981) note, for example, that a potent carcinogen such as aflatoxin B_1 can clearly be termed "carcinogenic," but it is difficult to make such a positive and conclusive assignment for weaker carcinogens. Available data from animal experiments leaves much to be desired for structural activity comparisons. The cost and time involved in animal testing limits the amount of data available. Data limitations result in all the data being used for model development, leaving none for validation (see Chap. 15). The number of animals that can practically be included in such experiments limits the reliability of the results. Differences among species create confusion; a compound may cause tumors in one species but not another or cause tumors in different tissues in different species. At least with current knowledge, SAR is oversensitive. There are structural characteristics which are common to most organic chemical carcinogens (Table 10-1). Presence of one of these characteristics in a compound is suggestive of carcinogenicity, but each characteristic also appears in noncarcinogens. So the suggestion is merely tentative and must be confirmed by bioassay (Ashby, 1985). SAR can prove a useful prescreening method, however, for identifying and setting priorities for the more expensive and lengthy bioassays.

Short-term mutagenesis tests (discussed below) provide a much larger data set with a better defined degree of reproducibility for studying SAR (e.g., Vance and Levin, 1984). This is a highly useful approach, but if the activity is mutation in bacteria, the SAR still includes the uncertainty of the relationship between that effect and the ability to produce tumors in the whole animal. Apparent carcinogens are often actually just metabolic precursors of the true carcinogen (see Chap. 7). Relating the structure of the compound administered to the animal to the carcinogenic response leads down a false path if the metabolite which actually evokes the response has a different structure. Variations in experimental protocol such as animal diet, dosing schedule, and route of administration all act to limit the number of consistent experiments that can be included in the analysis. SAR can also be of use here. There are structural features which may prevent absorption or facilitate detoxification or rapid excretion of a compound (Table 10-2). A chemical which does not reach sensitive

TABLE 10-1 Structural Features of
Molecules Suggesting Carcinogenicity

Arylamine functions
Ring epoxides
Alkane sulphonate esters
Arylnitro functions
Azo groups, ring N-oxides and -NMe2 groups
Methylols and aliphatic aldehydes
Ring vinyl groups
Aziridines, nitrogen mustards, and chloramines
Benzyl halides
Alkylnitrosamines
Alkylurethanes

Source: From Ashby, 1985.

TABLE 10-2 Structural Features of Molecules
Which May Lead to Non-absorption, Detoxification, or Rapid Excretion in Mammals

Sulfonic or carboxylic acids
Hydroxymethyl
Alkylketones
Ionic groups
Thiophene ring

Source: From Ashby, 1985.

tissue in its mutagenic form does not cause cancer. Even a reduced dosage
at the sensitive tissue will appear as a reduced potency in animals.

An application important for risk management is the use of SAR to
find noncarcinogenic substitutes for carcinogenic industrial chemicals or
to treat carcinogenic pollutant emissions before release. As in developing
new drugs, the molecular structure is the link between the biologist and
the chemist. As an example, dye manufacturing has historically been an
industry associated with carcinogens and increased cancer risk to workers.
Phenylenediamines are one of the chemical classes used in this industry
thought to contribute to this risk. Milman and Peterson (1984) found
several structural changes that could reduce carcinogenicity. One was
oxidation of one of the NH_2, groups in the molecule to NO_2, which
substantially reduced the carcinogenicity of 1,3,-phenylenediamines in animal bioassays.

Several approaches to SAR have been developed. These are described briefly below. A more detailed description is provided by Craig
and Enslein (1981). The first was an intuitive approach. This uses the so
called additivity model which assumes that each structural feature of a
molecule has a consistent role in the overall biologic activity. Given
enough examples one can determine the role of each feature. The activity
of molecules with various combinations of features can then be determined. Data on a large number of compounds are required, however.

Another approach is multiparameter analysis. In this, biologic activity
is correlated with one or more physical chemical properties of the compound. A common property is the n-octanol/water partition coefficient.
The relationship is derived empirically and can hold only for closely
related compounds.

A third approach is substructural analysis. This involves small fragments of a few connected atoms and bonds with computer searching of
a large database with detailed structural data on thousands of compounds.
Pattern recognition methods have also been used.

Finally, quantum chemical approaches use quantum chemistry calculations to obtain electronic indices representing the structure of the compounds.

To give some examples of results of SAR analysis, Craig and Enslein (1981) reported on a study of 416 compounds. Since no uniform endpoint was available, the analysis aimed to predict the probability that a substance was mutagenic. The relationship of various structural properties of these compounds were compared to the qualitative finding of mutagenicity for the compound. The most important properties predicting mutagenicity (in terms of their statistical significance) were: one benzene ring, branching terminal nitro group, generic halogen chain fragment, more than two carbocyclic or aromatic rings, more than one single heterocyclic ring unfused to any other ring, three-branch nitrogen atom, single occurrence of carbonyl in more than one ring, two benzene rings, single occurrence of carbonyl in a ring, one single heterocyclic ring unfused to any other ring, and a generic halogen substitute fragment. In all, 48 properties were included in the predictive equation. A score was calculated for mutagenicity and one for nonmutagenicity and the probability of mutagenicity was calculated from these scores. Taking a predicted probability of over 60% as mutagenic, a probability of less than 40% as nonmutagenic, and a predicted probability between 40 and 60% as indeterminate, the model had a false positive rate of 11% and a false negative rate of 8%.

Using a similar set of descriptors of structural properties, they (Craig and Enslein, 1981) analyzed a set of 99 mutagens for which mutagenicity could be quantified in terms of revertants per nanomole (R/nmol). An equation of 15 structural parameters was able to explain 75% of the variance in the quantitative values of mutagenic potency of the compounds. An enhanced version of this model (Enslein and Craig, 1982) provides a capability of calculating the probability that a compound is carcinogenic, based on substructural compounds or "fragment keys."

Rosenkranz and co-workers (1984) described an application of their Computer-Automated Structure-Evaluation (CASE) program. Drawing on a large database of coded information on molecular structure and a ranking (1 through 10) of the biologic activity of each in several different assays, the model will analyze any molecule submitted and predict its expected biologic activity based on evaluation of molecular fragments. The usefulness of such a method is illustrated by the case of nitrated polycyclic aromatic hydrocarbons (nitroarenes). Compounds of this class have been identified in diesel exhaust emissions, side-stream cigarette smoke, photocopy toners, and ambient air. While over 200 compounds in this group have been identified, only about 50 have been bioassayed. Many of those have been shown to be potent mutagens. Because of technical difficulties with preparation and purification and the associated costs, systematic bioassay of the remaining 150 compounds is impracticable. Two molecular fragments were found to be associated with mutagenicity in this class of compounds and two were deactivating. A nitroarene which includes one of the former but neither of the later would be predicted to be mutagenic. Verification of the accuracy of these predictions is incomplete, but the results can help to prioritize the testing of the remaining 150 compounds. Because CASE can compare among data from several bioassay systems, information can be obtained on which bioassays are sensitive to each structural fragment associated with mutagenicity. Thus, the method not only can identify which chemicals should be tested first, but can aid in selecting the specific bioassays that would be most effective. Beyond this role of guiding further bioassay for a class of compounds, CASE can be used to advance overall understanding on carcinogenesis by determining to what extent the various biologic indices used all respond to the same aspects of molecular structure. For example, induction of DNA adducts, of specific mutations, of chromosomal aberrations, and of tumor development are all taken as indicators of carcinogenic potential. Understanding of their relationship and reliance on the simpler bioassays would be greater if it could be demonstrated that the same structural characteristics of a chemical agent affected them all. On the other hand, if they were affected by different structural characteristics, identification of the differences could lead to better understanding of the relationships among them.

Summary

Methods of defining the molecular structure of a chemical compound are advanced and large databases are available. Several approaches to SAR and QSAR have been developed and tested, demonstrated, and used extensively in development of pharmaceuticals. The methods rely on large amounts of empirical data, however. In the case of chemical carcinogenesis, reliable data from whole animal bioassay is scarce and subject to uncertainties. This has limited the success of SAR in carcinogenic risk assessment. The increasing availability of data from bacterial mutagenesis testing has allowed considerable advances in applications of SAR. These results, of course, are subject to the same limitations as the mutagenesis bioassays themselves in their application to cancer risk assessment (discussed further below). For now it appears that SAR is in a strong position to aid in the hazard assessment process and to help to guide further biologic testing in the dose-response assessment process. It has an important additional role in the development of better basic understanding of the underpinnings of chemical carcinogenesis. The further along this latter role is pushed, the greater the role which will be available to SAR in the QCRA process.

SHORT-TERM BIOASSAY

There are over 100 short-term bioassay systems. A few of the more frequently used bioassays are listed in Table 10-3. Reviews describing individual test systems are available (Hollstein and Ashby, 1979; de Serres and Ashby, 1981). These test systems are based on four principal biological endpoints: gene mutation, chromosomal effects, general DNA damage, and neoplastic transformation. Each of these are discussed below (based largely on OSTP, 1984).

Gene Mutation Tests

The most widely known and practically reliable short-term in vitro genotoxicity bioassay is the Ames test (Ames et al., 1973). This is also the system for which the largest number of chemicals have been evaluated. A strain of the bacteria *Salmonella typhimurium* is genetically altered to require histidine. The sensitivity of the bacteria to mutation is then increased by removing normal cell defense mechanisms and modifying the outside of the bacteria to allow large molecules to get through its cell membrane. When exposed to a mutagen, the bacteria undergoes reverse mutation back to its normal state. This exposure is made in a culture with just a trace of histidine so that only colonies of the revertants grow. These can be counted in 48-72 hours.

Many environmental chemicals are not themselves mutagenic, but have metabolites which are. Thus, a bioassay which tests only the mutagenicity of the original chemical would not be very useful. This problem was solved by including a mix of homogenized rat liver microsomal enzymes in the test system. This is called the S9 fraction, and the Ames test is usually done with and without S9 to determine the direct and indirect mutagenic potential of the chemical. Liver cells are an appropriate choice since much of the metabolism of environmental chemicals takes place in the liver. Of course, an environmental chemical taken into the body is metabolized by various enzyme systems in different organs. Moreover, S9 preparation in a Petri dish may yield different metabolites than would be produced in vivo. Because of its ease of preparation, capability to activate many chemical classes, and its relative nontoxicity to the bacterial test strain, S9 remains the most commonly used activating agent in bacterial gene mutation bioassay. Efforts to obtain more realistic metabolites in the tests, however, led to the development of two additional approaches. One is to replace the liver homogenate with intact cells.

TABLE 10-3 Commonly Used Short-Term Bioassays for Potential Carcinogens

Type of assay	Endpoint	Reference
Mutation:		
Salmonella typhimurium	Histidine reversion	Ames et al., 1973
Escherichia coli	Tryptophan reversion	Brusick et al., 1980
Mouse lymphoma	Thymidine kinase (TK)	Clive et al., 1983
Chinese hamster ovary (CHO)	Hypoxanthine guanine phosphoribosyl transferase (HGPRT)	Hsie et al., 1981
Chinese hamster lung	HGPRT	Bradley et al., 1981
Human lymphoblasts	TK, HGPRT	Thilly et al., 1980
Chromosome effects:		
Many cell types in vitro and in vivo	Chromosomal aberrations	Latt et al., 1981
		Preston et al., 1981
	Sister chromatid exchanges	
	Micronuclei	
	Chromosoma gain or loss	
	Translocation	
DNA damage:		
Unscheduled DNA synthesis (UDA)	Radioactive nucleoside incorporation	Mitchell et al, 1983
Repair deficient bacteria	Differential growth inhibition	Leifer et al., 1981
Mammalian cell transformation:		
Syrian hamster embryo (SHE)	Altered cellular morphology and growth pattern, growth in soft agar, tumorigenicity	Heidelberger et al., 1983
Viral-enhanced-mediated Syrian hamster embryo		Heidelberger et al., 1983

Source: From OSTP, 1984.

These may be more likely to produce realistic metabolites, but have other difficulties. The chemical being tested may not be taken up by the cells or the metabolite may not make the transfer from the activation cell to the test bacteria. Homogenization makes this process smoother. Also, the cells often lose their metabolic capability over time and fresh cultures must continually be prepared. The second approach is much more ingenious, but involves even greater difficulty. The indicator organism is actually introduced into a live animal's body (e.g., into the blood stream). The chemical to be tested is then administered to the animal and sometime later, samples of the test organism are taken and tested for mutation.

Different salmonella tester strains are specific for a particular mutagenic action, and therefore to a specific class of mutagenic agents. Some classes of chemicals do not respond at all in the Ames test, although they have been shown to be mutagenic in other test systems or in humans. These include halogenated hydrocarbons and metals. A recent analysis by the International Program on Chemical Safety identified eight organics (Table 10-4), known to be human or animal carcinogens, which tested negative in the Ames test (Ashby et al., 1985). Some materials are difficult to test (i.e., gases) and the assay is made on extracts rather than the original material.

Qualitative reproducibility of the Ames test is reasonably good. In a test involving seven laboratories and a total of 756 samples, there was about 85% agreement between the Ames test results (mutagenic or nonmutagenic) and expected results based on consensus in the literature (Myers et al., 1987).

Many other microbial systems and cultured mammalian somatic cell systems have been developed which can detect either forward or reverse mutation (see Table 10-3 for examples). Mammalian cell assays are not as simple, rapid, and efficient as the Ames test. They require weeks rather than days to complete. Another disadvantage of tests using mammalian cells, such as the Chinese hamster ovary (CHO) assay, is that their results do not always show the precision characteristic of bacterial tests.

TABLE 10-4 Chemical Carcinogens Which Test Negative in the Ames Test

o-Toluidine
Safrole
Diethylstilbestrol
Benzene
Acrylonitrile
Diethylhexylphthalate
Phenobarbital

Source: From Ashby et al., 1985.

This seems, however, to reflect only methodological difficulties (Frazier and Samuel, 1985). Their advantage is that, although the chemical substance of the DNA is the same, mammalian cells are different structurally than bacterial cells and so may provide results more meaningful for people.

All are tests of the ability of the chemical being tested to interact with DNA in a way which will result in mutation. None of the specific gene loci and mutation types used in these systems are believed to be related to specific mutations which are involved in tumor initiation. In vitro gene mutation bioassays remain useful to predict the potential of a chemical pollutant to cause cancer, but require one to assume that in vitro metabolic conditions successfully mimic metabolism in vivo and that a somatic mutation can result in formation of a tumor. The performance of these bioassays can be tested by comparing them with the results of long-term animal bioassays. Early studies showed concordances (percentage of qualitative agreements between results and rodent carcinogenicity tests) of over 90%, particularly for the Ames test (McCann et al., 1975). A difficulty in making such a comparison, however, was that, since animal bioassays are so expensive, they were mostly done on chemicals that proved positive on simpler tests or otherwise are strongly suspected of being carcinogens. There were too few animal bioassay results on noncarcinogens to provide a good test that negative results in an in vitro test correlate well with negative results for tumors in whole animals. A new study (Tennant et al., 1987) compared four short-term, in vitro assays (the Ames test, the mouse lymphoma cell mutagenesis assay, and chromosome aberrations and sister chromatid exchange in Chinese hamster ovary cells) with 2-year rodent carcinogenicity studies conducted with the standard National Toxicology Program protocol. Of 73 chemicals tested, 60 were tumorigenic in at least one site in one of the four sex and species combinations in the rodent studies. The other 40% were nontumorigenic in the rodent studies. Concordance ranged from 60 to 62% for the four short-term assays, much lower than earlier studies. Disappointingly, no combination of the short-term tests could do much better; the concordance of the best combination was only 67%. It had been hoped that a battery of two or more tests would be much better, one test making up for the shortcomings of another. As a reference point, however, it is noteworthy that the concordance between rat and mouse carcinogenicity data for the 73 chemicals was also only 67%.

Short-Term In Vivo Assays

In vitro tests can show that a chemical has the potential to initiate a process leading to cancer, but this is only one requirement for the chemical actually to produce an increase in cancer in live animals. It is important to distinguish between materials that can cause mutations in some organism and those that actually do pose risks to people. It may not be necessary to immediately jump to long-term animal studies, however. One recommendation is " . . . that mutagenicity tests should be selected not for their association with carcinogenicity per se, but for their ability to detect the different classes of mutations in vivo . . . " (Guidelines, 1986).

Ashby (1983) proposed that two short-term genotoxicity assays conducted in whole animals be used to follow-up positive in vitro tests. The first was a rodent bone marrow micronucleus assay (Ashby, 1983) and the second the liver UDS assay (Mirsalis and Butterworths, 1980). Agents inactive in both in vivo assays would be judged to be unlikely to pose a significant human carcinogenic hazard. These two assays are able to effectively discriminate between those carcinogens and noncarcinogens that give positive results in vitro (de Serres and Matsushima, 1987); that is, they could act effectively as a second-round screen to eliminate false positives produced by in vitro bioassays.

Short-term in vivo bioassays take advantage of model systems which have a high background cancer rate, and thus a presumed high sensitivity to cancer induction. This leads, however, to the possibility that the effect being measured may be a decrease in latent period rather than an increase in tumor incidence. Other-short term in vivo assays (de Serres and Matsushima) include: (1) the well-known mouse skin model, widely used for initiation-promotion experiments. Tumorigenic effects can be detected in as little as 10 weeks in this test. (2) Breast cancer induction in female Sprague-Dawley rats. An injected carcinogen produces a high incidence of multiple mammary tumors in 9 months. (3) A rat liver initiation-promotion assay. One group of rats are used to test cancer promotion properties of a chemical. They are given a dose of diethylnitrosamine (DEN) to initiate hepatocarcinogenesis, and then given the test chemical. A second group of rats tests for initiation. They are injected with NaCl instead of DEN, followed by the test chemical. The third group of rats serves as the control; they are given only DEN. The livers of all three groups are assayed after eight weeks. Of the 18 known hepatocarcinogens, 16 scored positive for promotion; 8 known nonhepatocarcinogens scored negative.

Other Short-Term Tests

Although no causal associations are known, specific chromosomal rearrangements (or aberrations) have increasingly been linked with cancer (Yunnis, 1983). Sister chromatid exchanges (SCE) are also believe to result from DNA damage, but no correlation between frequency of SCE and heritable changes in cells has been demonstrated. Tests based on chromosomal effects are highly attractive since they can be done on cultured cells or on cells easily obtained from live animals or people. SCE do not occur in bacterial cells. Direct measures of DNA damage and repair include tests of unscheduled DNA synthesis (UDS), techniques to measure DNA strand breaks, and DNA- adducts (the binding of chemicals to DNA, presumably with associated damage). Finally, test systems using cells derived from rodent embryos have been developed to take advantage of findings that specific morphological changes in cultured cells increase the likelihood that these cells will induce tumors when inoculated in animals.

Non-Genotoxic Tests

While the predominant notion of carcinogenesis involves damage to DNA as an initiating factor, some chemicals appear to induce cancer without involving DNA, perhaps through interruption of cell-to-cell communication or simply by increasing cell proliferation. Short-term tests such as the cell transformation assay (Heidelberger et al., 1983) have been developed to detect such chemicals. There is still a need for further improvement in detecting promoting activity in short-term tests (NAS, 1986).

Limitations on Interpretation and Direct Quantitative Application

Despite the success of in vitro bioassays, and the ease with which their results can be expressed quantitatively, Ashby (1986) marks them inherently ill-suited for estimating quantitative carcinogenic potency. One difficulty is the lack of quantitative consistency between these bioassays and results in long-term animal studies and human epidemiology, although quantitative comparisons are difficult and little evidence is available to support a conclusion. One such comparison for roofing tar, coke oven gas, and cigarette smoke condensate is shown in Table 10-5.

Direct use of quantitative estimates from short-term bioassays depends in part of their reproducibility. Following an extensive multilaboratory test of reproducibility of quantitative results, Myers et al. (1987) warns that, "Scientists must be aware that individual single assays of different chemicals do not contain the information needed to compare the chemicals unless concurrent assays are done under identical conditions (same day, same laboratory, same analyst or team, same preparation, same batches of cells and S9, and so forth). Unfortunately, this is not practical in most cases." For single assays in different labs, the ratio of dose-response slope (revertants/μg) must be greater than 16 to have only an even chance of

TABLE 10-5 Comparison of Relative Potencies of Emission Extracts in Several Bioassay Systems

	Human lung cancer	Mouse skin tumor initiation	Mouse skin cancer	Mouse lymphoma cell mutation	Ames TA98
Coke oven	1.0	1.0	1.0	1.0	1.0
Roofing tar	0.39	0.20	0.20	1.4	0.78
CSC	0.0024	0.0011	–	0.066	0.52

Source: From Albert et al., 1983.
CSC is cigarette smoke condensate.

finding a statistically significant difference at the 5% level, and over 100 to assure an 80% power of detecting the difference. There are other sources of artifactual differences in results which must be considered. Modifications of standard protocols, differing procedures within protocols, or even properties of the test compound can have critical effects on the results. This not only implies that results may be faulty in assays done by less-than-experts, but that, even done expertly, there may be differences among laboratories testing the same substance or artifactual quantitative differences among different substances. These are explored by Gatehouse (1987): (1) Relatively small changes in pH or osmotic pressure can cause significant changes in mutation frequency and chromosomal damage in mammalian cells. Bacterial assays are less sensitive to such environmental changes. (2) Solvents used to dissolve materials being tested can affect the results. A commonly used solvent (dimethylsulfoxide) decomposes to form toxic and mutagenic products. (3) The size of the bacterial inoculum is generally not reported, but can influence the results. Very large numbers of bacteria may be necessary to detect weakly mutagenic agents. (4) Cells in a logarithmic growth phase are more sensitive to mutagens. (5) The stability of different enzymes in the S9 fraction varies with storage. (6) The concentration of S9 fraction must be optimized to the compound being tested, a complex procedure. (7) Presence of histidine in biologic fluids can increase the number of revertants, creating problems in testing of urine and fecal samples.

Complex Mixtures

Short-term bioassays have frequently been used to examine mutagenicity of complex mixtures. Despite the difficulties in interpreting test results discussed above, much useful information can be gained. For example, comparison of Ames test results with and without a metabolizing agent on extracts from increasing volumes of air outdoors and at various locations under different conditions indoors showed mutagenic components of indoor air particles to be different from those of outdoor particles, and to be heavily dominated by cigarette smoke and cooking products (van Houdt et al., 1984).

The simplicity and speed of short-term bioassays make them ideal for "taking apart" the mixture to find the key mutagenic agents and to examine the relative contribution of each component and the interactions among components. They are probably the only indicators of cancer risk which have the characteristics of speed, low cost, and capability of producing results with small samples of material which are necessary to couple with extensive chemical fractionation needed to directly examine interactions within complex mixtures.

An ideal example is a detective story with a gratifying ending (Mermelstein et al., 1982). Extracts of xerographic copies were found to be mutagenic in the Ames test. The source of the mutagenicity was traced to a toner, and then to a specific type of carbon black used in the toner. Repeated chemical fractionation combined with Ames testing of the fractions identified a neutral polar fraction containing only 3% of the mass but 85% of the mutagenicity. The particular compounds responsible for most of this were identified as 1,6- and 1,8-dinitropyrene. The manufacturer of the carbon black was able to reduce the amount of nitropyrenes, and copies made with toners using the modified carbon black did not test as mutagenic.

Extensive work sponsored by the Department of Energy and the Environmental Protection Agency have advanced the coupling of chemistry and mutagenic bioassay in evaluating difficult complex mixtures such as air pollution, diesel exhaust, and synthetic fuel products and byproducts (Albert et al., 1983; Wilson et al., 1981; Wright et al., 1983; Haugen and Stamoudis, 1986; Gray, 1986). Although several different schemes have been developed, all have the same basic approach. In this approach, the complex material is tested in short-term bioassay, then fractionated by some relatively standard chemical methods such as filtering, extraction, gas chromatography, and liquid chromatography. Each fraction is then screened by one or more short-term mutagenic bioassays. Fractions shown to contain biologically active agents are further fractionated and the subfractions bioassayed. Additional fractionation, chemical analysis, and bioassay may be done. The result is that the subclasses of material in the complex mixture, which contain the mutagenic agents, and possibly the specific mutagenic chemical compounds themselves, can be identified.

Furthermore, by comparing the quantitative results of bioassays at each stage, one can explore the nature of synergisms and antagonisms in the mixture. This is limited by the uncertainties in quantitative results of the tests. Even rough explorations along these lines, however, can be useful in furthering general understanding of toxicological properties of complex mixtures and projecting the changing toxicity as the mixture changes with time and environmental exposure or identifying possible methods of reducing the mutagenicity of the mixture in a specific case. The same procedure can then be used to explore the effectiveness of various control options. For example, in a synthetic fuels process, modification of process temperature produces a different complex mixture. In the case of a specific coal liquification process, the principal mutagenic activity was identified with polycyclic primary aromatic amines with some additional contribution from azarenes and polar-substituted aromatics (Gray, 1986).

SUMMARY

Short-term bioassays, primarily in vitro, provide valuable tools for research and prescreening of potential carcinogens. Their quick turnaround and relatively low cost make possible studies which simply could not be done with long-term animal bioassay such as detailed analysis of complex mixtures. They are not designed for amateur use, however. They are complex, technically and professionally demanding procedures, and require skilled scientists to perform them properly and to interpret results. They cannot provide the final determination of the question of carcinogenicity nor have they been acceptable for quantitative dose-response functions, although many short-term tests can provide quantitative results. They do provide additional information that can be used in conjunction with animal or epidemiological results in both qualitative and quantitative interpretation (see Chap. 12). As an example, they can aid in determining whether an agent causes cancer by directly affecting genetic material, or if it has a more peripheral role.

REFERENCES

Albert, A.E., J. Lewtas, S. Nesnow, T.W. Thorslund, and E. Anderson. 1983. Comparative potency method for cancer risk assessment: application to diesel particulate emissions. *Risk Analysis* 3:101-117.

Ames, B.N. W.E. Durston, E. Yamasaki, and F.D. Lee. 1973. Carcinogens are mutagens: a simple test system combining liver homogenates for activation and bacteria for detection. *Proc. Natl. Acad. Sci.* 69:3128-3132.

Ashby, J. 1986. Genetic toxicology in industry: perspectives and initiatives. In P. Ofteldl and A. Brogger (eds.), *Risk and Reason: Risk Assessment in Relation*

to Environmental Mutagens and Carcinogens. Alan R. Liss, Inc., New York,
pp. 89-94.

Bradley, M.O., B. Bhuyan, M.C. Francis, R. Langenbach, A. Peterson, and E.
Huberman. 1981. Mutagenesis by chemical agents in V79 Chinese hamster
cells: a review and analysis of the literature, a report of the Gene-Tox Program. *Mutat. Res.* 87:81-142.

Brusick, D.J., V.F. Simmon, K.S. Rosenkranz, V.A. Ray, and R.S. Stafford.
1980. An evaluation of the *Escherichia coli* WP 425 and WP425 urvA reverse
mutation assay. *Mutat. Res.* 76:191-215.

Claxton, L.D. 1982. Review of fractionation and bioassay characterization tech-
niques for the evaluation of organics associated with ambient air particles.
In R.R. Tice, D.L. Costa, and K.M. Schaich (eds.), *Genotoxic Effects of
Airborne Agents.* Plenum Press, New York, pp. 19-34.

Clive, D., R. McCuen, J.F.S. Spector, C. Piper, and K.H. Mavournin. 1983.
Specific gene mutations in L5178Y cells in culture, a report of the U.S. EPA
Gene-Tox Program. *Mutat. Res.* 115:22-251.

Craig, P.N. and K. Enslein. 1981. Structure-activity in hazard assessment. In
J. Saxena and F. Fisher (eds.), *Hazard Assessment of Chemicals: Current
Development*, vol. 1. Academic Press, New York, pp. 389-420.

de Serres, F.J. and J. Ashby (eds.). 1981. *Evaluation of Short-term Tests for
Carcinogens: Report of the International Collaborative Program.* Elsevier/
North Holland Publishers, New York.

de Serres, F.J. and T. Matsushima. 1987. Deployment of short-term assays for
environmental mutagens and carcinogens. *Mutat. Res.* 182:173-184.

Enslein, K. and P.N. Craig. 1982. Carcinogenesis: a predictive structure-activity
model. *J. Toxicol. and Environ. Health* 10:521-530.

Frazier, M.E. and J.E. Samuel. 1985. Genotoxicity of complex mixtures: CHO
cell mutagenicity Assay (PNL-5337). Battelle Pacific Northwest Laboratory,
Richland, WA.

Gatehouse, D. 1987. Guidelines for testing of environmental agents, critical features of bacterial mutation assays. *Mutagenisis* 2:397-409.

Gray, R.H. 1986. Coal liquefaction process development: solving potential health
and environmental problems. *Energy* 11:1337-1346.

Guidelines. 1986. Guidelines on the use of mutagenicity tests in the toxicological
evaluation of chemicals, a report of the Environmental Contaminants Advisory Committee on Mutagenesis. Department of National Health and Welfare,
Ottawa, Canada.

Haugen, D.A. and V.C. Stamoudis. 1986. Isolation and identification of mutagenic
polycyclic aromatic hydrocarbons from a coal gasifier condensate. *Environ.
Res.* 41:400-419.

Heidelberger, C., A.E. Freeman, R.J. Pienta, A. Sivak, J.S. Bertram, B.C. Casto,
V.C. Dunkel, M.W. Francis, T. Kakunaga, J.B. Little, and L.M. Schechtman.
1983. CEil transformation by chemical agents - a review and analysis of the
literature. *Mutat. Res.* 114:283-385.

Hollstein, M., J. McCann, F.A. Angelosanto, and W.W. Nichlos. 1979. Short-
term tests for carcinogens and mutagens. *Mutat. Res.* 65:133-226.

Hsie, A.W., D.A. Casciano, D.B. Couch, D.F. Krahn, J.P. O'Neill, and B.L. Whitfield. 1981. The use of Chinese hamster ovary cells to quantify specific locus mutation and to determine mutagenicity of chemicals, a report of the Gene-Tox Program. *Mutat. Res.* 86:193-214.

Kland, M.J. 1977. A priori predictive methods of assessing health effects of chemicals in the environment. LBL-6372. Lawrence Berkeley Laboratory.

Latt, S.A., J. Allen, S.E. Bloom, A. Carrano, E. Falke, D. Kram, E. Schneider, R. Schreck, R. Tice, B. Whitfield, and S. Wolff. 1981. Sister-chromatid exchanges: a report of the Gene-Tox Program. *Mutat. Res.* 87:17-62.

Leifer, Z., T. Kada, M. Mandel, E. Zeiger, R. Stafford, and H.S. Rosenkranz. 1981. An evaluation of tests using DNA repair-deficient bacteria for predicting genotoxicity and carcinogenicity, a report of the U.S. EPA Gene-tox Program. *Mutat. Res.* 87:211-297.

McCann, J., E. Choi, E. Yamasaki, and B.N. Ames. 1975. Detection of carcinogens as mutagens in the salmonella/microsome test: assay of 300 chemicals. *Proc. Natl Acad. Sci.* 72:5135-5139.

McKinney, J. 1984. The molecular basis of chemical toxicity. In *Proceedings of the DOE-OHER Workshop on Monitoring and Dosimetry* (CONF-8403150). U.S. Department of Energy, Washington, D.C., p. 91.

Mermelstein, R., H.S. Rosenkranz, and E.C. McCoy. 1982. The microbial mutagenicity of nitroarenes, in R.R. Tice, D.L. Costa, and K.M. Schaich (eds.), *Genotoxic Effects of Airborne Agents*, Plenum Press, New York, pp. 369–396.

Milman, H.A. and C. Peterson. 1984. Apparent correlation between structure and carcinogenicity of phenylenediamines and related compounds. *Environ. Health Perspect.* 56:261-273.

Mirsalis, J.C. and B.E. Butterworth. 1980. Induction of unscheduled DNA synthesis in hepatocytes isolated from rats treated with genotoxic agents: an in vivo/in vitro assay for potential carcinogens and mutagens. *Carcinogenesis* 1:621–625.

Mitchell, A.D., D.A. Casciano, M.L. Meltz, D.E. Robinson, R.H.C. San, G.M Williams, and E.S. von Halle. 1983. Unscheduled DNA synthesis tests. a report of the U.S. EPA Gene-Tox Program. *Mutat. Res.* 123:363-410.

Myers, L.E., N.H. Adams, T.J. Hughes, L.R. Williams, and L.D. Claxton. 1987. An interlaboratory study of an EPA/Ames/Salmonella test protocol. *Mutat. Res.* 182:121-133.

NAS. 1986. *Drinking Water and Health*, Vol. 6. Safe Drinking Water Committee, National Research Council. National Academy Press, Washington, D.C.

Nesnow, S. and J. Lewtas. 1981. Mutagenic and carcinogenic potency of extracts of diesel and related environmental emissions: summary and discussion of the results. *Environ. Int.* 5:425-429.

OSTP. 1984. Chemical carcinogens; notice of review of the science and its associated principles. Office of Science and Technology Policy. *Fed. Reg.* 49:21594-21661.

Preston, R.J., W. Au, M.A. Bender, J.G. Brewen, A.V. Carrano, J.A. Heddle, A.F. McFee, S. Wolff, and J.S. Wassom. 1981. Mammalian in vivo and in vitro cytogenetic assays: a report of the U.S. EPA Gene-Tox Program. *Mutat. Res.* 87:143-188.

Rosenkranz, H.S., G. Klopman, V. Chjankong, J. Pet-Ewards, and Y.Y. Haimes. 1984. Prediction of environmental carcinogens. *Environ. Mutagen.* 6:231-258.

Tennant, R.W., B.H. Margolin, M.D. Shelby, E. Zeiger, J.K. Haseman, J. Spalding, W. Caspary, M. Resnick, S. Stasiewicz, H. Anderson, and R. Minor. 1987. Prediction of chemical carcinogenicity in rodents from in vitro genetic toxicity assays. *Science* 236:933-941.

Thilly, W.G., J.G. DeLuca, E.E. Furth, H. Ohppe, D.A. Kaden, H.L. Kralewski Liber, T.R. Skopek, S.A. Slapikoff, R.J. Tizard, and B.W. Penman. 1980. Genelocus mutation assays in diploid human lymphoblast lines. In F.L. de Serres and A. Hollaender (eds.), *Chemical Mutagens*, vol 6. Plenum Press, New York.

Wilson, B.W., M.R. Petersen, R.A. Pelroy, and J.T. Cresto. 1981. In-vitro assay for mutagenic activity and gas chromatographic-mass spectral analysis of coal liquefaction material and the products resulting from its hydrogenation. *Fuel* 60:289-294.

Wright, C.W., W.C. Weimer, and W.D. Felix. 1983. Advanced Techniques in Synthetic Fuels Analysis (PNL-SA-11552), Technical Information Center. U.S. Department of Energy, Washington, D.C.

Yunnis, J.J. 1983. The chromosomal basis of human neoplasia. *Science* 221:227-236.

van Houdt, J.J., W.M.F. Jongen, G.M. Alink, and J.S.M. Boleij. 1984. Mutagenic Activity of airborne particles inside and outside homes. *Environ. Mutagen.* 6:861-869.

Vance, W.A. and D.E. Levin. 1984. Structural features of nitroaromatics that determine mutagenic activity in *Salmonella typhimurium*. *Environ. Mutagenesis* 6:797–811.

11

Epidemiology

INTRODUCTION

As the name suggests, epidemiology started as the study of epidemics in an attempt to find out what caused them and how to control them. Every epidemiologist studies John Snow, who stopped a London cholera epidemic by removing the handle of the Broad Street pump. He plotted the location of cholera cases house by house and found the common factor to be the water supply (Snow, 1855). Snow's basic methods are still used today. More important for our purposes, however, is Snow's philosophical approach. He used epidemiology as a pragmatic tool for protecting public health. John Snow didn't know about the germ theory of disease. He didn't know about disinfection. Chlorination and immunization hadn't been discovered. What he did know was that his cases all drew water from the Broad Street pump, and he could change that. The infectious disease epidemiologist today is backed up by the armamentarium of the bacteriologist, the virologist, the immunologist, the biochemist, and others. All of that and more is also available to the cancer epidemiologist. The epidemiologist, together with laboratory scientists and others, contributes to the scientific base that one day may bring a full understanding of cancer. Today our view of cancer is still somewhat akin to Snow's view of cholera. The cancer epidemiologist essentially is still in the phase of looking for common factors. Laboratory-based aides, however, are growing in importance.

Snow was a risk manager. He took an epidemiological approach to defining the hazard and used the knowledge directly to intervene. There was no need to quantify the risk; people were dying left and right. Risk analysis today examines more subtle risks. Here we will deal with epidemiology as one method for deriving dose–response relationships. In comparison with animal toxicology, epidemiology has the advantage that it deals

243

directly with people. There is no need to play guessing games about interspecies extrapolation. What you see is what you get. Moreover, your arena is a real-world situation where the population is exposed to all the chemical, physical, biological, and psychological stresses that real people are exposed to. The animal toxicologist exposes mice to a single substance and gets a clear-cut dose–response function, but how is that dose–response function modified by the million other exposures and host factors affecting the human population but not affecting the laboratory mouse?

There is another side, of course. The epidemiologist sees the end result, but because of the heterogeneity in the population may not recognize exactly what it is, or how big it is. Because of the million different factors affecting the population, including thousands of different chemical exposures, each person is exposed to a slightly different mix. It is difficult to sort out which exposures are the important ones. Some exposures or other factors may not even be known. This is particularly difficult in the case of cancer where the key exposure may have occurred 20 years or more before diagnosis. When you do find a common factor or a statistical association between a particular exposure and an increased incidence of cancer, how do you know it is a causative relationship, not just a statistical fluke?

Like toxicology, epidemiology as a science can stand on its own. It can provide dose–response results just as valid as those from animal studies and perhaps more so. The strengths and weaknesses of the results from the two fields are just in different places. The conclusion is obvious. By drawing on both, each complements the weaknesses of the other, and the overall result is much strengthened. How to combine the strengths of each field is a question for which there remains wide open opportunities for new answers. Some approaches are discussed in the next chapter.

When comparing epidemiology and toxicology, there are some similarities which should be noted. Animal studies often use unrealistically high doses to overcome the small numbers of animals that can be accommodated in a study. In principle, epidemiology deals with the doses which people actually receive. Lower doses are compensated by large numbers. In practice, however, larger numbers must also compensate for heterogeneity in the population (people are not genetically pure-bred laboratory animals), variability in extraneous exposure factors, and variability in measured exposures within groups. Very large study populations usually involve tradeoffs in the amount of individual information that can be obtained. Moreover, there are usually cost and other limitations on sample size. The result is that epidemiological studies which produce the best dose–response results usually involve special populations of one to a few thousand who have inordinately high exposures. Studies of coke-oven workers have provided some of the most useful dose–response information for exposure to airborne polycyclic organic material. The exposure levels of these workers, however, was similar to the levels used in animal experiments and 10,000 times general population exposures. Similarly, studies of the survivors of the atomic bomb blasts in Hiroshima and Nagasaki provide the best available data on dose–response for radiation-induced cancer. The exposure groups in these studies, however, received doses of 10 to over 300 rads, far higher than environmental exposures of the order of 0.1 rad to which these dose–response functions are applied today. Epidemiology removes the interspecies problem, but does not necessarily solve the high-dose to low-dose extrapolation problem.

In addition to higher doses, these special human populations, like animal studies, often have different *patterns* of exposure than general populations exposed to low doses. The atomic bomb survivors, for example, received an acute, one-time exposure. The coke-oven workers received an 8-hour/day, 5-day/week exposure. The importance of differences between these exposure patterns and 24 hour/day, 365 day/year exposure to more general, low-level, environmental pollution is not completely understood.

Epidemiology inherently focuses on comparisons between two or more groups. The epidemiologist wants to know, for example, whether coke-oven workers have a higher lung cancer incidence than workers in other parts of a steel mill (Redmond et al., 1972). Coke-oven workers are exposed to the organic and irritant gases and particles emitted from the coke ovens. The finding that coke-oven workers indeed had a higher lung cancer rate marked them as a high risk group. The gradient of exposure, in which workers on the top of the ovens, where the exposure is highest, had a higher rate than those at the side of the oven, who in turn had a higher rate than those who worked away from the ovens, clearly pointed at the coke-oven emissions as the source of the risk. This ordinal dose–response relationship was enough to demonstrate the causative nature of the findings. In the coke-oven case, it was sufficient proof for the Occupational Safety and Health Administration to establish controls on coke-oven emissions. The most exposed workers had a lung cancer rate 2 to 7 times that of the control group; like the Broad Street pump, there was a clear problem and OSHA intervened to protect the workers. Although a quantitative risk assessment was made (Land, 1976), OSHA did not use it as a basis of their proposed regulation. The regulations were the strictest that could be imposed.

Now comes a different problem. What about public exposure to coke-oven emissions in nearby communities? What about public exposure to diesel exhaust, smoke from wood and coal stoves, or emissions from new synthetic fuel plants? These differ from coke-oven emissions, but were close enough that in the absence of other information the coke-oven epidemiology looked like it might be helpful. In these situations the exposure and the health risk are much lower; it has been debated whether there is a health risk at all. Under these circumstances, there is more room for trade-offs in deciding on an appropriate level. To make rational trade-offs, there is a need for quantitative estimates of the cancer risk. How many cancers are caused by this exposure? How many cancers will be averted by a given level of reduction in exposure? To be of use in quantitative risk assessment, epidemiology must focus on dose–response in a quantitative way. The dose (or exposure) must be measured in each group in the population. Dose-response must be expressed in cancers per mg/m^3 of an index substance or some similar units which will allow the effects in the population to be calculated for various exposure levels. In the coke-oven worker case, an older data set provided exposure levels for various job categories at the coke ovens in terms of concentrations of coal tar pitch volatiles (CTPV). This allowed the top-to-side-to-away from the ovens gradient to be transformed into annual excess cancers per mg/m^3 CTPV (Mazumdar et al., 1975).

The need for quantitative dose–response functions is the most important lesson for epidemiologists who want their results to be useful for quantitative risk assessment. Expressing dose–response in terms of an index of exposure, however, is only the bare minimum. To extrapolate results to other situations and other populations, it is important to know how close the total exposure mix in the epidemiology study is to that in the population to which the results of the study are to be applied. To carry through the coke-oven example, the coke-oven quantitative dose response function proved a useful one for evaluating a wide variety of exposures to organic mixtures such as diesel engine exhaust, wood smoke, and exposures to workers at planned coal liquefaction and coal gasification plants, (e.g., Cuddihy et al., 1981; Cuddihy, 1982; Myeus et al., 1982). The CTPV index was simple to apply in each case, but while there were many qualitative similarities in the total exposure mix of all cases, there were both qualitative and quantitative differences. No completely reliable method is available to adjust the dose–response function to reflect such differences in total mix, although some attempts have been made using animal data. It is ironic that while reasonably detailed chemical exposure characteristics were available for the new technologies to which risk analysts hoped to apply the coke-oven dose–response function, there existed no detailed chemical exposure characterization for the coke-oven workers for the period prior to implementation of control technologies. An important point for epidemiologists (and those who fund epidemiology studies) to remember is that risk assessment provides the means to make the results of an epidemiological study useful far beyond the population studied. The expectation of a broader application is often the primary justification for doing the study. This application, and the value of the study, can be greatly enhanced by making a greater effort in exposure characterization than is immediately needed or that can ever be used in the epidemiological analysis itself. It is frequently impractical and often impossible to make these additional exposure measurements later. In the Kosovo Coal Gasification Plant Health Effects Study (Morris et al., 1987), detailed exposure characterization was done in part against the possibility that useful dose–response information would be derived that could be applied to assess risks of newer coal gasification plants which have a somewhat different pollutant mix.

It is important that risk analysts understand the strengths and weaknesses of different epidemiological designs, how to determine the validity of the results in their own context and their applicability to the problem the risk analyst must address. It is first useful to understand some basics about the kinds of data epidemiologists deal with. Epidemiologists must consider both exposure and effects data, but the emphasis here will be on disease and health status data, since exposure data were covered in earlier Chapters. Then different epidemiological designs will be described and the merits of each discussed from the standpoint of risk assessment. Finally some general considerations applicable to all designs will be covered.

EPIDEMIOLOGICAL DATA

Epidemiology is the study of health and illness in human populations (Kleinbaum et al., 1982). The epidemiologist studies populations, as opposed to the clinician who studies individuals. Of course, populations are composed of individuals. In the usual situation, the epidemiologist collects the data on individuals directly, either through direct contact or indirectly by looking up their death certificates, hospital records, and similar information. Thus, medical data the clinician collects on individuals become epidemiological data when they are compiled for a "population" or group of individuals. At times the epidemiologist draws on data already compiled by others at the population level. Mortality rates by city or county and demographic information from the census are examples. Nomenclature of epidemiological data varies. The definitions below are drawn largely from Kleinbaum et al. (1982), who use what is perhaps the most precise terminology. Risk analysts are generally interested in quantifying the cancer risk. In epidemiological terms, risk is the probability that a disease-free individual develops a given disease over a specified period, conditional on that individual not dying from another cause during the period. As a probability, risk is dimensionless and must be between zero and one.

Mortality Data

Mortality data are generally easier to obtain and are more reliable than disease incidence data. There is little question of whether someone is dead or not, and virtually every death is accounted for due to the legal ramifications. Two sources of error associated with mortality data are place and cause of death. Deaths are recorded by place of residence, but the elderly or chronically ill may move to a more favorable climate or closer to medical care facilities. Such places may have an elevated death rate completely unrelated to any environment agents. While the fact of death is well established, the cause of death often is not. Autopsy rates are low, and even when autopsies are done the results may never catch up to the mortality record. Different diagnoses may become popular during different time periods or in different regions, confusing temporal or regional comparisons. The accuracy of the assigned cause of death may vary considerably depending on the level of medical care in the area. More and better information is likely to be included in the death certificate of a person who has been under regular medical care than someone who has not seen a physician in some time. In general, cancer deaths are better defined than other causes.

Mortality rates by cause are generally expressed in terms of the underlying cause of death. The attending physician or medical examiner may write the underlying cause on the death certificate, but for statistical and research purposes underlying cause should be determined by a trained nosologist and classified according to the International Classification of Diseases (WHO, 1975).

Summary U.S. mortality data are published by the National Center for Health Statistics (e.g., NCHS, 1987) which also makes available computer tapes of the complete data set through the National Technical Information Service of the Department of Commerce. The summary data do not include detailed age-, race-, sex-, and cause-specific mortality rates at the local level. The generation of these rates involves considerable difficulty because of the problems of changing geographical definitions of local political districts such as counties, but several research institutions have developed computerized data retrieval and rate generating systems (e.g., see Marsh and Caplan, 1986; Grimshaw, 1987).

Incidence Data

Disease incidence is the usual, and most desirable way to express disease rates. Formally, the disease rate is the instantaneous potential for new cases per unit of time relative to the size of the disease-free population, expressed in units of 1/time. Incidence rates are generally given as the average rate over a specified period. This is formally called incidence density. While in a cohort study they may be expressed in terms of the disease-free population, when national or state rates are given it is generally in terms of the entire population. In the case of chronic disease such as cancer, incidence rates are usually expressed in terms of the first diagnosis of the disease in an individual, for example, 60 new cases per year per 100,000 people. Including only the first diagnoses avoids double counting, i.e., the same person may be diagnosed with the same tumor more than once. This is in contrast to acute diseases such as viral infections which may be expressed as total cases in a given period and population. Since one person may have several different episodes of the same disease during the period, the rate can even exceed one. For example, the incidence rate of the common cold in school children could exceed 1000 cases per year per 1000 children.

Since the size of the population at risk may vary during the time over which average incidence rate is calculated, average incidence, especially in cohort studies, is frequently expressed in terms of new cases per person-years. This rate may be broken down by age, sex, race, exposure, and other categories. An individual can move from one category to another during the course of the study. For example, an individual may contribute 5 person-years to the population at risk in the 25-29 age category, 5 person-years in the 20-34 age category, and 2.5 person-years in the 35-40 age category, at which point he develops the disease. The case is counted in the latter category.

In a cohort study, incidence data are directly obtained by the epidemiological researcher. For cross-sectional studies, incidence data are usually derived from cancer registries or through specific collections such as the National Cancer Institute's Surveillance, Epidemiology, and End Results (SEER) program (NIH, 1984). Unlike mortality data, these are geographically and temporally limited. It is important to recognize the difference between incident *cases* and incidence *rates*. Cancer registries, for example, collect incident cases. Rates are then calculated by dividing by the population at risk. This is a more complicated business than it may seem, since, for example, even in a large area such as a state, people actually living in an adjoining state may be diagnosed in large medical centers in the state. For case data from hospital registries, the population to use as the denominator of the rate is even harder to determine. The only reasonable accuracy is obtained by combining cases from all hospitals within a given "catchment" area so that there is reasonable assurance that all cases in the population have been included. Even this is not perfect. Sometimes incidence rates are established from insurance, Health Maintenance Organization, or trade union data. Here the base population belonging to the health plan is known, but there is the problem of people entering and leaving during the course of the study period. There is a similar problem when using occupational data from company medical department records. People who quit, and often also those who retire, are no longer included, yet these can be the key to unlocking the dose–response effect. Because of the importance of occupational studies in developing dose–response functions, this problem is discussed further below in the section on cohort studies. In countries with socialized medicine, incidence rates are theoretically more easily available, yet migration within the country can still create difficulties.

Prevalence Data

As opposed to incidence, which is the number of new cases developing in a period in a given population, prevalence is the number of people with the disease at a given time in a given population. The cancer prevalence rate is always larger than the cancer incidence rate, since it includes not only those cases which have developed in the immediate year, but all the cases developed in past years who are still alive and in the population. Since it incorporates factors affecting the survival rate following diagnosis and well as possible in-or out-migration from the area following diagnosis of the disease, prevalence rates are more difficult to translate into risk than incidence rates and so are not as useful for risk assessment. The advantage of prevalence rate is that it is easier to ascertain than incidence rates in surveys.

EPIDEMIOLOGICAL DESIGNS

Several kinds of epidemiological studies have been developed. Each is designed to take advantage of a particular kind of situation from which the etiology of a disease can be studied. Different designs have different advantages and weaknesses. In selecting a design, or in evaluating the validity and appropriateness of a study, it is important to classify the design type and recognize its characteristic strengths and weaknesses.

There is frequently confusion in the terminology of classifying epidemiological studies. The terms "retrospective" and "prospective" are used in different ways by different people. Some people refer to any study looking back in time as retrospective. A case-control study which looks back to find differences in exposure between people who now have a disease and those who do not is obviously retrospective. A cohort study which identifies a healthy group of people (a cohort) in the present which has varying exposures, and follows them for some time into the future to see whether there is a difference in disease incidence associated with differences in exposure is prospective. What about a study which identifies a group of people with different exposures based on some past documentation, for example, a group of people who began work at a given factory 30 years ago, who received a pre-employment physical examination at that time, whose exposure has been regularly monitored, and who have received annual physical examinations. This group could be "followed" over the 30 years between that time and the present to determine differences in disease incidence with exposure. Although this has all the characteristics of a prospective study, some would call this retrospective, since the entire study looks into the past. Others would call it an historical prospective study. They use the terms retrospective and prospective to describe the direction in time in which the study progresses, rather than the time of the study in relation to the present time.

Study designs can then be described in terms of their *directionality* and their *timing* (Kleinbaum et al., 1982). Directionality refers to the temporal relationship between observation of exposure and disease incidence. A prospective study, in which exposure is measured first and the population is followed to observe disease incidence, has *forward directionality*. A case-control study, in which the disease is observed first, and exposures are then investigated through individual histories, has *backward directionality*. Some would use the terms prospective and retrospective to describe directionality, instead of forward and backward. In reading the report of a study, it is important to look behind the terms used and understand the nature of the design. A study may also have *nondirectionality*, in which exposure and disease are observed simultaneously. A cross-sectional study, for example, in which cancer mortality rates and concentrations of carcinogens in air are determined in several different cities and correlations then analyzed, would be nondirectional. Both exposure and disease are observed at a single point or interval in time. Especially for a cancer study, of course, there is an implicit assumption in such a cross-sectional study that the current exposure is an indication of past exposure, since current cancer incidence could not have been caused by current exposure levels.

Timing refers to the chronological relationship between the onset of the study and observations of both exposure and disease (Kleinbaum et al., 1982). Some epidemiologists use retrospective and prospective to describe timing. Others might use historical and contemporaneous. Timing can be an important factor. Studies relying entirely on historical data are "stuck" with the kind and quality of data that exists. The design of the study must depend on that existing data. This contrasts with studies which move into the future. There, epidemiologists can theoretically collect whatever data they think is important. In practice, however, epidemiological studies are usually heavily constrained by various circumstances in the amount and kind of data that can be collected, so the difference is not as important as it may at first seem.

Considering that timing refers to observation of both exposure and disease, most studies have some historical aspects. In a typical prospective study, the design begins with exposed and nonexposed groups which have been identified in the present or past, but which generally have a pre-existing (past) exposure history. They are then followed into the future with contemporaneous observation of disease incidence and continued exposure measurements. Kleinbaum et al. (1982) use the incredible term "ambispective" to describe these mixed studies.

The advantage of the historical study, of course, is that one does not have to wait 20 or 30 years to get results. The disadvantage is that techniques used to measure exposure and disease may not be up to modern standards, may omit newly developed tests, or simply may not have measured some parameters of current interest. Of course, in a forward looking, contemporaneous study, by the time data become available years in the future, the techniques used at the beginning will seem antiquated and inadequate. This is not to argue against forward looking prospective studies. The atom bomb follow-up studies, for example, have been continuing for almost 40 years and are by far the most valuable source of information available today on health risks of exposure to ionizing radiation. Their major weakness is in their historical part, the exposure estimates, which by necessity were developed after the fact based on reconstructions of where each individual was at the time of the blast and what the estimated radiation levels were at that location.

In examining or interpreting an epidemiological study, its characteristics in regard to directionality and timing are important design features that must be understood.

Another way to classify epidemiological studies is the degree to which they meet classical statistical requirements of experimental design. Kleinbaum et al. (1982) divide the types of epidemiological research into three classes: (1) experimental, (2) quasiexperimental, and (3) observational. They use two criteria for this design classification: (1) is the study factor, generally the exposure, artificially manipulated by the investigator. That is, does the investigator have control over who is exposed and who is not and when the exposure begins and when it ends. (2) If exposure is manipulated, are the study subjects randomly allocated to various exposure categories. These, of course, are basic design principles for laboratory experiments. Laboratory experiments using people as subjects must necessarily be of short duration, and so are not suitable for cancer studies. Strict experimental methods are, however, used in *clinical trials*. While clinical trials are generally not used for studies of environmentally induced cancer, they are used in the testing of cancer chemotherapy drugs. In these studies, cancer patients are assigned randomly to different chemotherapy drugs and followed to determine which ones work better in the same way that other kinds of drugs are tested. One aspect of such testing is double-blindness. Neither the subjects of the study nor the investigators evaluating their progress know which subjects are using which drug until after the analysis is completed. This avoids any subjective bias on either side. Many chemotherapy drugs are themselves carcinogenic. These clinical trials thus provide an experimental approach to the study of cancer dose–response for these agents. Assessing the risk of cancer from chemotherapy drugs is an appropriate role for QCRA, but a rather specialized application. The implications may be broader, however, since knowledge gained may provide a better understanding of cancer dose–response in general.

Another experimental epidemiological method which might, under certain circumstances, have application to cancer risk is community intervention. Intervention is the breaking of the chain of events leading to disease, generally stopping the exposure. Subjects might be randomly selected and given an incentive to stop smoking, for example, and the cancer incidence rate in the population followed. There could be no control group; no one would provide a control group an incentive to continue smoking. One could imagine community intervention experiments, but it would be politically difficult to randomly select communities for environmental intervention.

Quasiexperiments require artificial manipulation of the study factor, but relax the requirement for randomization. Into this category fall *natural experiments* where "the allocation process appears random, although no deliberate attempt was made to randomize." Different geographical areas may have different pollution levels due to the seemingly chance location of industries or availability of different home heating fuels. Similarly, governments in different cities or different countries may take radically different approaches to environmental control, leading to differences in exposure character. For example, in the 1950s and 1960s, London focused on removing particles from the air while New York focused on removing sulfur dioxide gas. The division between such a natural experiment and an observational study seem more one of degree than any sharp definition. Observational studies range from *descriptive* studies which simply estimate the disease frequency, time trend, or geographical variation in a population, to *analytic studies* which test specific a priori hypotheses or estimate a dose–response function.

The weaknesses of these latter designs should be evident. Populations may seem "naturally" randomized among different exposure levels, but may not be. Wealthier people with jobs where they are less likely to be exposed to carcinogens may be more likely to live in the less polluted area. In the area with the polluting factor located by "chance," a higher fraction of the population may work at that factory and have high occupational exposure to the same pollutants that are emitted to the environment. Such possibilities should be hypothesized and investigated as part of the study to determine if biases exist. Blindness is harder to achieve in these studies than in true experiments. Usually there is no way to avoid both the investigators and the subjects knowing who is the case and who the control or, in a cohort study, who is the exposed and who the nonexposed comparison.

Epidemiological designs include cross-sectional, cohort, and case-control. Each of these is discussed below. Case-control and cohort studies are the real mainstays of epidemiology and the sources of the best dose–response functions. Special attention is given to two design subcategories, ecological and proportional mortality studies, which are simple to do, but create great problems in interpretation. Epidemiologists view these designs as useful for suggesting subjects for more in-depth study with cohort or case-control designs. To risk analysts, they are an attractive source of preliminary dose–response function for risk assessment, but their weaknesses and associated uncertainties must be clearly understood. Their use can lead to results far from reality.

Cross-Sectional Studies

Cross-sectional studies compare disease information among two or more populations at the same time. They are thus nondirectional and their timing is the present, although historical data such as smoking and occupational histories are often collected. Many ecological studies (see below) are cross-sectional in form, although a cross-sectional study need not be ecological. Because they are carried out at one time, they generally deal with prevalence rather than incidence of disease. They suffer from the frequently erroneous assumption that present exposure is representative of past exposure. If current effects were due to past exposures and the latter were higher then current exposures, constructing dose–response functions from current effects and current exposures would result in a higher than appropriate dose–response function (Higgins, 1983). Cross-sectional studies suffer especially from migration effects because they often collect data on prevalence rather than incidence. If either diseased people or healthy people have tended to migrate out of the area, the current disease prevalence will misrepresent the true prevalence associated with the exposure.

Cross-sectional studies of prevalence rates, however, have the advantage that they can be done relatively quickly. All the information needed can be collected in the present, without the need to study past records or to wait for future events. That is also, of course, the key to their weaknesses. They make a good starting point, however, for a community-based case-control or cohort study. The cross-sectional study provides baseline information which can be useful in designing other studies and selecting cohorts or cases and controls. Higgins (1983) describes cross-sectional studies as "good for telling us how things are but they may not always tell us how they got that way." Quantitative dose–response functions can be developed from "how things are," but such functions can prove misleading. It is better to derive dose–response functions from a knowledge of how things got that way.

Ecological studies, also called aggregate or correlational studies, compare aggregated disease data with spatial data on exposure. Most ecological studies are crosssectional in design, but they can be done longitudinally, comparing aggregated disease data in the same location in different time periods. In a classic example, Lave and Seskin (1977) compared mortality rates in U.S. Standard Metropolitan Statistical Areas (SMSA) with air pollution levels in those cities in a multiple regression analysis which also included population density and factors accounting for age, race, and income. Significant correlations were found between air pollution and total mortality and total cancers. The primary weakness of such a study design has been described as the *ecological fallacy* which results from drawing causal inferences about individual phenomenon from observations of groups. The study tells us that mortality rates were correlated with air pollution levels, but the air pollution levels were based on central city monitoring stations. We do not know whether the individuals who died were exposed to those levels. Put another way, "we do not know the joint distribution of the study factor(s) and the disease within each group" (Kleinbaum et al., 1982). The correlation between two ecologic variables can be markedly different from the corresponding correlation using individual data from the same populations.

There are other difficulties. One is the problem of *multicollinearity*.

Many different factors will be correlated among themselves to some degree in a population. Income, dietary habits, age of housing, level of employment in hazardous industries all might be correlated with air pollution levels and with mortality. Strictly speaking the independent parameters in a multiple regression should be independent, not correlated. To the extent that they are correlated, it is possible that the importance given to one variable in the analysis (say air pollution) can be misleading. Variations in the way the parameter is expressed (e.g., annual average or peak values) can shift its importance in the analysis. Omitting a correlated variable from the analysis can shift greater importance to the air pollution variable. Inclusion of different life-style factors in ecological analyses have been shown to drastically affect the influence of environmental pollution coefficients. Deleting specific locations from the analysis or varying the choice of geographic unit (e.g., city, county, standard metropolitan statistical area) can affect the pollution coefficients (Lipfert, 1985). Ecological studies must rely on data that is already available, and so frequently use mortality rates rather than disease incidence data or other more specific measures.

Because of their weaknesses, ecological studies must be interpreted with caution. Even numerous independent studies might suffer the same internal problem and come to similar but misleading results. Biological reasonableness can be a useful test. Although the Lave and Seskin study found a correlation between air pollution and total cancer mortality, for example, when specific cancers were examined the correlation was with cancers of the digestive system rather than of the lung. This suggests the effect may have been related to socioeconomic factors rather than air pollution (Lave and Seskin, 1977).

One database which proved an especially useful source for ecological studies was a set of average annual age-adjusted cancer mortality rates by sex and race for each county in the U.S. over the period 1950-1969 (Mason and McKay, 1974). These rates were graphically presented in color maps of the United States, often called the *Cancer Atlas* (Mason et al., 1975), but more importantly formed the basis of several ecological studies which explored the relationship between cancer rates and various potential sources of environmental carcinogens. By grouping counties with given characteristics, cancer rates associated with given levels of those characteristics could be compared. For example, possible links between air pollution emissions from the paper, chemical, and petroleum industries were explored by grouping counties with no employment in these industries, counties with 0.1–1% of the workforce employed in these industries, and counties with over 1% of the workforce employed in these industries. Each was then subgrouped by the percentage of the population living in urban areas to avoid bias from the well-known urban–rural gradient in lung cancer, and lung cancer rates were calculated for each subgroup (Blot and Fraumeni, 1976). The pitfalls of the ecological fallacy are clearly evident in such a study. Counties can cover a fairly large area; depending on the location of the industry in a county, a larger or smaller fraction of the population might be exposed to its pollution. The vagaries of geography and meteorology may be such that the pollution exposure falls in a different county than supplies the industries' workforce. These studies were exploratory analyses, to be followed by more detailed studies using more rigorous designs. For example, the *Cancer Atlas* indicated parts of Georgia exhibited high cancer rates. A subsequent case-control study established that occupational exposure in shipyards incurred by some 35,000 people during World War II was the basis of the apparent environmental variations seen in the ecological analysis (Blot et al., 1979).

The potential for misinformation from ecological studies can also be seen in another example. An ecological study compared measured levels of benzo[a]pyrene (BaP) with lung cancer mortality rates in different subdivisions of Los Angeles (Menck et al., 1974). The results showed an increased rate of lung cancer in parts of the city where BaP levels were as much as five times that expected from automobile emissions alone, presumably as a result of local petrochemical industries. A subsequent case-control study which examined the exposure of the lung cancer cases on an individual basis, however, demonstrated that essentially all of the excess cancer rate could be accounted for by considering occupational exposure (Pike et al., 1979).

Despite their weaknesses, ecological studies have a place. Their principle advantage is cost and time. They can be done faster and cheaper than studies which require the collection of individual information. They can be helpful in developing or refining hypotheses about carcinogenic risk and they can provide supporting evidence in evaluating relationships found in other study designs.

Case-Control Studies

Case-control studies first identify people with a particular disease (the cases) and another group of people without the disease (the controls). Then information on past exposures and other factors is collected from interviews, questionnaires, medical records, work records, and other sources. If a higher proportion of cases were exposed, then a link between exposure and disease is suggested. This is a uniquely epidemiological design which has no parallel in the classic experimental approach as used in toxicology. It is, in many ways, the most powerful design in the armamentarium of the epidemiologist. Comparing it to prospective studies, Sartwell (1983) describes the advantages of the case-control design as (1) enormously more efficient in requirements of manpower, cost, and time; (2) not requiring follow-up; (3) permitting careful examination of a wide array of factors; (4) the ability to take into consideration changes in the amount of exposure over time up to the onset of the disease. Its efficiency and ability to examine exposure and other factors more closely for each subject is because one only must be concerned with, say, 300 cases and 600 controls when in a prospective study it might be necessary to deal with 10,000 subjects to ultimately end up with the same number of cases. There are three key areas to look for in a case-control study: (1) selection of cases; (2) selection of controls; and (3) ascertainment of exposure and other cofactors.

Selection

Cases may be selected from hospital patients, cancer registries, death certificates, hospital discharge data, health insurance claims, or clinical examinations (Smith, 1983). Case-control studies are limited to examining a single outcome. The same exposure may cause several diseases, but because of its nature, a case-control study can only look at one; that is the one identified as a case. Case definition can have an important influence on the results. Few exposures cause "cancer." They cause one, or perhaps a small number, of particular cancers at particular sites. An exposure may even be related to a particular cell type (Smith, 1983). The definition of a case may thus be very specific. If a case is defined too broadly, the effect sought may be lost in the overwhelming noise of all the other nonrelated cancers included in the study. If the case is defined too specifically, it may demonstrate the effect precisely but risks missing the effect if the hypothesis is wrong on the specifics.

Where the study is focusing on a dose–response relationship that is already known or suspected, it is possible that the presence of the exposure might itself increase the likelihood that a person would be hospitalized for the disease. Sartwell (1983) gives the example of oral contraceptive use and thromboembolism. Since the possibility of this relationship was known, a physician might have been more likely to hospitalized a patient using oral contraceptives than one not using them. This would bias the results in favor of the hypothesis. Such a bias was not found in this case, but must be considered. If cases are all selected from the same hospital, one must consider the population served by that hospital to assure there are no exposure-related biases.

Selection of Controls

Selection of appropriate controls is more difficult. If cases are selected from a particular hospital, controls are often selected from the same hospital. Hospital controls have the advantage that the same selective factors that brought the cases to the hospital may have brought the controls to the same hospital. Also, interviewing controls in the same setting enhances comparability, and selection and interviewing controls is simplified (Sartwell, 1983). The disease state of the controls must be considered, however. Sartwell points out that diseases in hospital controls may correlate with the exposure of interest. He gives two examples: (1) early studies linked coffee drinking to myocardial infarction, but it was later shown that controls with chronic diseases drank less coffee because of their disease. (2) In studies of smoking and lung cancer, using controls with myocardial infarction or chronic respiratory disease would bias the results, since these diseases are linked to smoking also.

When cases are selected from cancer registries, selection of controls is even more difficult. There is no comparable list from which to select controls. They might be selected at random from people who live in the same area, work in the same occupation, or other consideration. The problem becomes even stickier when the cases are dead. Does it bias the study to select living controls for dead cases?

Controls should be selected to avoid bias in the risk factor and in various confounding factors as much as possible. Age is an important confounding factor that must be considered, for example. In some case-control studies, controls are matched with cases. For each case, one or more controls is selected by matching under preestablished criteria. These might be: within two years of the same date of birth, began work in the same year, and similar smoking habits.

Because of the importance of controls, and the biases that can be introduced by different methods of selecting controls, studies often include two or more control groups selected in different ways. Thus, a study might have hospital controls and healthy neighborhood controls.

Since all exposure data are obtained retrospectively, there is no opportunity to make new measurements; existing data must be relied upon. Often, information on exposures and cofactors is obtained through interviews with the subjects or their relatives. Historical data obtained this way are naturally less accurate than data obtained contemporaneously. Moreover, there is the possibility that cases, because they have a natural incentive to be aware of exposures or other factors possibly related to their disease, will exhibit greater recall than controls, thus biasing the results. Uncertainty in estimating past exposures is the principle drawback to use of case-control designs when the aim is to estimate quantitative dose–response information.

Because the actual disease rates in the underlying population at risk, from which the cases and controls are both presumably drawn, are not a part of the study design, relative risk cannot be determined directly, but can be inferred indirectly using the odds ratio. This is the odds of having the disease among the exposed divided by the odds of having the disease among the nonexposed.

Cohort Studies

Cohort studies have a design similar to animal experiments. An exposed group and a nonexposed group (or two or more groups with varying levels of exposure) are selected and followed over time to determine subsequent health outcomes. These are also called prospective or longitudinal studies. Cohort studies with forward progression are generally considered to provide the strongest epidemiological evidence, since they give the investigator the greatest degree of control over the design. They are expensive and take decades to achieve results. Looking back in time, however, one wonders if a well-funded, long-term prospective cohort study for environmental cancer begun, say, in the early 1950s, might not have produced more information at the same cost as the many shorter-term studies that were conducted over the same period. Compare, for example, the much greater information on radiation carcinogenesis that has come from the longterm follow-up of atomic bomb survivors in Japan compared to other studies. Will the judgment looking back be different 30 years from now?

Rare diseases, the case-control design's strength, are the cohort study's weakness. Cohort studies are not generally suitable for studying rare diseases, since the sample size must be very large to assure an adequate number of cases will develop within the population. Cancer is not a rare disease; it affects more than 25% of the American population. Environmental exposures do not simply cause "cancer," however; specific exposures cause specific cancers. Some of these cancers may be relatively rare. In one way, this problem might seem to have its own solution. the rarer a cancer is, the less it is likely to be of concern for risk assessment. There are two reasons the rare cancer is often still of interest. First, evidence of a rare cancer is often the first indication of a carcinogenic risk to the population. The cancer risk of asbestos exposure was first linked to mesothelioma, a rare cancer, although the risk of lung cancer later proved greater. The second reason is that a "rare" cancer in the context of design of a cohort study may still take a substantial toll in the national population.

Cohort studies make up for this in their ability to follow many different diseases in the cohort simultaneously with little increase in cost. Thus, the specific type of cancer caused by an exposure can be determined as part of the study and does not have to be hypothesized beforehand. Cohort studies also estimate incidence rates and relative risks directly.

The primary drawback of cohort studies is the length of time required. For cancer assessment, cohorts ideally should be followed to extinction, that is, until the last individual in the cohort dies. This is important in studying cancer for two reasons: (1) the long latent period between first exposure and ultimate manifestation of the disease; (2) cancer increases exponentially with age. While it is not certain that environmentally induced cancers follow this same pattern, some age relationship appears to exist. Thus, for the first 20 or more years a cohort study would not be expected to show any increase in cancer in the exposed group. In the third decade an increase might appear, but risk estimates based on this might underestimate the true risk, since the excess cancer rate might well increase with more time. The opposite can also be the the case, however. There is some reason to believe that the risk of environmentally induced cancer decreases with increasing time since exposure. The excess lung cancer risk of ex-cigarette smokers, for example, decreases after they quit smoking and their cancer rates begin to return toward those of non-smokers. Some believe that if a cancer does not express itself within 40 years following exposure, it never will. The National Council on Radiation Protection (NCRP, 1984) includes an exponential decrease in the lung cancer risk due to exposure to radon progeny with a half-time of 20 years. Yet a popular risk assessment model is based on relative risk, predicting a flat percentage increase in the background cancer rate from a given exposure. If the effectiveness of the exposure decreases with time, such a model would substantially overestimate the risk because of the sharp increase in background cancer rates with age. The subsequent risk after exposure ceases may depend on the mechanism of effect. If the carcinogen is complete (i.e., is both an initiator and a promoter) then risk probably decreases after exposure ceases.

Some of the difficulties in carrying out long-term surveillance on a cohort include name changes, social and geographic mobility, maintenance of long-term study management, and cost (Brown, 1980). Registration in labor unions and medical insurance plans, and national facilities such as the National Death Registry and Social Security can help greatly.

While the design of cohort studies is directionally forward, they most commonly have at least some historical roots in their timing, and many are entirely historical. Because of the ease in identifying groups with specific exposures, cohort studies are frequently occupationally based. Results of these studies are often extrapolated to general populations with much lower exposure levels. Because of the importance of occupational cohort studies, some attributes of these studies are discussed.

Occupational Studies

The most difficult problem in occupational studies of cancer is a result of the long latency period. Many people do not develop cancer until after they retire or otherwise leave the company. Most occupational studies, however, deal with the active workforce. O'Berg (1983), speaking for a large chemical company, reports, "We have no systematic way of learning about medical diagnoses among former employees or pensioners." Often if workers leave for reasons other than retirement, they are simply lost to follow-up. When cancer deaths are being studied, it is possible to track down a very high percentage of the deceased members of the cohort using the National Death Index, Social Security records, and other sources. This is the approach used in the Pittsburgh Steelworkers Study (Redmond, 1983) which included 58,828 men employed in Allegheny County, Pennsylvania, steel mills in 1953. By 1966, 10,800 of these had reached age 65 of which 9,688 had retired, 391 had left before retirement, and 721 were still employed. Standard mortality ratios for deaths from all causes and for lung cancer were higher for retirees than for all steelworkers, and higher yet for those over 65 who left employment at the steel mills before retirement. The latter had a relative risk of lung cancer twice as high as all steelworkers. The unanswered question is, what are the factors which lead to people leaving the steel mill before retirement and do these involve possible biases which affect the rates? Redmond's conclusion is that one must take care when studying retired populations alone, but the broader conclusion is that occupational cohort studies which do not include follow-up of retired workers and workers who leave before retirement are missing important information which affects the dose–response estimate and may seriously underestimate dose–response relationships. Enterline (1983) notes that, if there is an effect, it is more likely to be detected in the retired population than in any other. Limitations on studies including retired workers are discussed by Mazumdar and Redmond (1982).

Comparison Group for Occupational Studies

Relative risk is calculated as a direct comparison between the exposed cohort and the control or comparison cohort. It is obvious that differences between the two, other than the exposure of concern, can affect the derived dose–response function. A common study design examines cancer mortality in an occupational population and compares the result to cancer in the general population on an age-, sex-, and race-specific basis. For cancer studies, smoking can be an important variable but, while detailed cancer mortality statistics are available for the general population, it is not broken down by smoking status. Sometimes smoking information is available for the exposed cohort, sometimes not. Lloyd (1983) shows the effect of comparing smoking-specific lung cancer rates in an occupational cohort with general population lung cancer rates in which smokers and nonsmokers are mixed. Assuming an occupational exposure that increases the lung cancer rate something less than smoking does, the rate among nonsmokers in the industrial cohort appears low, and among smokers high, in comparison to the rate in the mixed general population. The erroneous conclusion is that the effect seen is due to smoking rather than to occupational exposure. If the occupational exposure produces a lung cancer risk much higher than smoking, the effect will be apparent despite the mixed comparison population, but the quantitative dose–response function derived will be in error. There are localized differences in cancer rates; some are understood; some are not. This raises the question of which general population should be used as a comparison population. Cancer mortality data are usually available on the national, state, and county level, but the more localized the data, the fewer the number of cases the rates are based on, thus increasing the error involved. Consideration also must be given to the degree to which the occupational population is representative of the local population. Certain industries may attract skilled workers from a regional or even national pool, and the local county or even state rates may be inappropriate. In the case of standard, general population rates, data are easily available and, when there is a question, separate comparisons should be made with data from different levels so differences among the results can be taken into account in any inferences drawn from the study.

In an occupational study, the comparison group is often another group of workers with lower levels of or no exposure. This is generally preferable to a general population comparison because it is likely to parallel more closely that of the exposed group and because data on exposure and disease similar to that on the exposed group are likely to be available. In selection of such a group, however, it is important to be aware of possible differences. The exposed group, for example, may be in a dirtier, less desirable job because of their exposure. This can mean socioeconomic differences between the exposed and nonexposed. In the Kosovo coal gasification plant worker study (Morris et al., 1987), surface coal miners were chosen as the nonexposed comparison population because:

1. Experience in the United States indicated that surface coal miners were not subject to excessive occupationally related disease.
2. As the gasification plant was largely exposed to the weather, both gasification plant workers and surface miners were believed to spend much of their workday outdoors.
3. The mines were less than 10 km from the gasification plant.
4. The surface miners were employees of the same organization which operated the gasification plant and all received primary health care in the same clinic so that medical care and medical record keeping were identical.

During the course of the study, however, it developed that a higher percentage of the miners lived in small villages than did gasification plant workers, and while both were allowed to bring coal home for heating and cooking fuel, the miners were more likely to do so. The result was that while the the comparison population had little exposure to coal chemicals at work, they were exposed to the products of incomplete coal combustion at home.

Exposure in Occupational Studies

When contemporary measurements can be made a part of the study, accurate and detailed exposure estimates can, theoretically, be included in the design. More commonly, in occupational studies, much of the exposure is historical, or exposure measures are limited by available funding or accessibility to whatever measurements are being made as part of routine industrial hygiene control. At the simplest scale, exposure is approximated by job title or workplace and length of time on the job. This can be adequate for demonstrating an effect associated with the work environment, but cannot point to any specific agent, likely means of control, or be used for development of a quantitative dose–response function useful outside the circumstances of the study without additional information. The simplest additional information is a general level of exposure associated with each job, ideally year by year, accounting for the effect of changes in technology and work practices. Use of broad categories can lead to a wide range of exposures within each group, often resulting in overlapping between exposure groups. This tends to reduce both the probability of finding a dose–response and the quantitative value of any dose–response function found.

Nested Case-Control Studies

As the name suggests, this design consists of a case-control study "nested" in a cohort study. It combines some advantages of both types. A single population is defined at the outset and followed for a given period, identifying incident cases or deaths. At some point in the study, often after an etiologic hypothesis emerges from the preliminary cohort study results, the cases are compared with a group of controls selected from the same cohort population on either a random or matched basis. This assures that the cases and controls are from the same well-defined population.

Proportional Mortality Studies

Like ecological studies, proportional mortality studies are discussed extensively here because they are so frequently seen in the literature and cited as evidence of excessive risk and because in the early stages of hazard identification they may be the only kinds of study available. The risk analyst must be able to interpret them and understand their shortcomings in order to avoid misusing them. Data on deaths are often easy to obtain, but linking them with the population at risk to form mortality rates is more difficult. Looking for links between occupation and cancer, for example, specification of the occupation of disease cases in hospital records or death certificates may not be consistent with occupational classifications in census data, making occupation-specific rates difficult to construct. Given only total deaths, nothing can be done. Given cause of death, one can compare the percentages of deaths from different causes in groups with different exposure, asking, for example, does the exposed group have a higher percentage of deaths from cancer than the nonexposed group? These proportions can be stratified not only by exposure level but by area of work, by age the exposure or work began, or on the number of years exposed or worked. The studies are subject to error introduced by misclassification of cause of death on death certificates (Percy et al., 1981). In addition, errors from extraneous risk factors are likely since stratified analysis, the most useful way of controlling for such errors, requires information on the size of the population at risk (Kleinbaum et al., 1982).

The "healthy worker effect" can have some influence on proportionate mortality. "Healthy workers" generally have lower mortality rates than the general public; this effect is much more pronounced for causes of death other than cancer. The result is that, even if there is no excess cancer rate in the population (something which cannot be known from these data), the proportion of deaths from cancer in workers would generally be expected to be 10-20% higher then would be expected based on data from the general population (Monson, 1980). The reverse can also result. If proportionate mortality analysis had been applied in the coke-oven worker study, a cohort study which demonstrated increased cancers in workers, mortality from heart disease would have been overestimated and mortality from cancer underestimated (Lloyd, 1983).

Another consideration is that, while standard mortality ratios (SMRs) are based on mortality rates and SMRs for different causes of death are independent of one another, proportionate mortality ratios (PMRs) for different causes of death are not independent of one another since they are based on death data alone and the proportions must add to 100%. Thus, a population that, for some reason, has a reduced mortality rate for a given cause will have a reduced percentage of deaths from that cause and therefore an increased percentage of deaths from all other causes, even though rates from all other causes may be exactly the same as in a standard population. Thus, an occupational group with a low rate of heart disease due to high job-related physical activity might have an increased PMR for cancer even though its cancer rate is not elevated and might even be lower than average.

PMRs may be useful for detecting unusual patterns of deaths which may be worth investigating; they are inadequate for assessment of risk. Two ways to make them more convincing by examining internal consistency and strength of association are to: (1) compute sets of PMRs defined by different characteristics that allow patterns of risks to be examined, e.g., different types, levels and lengths of exposure, and (2) compute PMRs from differing standard population data (Wong and Decoufle, 1982).

One controversial area in which proportionate mortality has been used is a hypothesized relationship between leukemia and electrical and magnetic fields. All deaths in the State of Washington from 1950 through 1979 were coded for occupation. Eleven occupations with presumed exposure to electric or magnetic fields produced an average PMR of 137 for all leukemia (136 cases) and 163 for acute leukemia (60 cases) (Milham, 1982). A similar study using 1970-1972 data from England and Wales, found average PMRs for all leukemia (85 cases) and for various subclasses of leukemia to be insignificantly different from a no-effect level of 100 (McDowall, 1983). Although some individual occupations had increased PMRs in the British study, there were inconsistencies between this and the Washington State Study with regard to which occupations were high and which low. Two additional studies did a similar analysis, but drew on cancer registry data instead of mortality records. Both showed elevated proportionate risk in leukemia incidence (Wright et al., 1982; Coleman et al., 1983). The results from different PMR studies, drawing on different kinds of data, were mixed. In this instance, case-control studies in general supported an effect (Wertheimer and Leeper, 1979; Slesin, 1987), although the implications remain controversial.

A less muddied example deals with radiation-induced leukemia in workers at the Portsmouth Naval Shipyard (PNS) in New Hampshire. Monitoring of workers for radiation exposure at PNS began in 1950 for workers using x-rays to examine welds, and expanded in 1958 when radiation work on nuclear submarines began. Najarian and Colton (1978) reviewed death certificates in New Hampshire, Maine, and Massachusetts for 1959-1977 and they identified 1,722 deaths as former PNS workers. They were able to contact next-of-kin of only 592; through these contacts they classified 146 as nuclear workers and 466 as nonnuclear workers. Proportionate mortality ratio, compared with expectations for total U.S. white males, were 5.62 for nuclear workers and 0.71 for nonnuclear workers. In addition to the unavoidable drawbacks of proportionate mortality studies, this study suffered from several additional problems: (1) the percentage of deceased PNS workers included in the study was unknown; (2) accuracy of information obtained from relatives regarding workers' radiation exposure status was uncertain; (3) no quantitative data on radiation exposure levels was included; (4) no information on other potential leukemogens to which workers were exposed (e.g., benzene) was considered. In addition, the study failed to consider the well-known phenomenon of a latent period between exposure and manifestation of cancer (Hamilton, 1983). To evaluate this reported 5-fold increase in leukemia, a historical cohort mortality study was done of all PNS civilian workers employed from 1952 to 1977 (Rinsky et al., 1981). These were divided into three subcohorts: (1) 7,615 workers with radiation exposure above 0.001 rem; (2) 15,585 nonradiation workers; and (3) 1,345 monitored workers with no measurable exposure (<0.000 rem). The exposed subcohort was stratified into seven dose categories chosen before data analysis and by time since initial radiation exposure. Of the total cohort, 19% (4,762) were dead. No excess leukemia deaths were found in the exposed subcohort compared to either U.S. white males or to the nonradiation worker subcohort. No significant trends by radiation dose were seen in leukemia deaths in the exposed group.

USE OF BIOMARKERS IN EPIDEMIOLOGY

Biologic markers are a subject of considerable interest and controversy in epidemiology. In the epidemiology of infectious diseases, field epidemiologists have long taken biological samples to be cultured in the laboratory. The role of the laboratory as a tool of the epidemiologist is thus well established. A similar role is now being established in the epidemiology of cancer and other chronic diseases. Many of the biomarkers are new and still experimental, so the risk analyst must exercise caution in using the results.

Biologic markers are categorized as exposure markers, effect markers, or susceptibility markers. Categorization can be ambiguous because specific markers may fall into different categories in different circumstances, markers may be insufficiently understood to know into which category they fall, or clear-cut lines may be difficult to draw between categories. Exposure markers were discussed in Chapter 5. Epidemiology involves measuring exposure, effect, and susceptibility. The latter is an important recognition of the heterogeneity in the population and the growing recognition of the need to emphasize sensitive or susceptible populations.

Biomarkers are especially attractive for cancer epidemiology because they may reduce the presently required long follow-up period. This is because markers can be detected sooner than overt disease. Other advantages of markers include: biomarkers may indicate subclinical changes which appear with exposures too low to produce measurable changes in disease rate in a population, allowing statistically significant relationships in smaller populations. Sensitivity markers may allow researchers to prescreen for susceptible individuals, limiting the size of the cohort to be followed. Biomarkers, by detecting early signs of cancer development, may provide clinicians the opportunity to prevent the disease. It should be noted that the latter is a side benefit, not a prerequisite. Epidemiology is different from mass screening programs and the same methods may not apply to both. The big benefit of epidemiology from the cancer risk assessment standpoint is that it provides the information necessary to prevent unnecessary cancers in a much wider population. If biomarkers can make that information better or more quickly available, the benefits of epidemiology are increased. Naturally, epidemiologists also want to make every advantage of the knowledge gained by the study available to the people studied, but the people actually involved in the study are usually a representative sample of a larger population which is the focus of the epidemiologists' concern.

Biomarkers are relatively new, however, and must be used and interpreted with caution. They currently offer more promise than help. Chromosome aberrations, for example, seem to be a good index of nonspecific exposure to mutagenic and potentially carcinogenic agents and may be useful as early markers of carcinogenic risk, but neither role (especially the latter) is well documented. There is a need for extensive field studies using epidemiology to determine and quantify the relationships between exposures and markers and between markers and cancer incidence. The latter relationship is the real key to wider acceptance and use of biomarkers in risk assessment.

INFERRING CAUSATION FROM EPIDEMIOLOGICAL STUDIES

Epidemiology is often disparaged on the basis that, unlike toxicology, it can only show associations and cannot demonstrate causality. The more controlled experimental conditions of animal studies do help in making an inference of causal effect in the test animals. There are two misperceptions in this viewpoint. First, the causation inferred in animal studies applies only under the restricted experimental conditions. When results are extrapolated to different dose levels in the presence of complex mixtures to estimate effects in a heterogeneous group of a different species than the one tested, much of the strength is removed from the findings of causality. Second, and more important, a finding of causality is not something which results automatically from a particular study design or statistical analysis. Causality is always inferred. The strengths and weaknesses of epidemiology are different than those of toxicology, but properly conducted epidemiological studies can be the basis of causal determinations. The philosophy and logic of causal inference has been the subject of considerable academic discussion (Maclure, 1985; Weed, 1986), but practical guidelines have been developed over the years to judge whether the associations seen in epidemiologic studies are spurious or causal. These guidelines are outlined below (Susser, 1986; NAS, 1985; Weiss, 1981).

Statistical Significance. Lack of statistical significance in an association is not sufficient by itself to reject a causal effect, particularly if the study had insufficient statistical power. Contrariwise, statistical significance alone does not make a causal relationship. In fact, the importance attributed to it is often overestimated in the interpretation of epidemiological studies. Nonetheless, a high level of statistical significance in an association contributes to a determination of causality.

Strength of Association. High relative risks are more likely to represent causal relationships because strong relationships are less common than weak ones, so there is less likelihood that a strong association is caused by some confounding variable. This does not mean findings of low relative risk are not causal, it just means it is harder to "prove" they are causal.

Consistency. Replication of the findings in different times, places, and circumstances is a strong indicator of causality. It is possible that the same error may exist in several studies, but if the studies are different in design or character it is less likely. Natural variability must, of course, be considered in evaluating consistency. One would not expect the exact same relative risk from several studies.

Predictive Performance. If a hypothesis drawn from an association predicts a hitherto unknown fact or consequence, which is later shown to be true, greater credence is given to the original relationship. As an example, Susser (1986) cites early defenders of the smoking and lung cancer hypotheses who predicted that lung cancer among women would increase as time caught up to the latent period following their later adoption of smoking. This, in fact, has happened.

Sequence of Events. Exposure must be shown to precede the health effect. In certain circumstances it may be possible to show that, not only does the effect follow the exposure, but when the exposure is eliminated or reduced, the effect is correspondingly reduced. Thus, those who stop smoking have been shown to have lower lung cancer rates than those who continue. Although it has been known for high exposures to reduce the latent period of cancer, these latent periods are fairly well established and a relationship which showed increased relative risk of cancer in a shorter time might be suspect.

Specificity. Strictly applied, this means that an effect has only one cause. This is true for infectious diseases; meningitis, for example, occurs only with infection of meningococcus (although not all those who carry meningococcus are stricken with meningitis so other factors are involved also). This situation does not generally exist in environmental carcinogenesis, but certain agents are frequently associated with a single cancer site. If an agent always seems to be associated with bladder cancer, for example, that would favor a causal relationship. If several studies each showed the agent associated with cancer at a different site, the case for causality would be weakened.

Dose-Response. If increasing levels of exposure are associated with increasing levels of effect, a causal relationship would be supported. "Increasing levels of exposure" may not always be represented on the one-dimensional scale in which it is expressed in most epidemiological studies. Intensity and duration of the exposure both are important. Moreover, a dose–response relationship may be modified or concealed by varying characteristics of the environment or susceptibility of the population.

Biologic Plausibility. The association is plausible given pre-existing biological knowledge. Plausibility may not be as useful a criterion as it may seem. It is quite often possible to find biologically plausible explanations for even contradictory findings. There is great subjective incentive to find justification for one's research results. Also, while causality must be judged on the existing body of knowledge, it is always possible that a new, seemingly implausible result is correct and reflects a flaw in pre-existing knowledge.

NEGATIVE STUDIES AND STATISTICAL POWER

A study of 30-year-old cigarette smokers who began smoking at age 20 shows no increase in lung cancer compared with nonsmokers of the same age. Does that prove that cigarettes do not cause cancer? Of course not.

Lung cancers below age 40 are extremely rare, even among those exposed to known carcinogens. Moreover, environmental lung cancers are known to take 15 to 20 years minimum to express themselves. This study could not have hoped to detect the effect of cigarette smoking on lung cancer.

Suppose the study continued until the cohort was age 60, and suppose the annual lung cancer rate among nonsmokers age 60 was 5 per 10,000, and among smokers of the same age ten times higher, or 50 per 1,000. If there were 10,000 smokers and 10,000 nonsmokers in the study, one would expect to see 5 cases versus 50 cases that year, quite an evident difference. If the exposure was something other than cigarette smoking however, say a low level of an organic carcinogen in the air which would cause a 10% increase in the cancer rate rather than a 10-fold increase, then one would expect to see 5 cases versus 5.5 cases. The number of actual cases in a population this size can vary markedly in a year. With this expectation, one might in a particular year see 6 cases in the unexposed population and 4 in the exposed. Does that prove there is no effect? Again, the answer is "certainly not." This study design does not have the statistical power to detect a 10% increase even if it existed. One can never completely prove "no effect." A study that could detect the 10% increase in cancer might not be able to detect a 1% increase, and so on. Negative results in epidemiological studies can be used to demonstrate that the effect is less than a given amount provided the study had the power to detect an effect of that level had it existed. More detailed discussion of this point is given by Wald and Doll (1985). Table 11-1 lists some factors which determine the statistical power of an epidemiological study.

TABLE 11-1   Factors Which Affect the Power of an Epidemiological Study

---

- Size of the study group and the control groups. Power tends to increase and the population size increases.
- Variability of the background cancer rate or other health outcome under study. Power tends to increase as variability decreases.
- Predetermined statistical significance level or Type I error that will be accepted as conformation of an effect (this assumes a specific probability model, of which more than one may be feasible). With all other parameters fixed, power is directly related to the significance level.
- Magnitude of the expected association between exposure and effect. With all other parameters fixed, power is directly related to this magnitude.
- Design of the study and the statistical techniques used for analysis.

Source: From Marsh and Caplan, 1986.

CLUSTERS IN SPACE AND TIME: ENVIORMENTAL HAZARD OR RANDOM

Clusters of disease cases in space or time are, of course, the epidemiologist's bread and butter. They suggest to the epidemiologist the possibility of an environmental etiology. The purpose of the *Cancer Atlas* (Mason et al., 1975), for example, was to identify such clusters. Clustering of cancer cases suggests the same thing to the layman, especially if a potential source of environmental carcinogens is, or is suspected to be, readily at hand. Such clusters can also occur completely at random, with no environmental inducement, but it is difficult to convince the workers in a factory which uses potentially carcinogenic chemicals or residents of a community next to a hazardous waste site that their cluster is random.

If the national annual cancer rate were 3 per 1,000, a rate of 9 per 1,000 would be unusual. But among 1,000 factories, each employing 1,000 people, quite a few might experience a rate of 9 in a single year, and some a rate of 12. How does one determine if this particular cluster is random or is associated with an environmental exposure? This is not a situation from which a dose–response function might be derived; the numbers are too small. It is included here because it is a situation which frequently happens, and which risk analysts are asked to address. There are lots of examples. A leukemia cluster in a community near a hazardous waste site in Massachusetts, an unusual number of cancers in a football team in the New Jersey Meadowlands. There are also cases of less obvious clusters which are discovered and related to environmental sources by researchers and which often lead to controversy over whether the relationship is real (e.g., Lyon et al., 1979; Shear et al., 1980).

Epidemiological methods are applicable. The first step is usually a survey of the site, to see if any sources of carcinogens are present. This should be thorough and work back in time as far as possible as well as looking at present conditions. It should include review of directories, maps, and aerial photographs to detect existing or past storage tanks, waste dumps, or similar potential sources of chemical carcinogens, evaluations of private and public water supplies, examination of building floor plans, investigation of heating, air conditioning, and ventilation systems, and samples taken for analysis of any suspicious chemicals or materials. Next, broad-range environmental samples are taken. Special attention should be given to the areas where the cases worked, to determine exposure there as well as to determine if there is any difference between their working situation and others. Recalling the lag time involved in cancer, changes in technology, work practices, personnel assignments, etc., must be investigated over past *decades*. If no exposure is identified which from available dose–response information could suggest the increased cancer rate, some support in favor of a random cluster has been established.

A parallel line of approach is to examine the specific cancers involved. Are the cases smokers? Are the cancers of the same site and of the same histologic type? Or is there a wide distribution of different cancers? Is there a pattern of cancers known to be environmental produced by environmental agents (e.g., lung, bladder)? What has been the cancer experience over past years? Is this year an isolated high point or part of a long-term trend? What is the background cancer rate in the local area? Workers likely reflect regional norms in cancer rate. What seems like a significantly high rate in comparison to the national average may not seem so extreme in a New Jersey population where the background rate is 20% higher than the national average. This line of investigation provides a second level either supporting or opposing a random cluster.

Such an investigation may lead to an important discovery of an unsuspected source of environmental cancer. More often, it leads to no explanation and no solution. The reasons are clear. Many such situations are unsuitable for epidemiological study. Populations are small and generally heterogeneous in terms of age, race, socioeconomic status, occupation, smoking, alcohol consumption, and other factors affecting health outcomes. Many of the health endpoints of concern are associated with long latency periods and the situation is then complicated by in-and out-migration. Actual exposures in the population from the suspected source are generally poorly defined. Finally, such episodes are generally characterized by extensive local publicity and a highly charged atmosphere of fear, anger, and distrust which affects the degree of cooperation with a study and could bias results (Marsh and Caplan, 1986).

QUANTITATIVE DOSE-RESPONSE ESTIMATES
FROM EPIDEMIOLOGY

Epidemiology is the primary source of several dose–response functions widely used in QCRA. An epidemiologic study must meet two minimum requirements to contribute to a quantitative dose–response assessment (Infante and White, 1985): (1) it must estimate the excess risk in an exposed population; and (2) it must include a reasonable characterization of exposure over the lifetime of the population studied. One must work with what is available or can be developed within available resources, of course, so these requirements are often bent. How epidemiology is used to develop dose–response functions for risk assessment is best described with examples. Perhaps most important and most widely used are the dose–response functions for low LET radiation (gamma and x-rays) derived from the follow-up studies of the survivors of the atomic bomb explosions at Hiroshima and Nagasaki. These are described in detail in several authoritative publications (NAS, 1972b, 1980; Preston et al., 1987). Since this book focuses on risks of chemical carcinogens, two examples in that area will be discussed in detail. The first involves exposure to a single chemical, benzene. The second involves dose–response assessment for a complex mixture, polycyclic organic matter (POM). The POM example sets the stage for a case study look at combining epidemiology, animal toxicology, and short-term in vivo studies in the development of a dose–response assessment for diesel exhaust. Both the benzene and POM examples draw on occupational studies. The first draws on studies in which benzene was the principal exposure and which generally met both requirements fully. The second examines a more complex, but less well characterized situation: the development of dose–response functions for organic particulate matter as part of a complex mixture. In both cases, the base studies and the dose–response assessment are described and the strengths and weaknesses of the resulting dose–response functions discussed.

Benzene

A relationship between leukemia and occupational exposure to benzene has been known since the 1920s, but detailed epidemiological studies were not begun until the 1970s (Infante and White, 1985). Because an animal model for benzene leukemogenicity was not available until the 1980s, risk assessment has been based almost entirely on epidemiology. Several epidemiology studies were initiated relying on historical data; three of these were the principal basis for EPA and OSHA standard setting in the late 1970s (Infante et al., 1977; Aksoy et al., 1974; Ott et al., 1978). These three studies and the EPA quantitative risk assessment are described by Bartman (1982). OSHA did not do a quantitative risk assessment, and its proposed regulation was invalidated by the U.S. Supreme Court when it was thus unable to estimate the cost per leukemia prevented. The basis for developing a quantitative dose–response function was sparse. Infante studied workers in a rubber film manufacturing process in Ohio. The study had limited exposure data, but showed a significant excess of leukemia in a population which had benzene as its principal exposure. The Aksoy study (1974) of Turkish shoe workers suffered similar problems to an even greater degree. There were few measurements of benzene in the workplace and since workers often lived in the same building as their shop, there may have been additional exposures outside of working hours. Furthermore, the cohort, although large, was not well defined. The Ott study

(1978) had the best defined exposure estimates, but workers were also exposed to a range of other chemicals. Its major limitation was its small population size which led to statistical inconclusiveness.

It should be noted that this was one of the earliest assessments of the EPA Carcinogen Assessment Group (CAG) and, moreover, there were few data available to work with. Their analysis of the Infante study gives an example of the state of quantitative risk assessment at that time. In addition to seven leukemia cases reported by Infante, CAG added two more that were "probably" in the cohort. Dividing by the 1.25 leukemias "expected" in the cohort based on U.S. white male mortality rates gave a relative risk of

$$RR = \frac{9}{1.25} = 7.2$$

Based on the vaguest estimate of pre-1946 exposures and the assumption that post-1946 exposures were at applicable standards of the time, CAG calculated average lifetime exposure levels over a period of 35 years of 40.36 ppm for those who started before 1946 and 23.7 ppm over 25 years for those starting after 1946. Although the cohort included workers who may only have been employed at the plant for 1 day, CAG assumed all were exposed the full time. CAG then calculated equivalent average lifetime exposure levels by multiplying by the ratio of time exposed on the job to total lifetime (240 days/year, 8 hours/day, for 25 or 35 years divided by 365 days/year, 24 hours/day for 70 years). This gave average lifetime exposure levels of 4.4 ppm for old workers and 1.8 ppm for new workers, with a geometric mean of 2.81 ppm. Taking the average lifetime risk of leukemia with no benzene exposure as 0.006732 and using a linear dose–response function, the increase in lifetime leukemia rate for an average lifetime benzene exposure of 1 ppm was then calculated as

$$\frac{0.006732}{2.81} \times (7.2 - 1) = 0.015$$

Similar calculations were done for the other two studies and the geometric mean taken to get a combined value for lifetime leukemia rate for an average lifetime benzene exposure of 1 ppm of 0.02.

A decade has passed since these risk calculations were made and an extended follow-up of an expansion on the cohort studied by Infante with much better exposure data has recently been reported (Rinsky et al., 1987). The study cohort included 1165 white men with at least 1 ppm-day cumulative benzene exposure who worked at least 1 day during the period from January 1, 1940 to December 31, 1965 at one of three Ohio plants which manufactured a rubber film by dissolving natural rubber in benzene and spreading it on a conveyor. The vital status of these men was acertained through 1981 with the exception of 16 (1.4%) who could not be traced and were assumed to be still living. Death certificates were obtained for the 330 known dead and cause of death coded by a qualified nosologist. Detailed job histories on each worker were obtained from personnel records, a system of job-title codes and exposure classes were developed. Extensive industrial hygiene data on exposure measurements made at the facilities were compiled from company records, state agencies, NIOSH, and a university. These data were not originally collected to estimate exposure for an epidemiologic study, but for industrial hygiene control and regulatory compliance. It was felt that they may overestimate average exposure because the industrial hygienists who made the measurements were looking for trouble spots rather than trying to document typical exposures. On the other hand, since the measurements were not continuous, nor even necessarily regular or systematic, short-term, high-exposure episodes might have been missed. Nonetheless, the exposure data were more extensive, more detailed, and of better quality than most historical-prospective occupational studies (Infante and White, 1985). A job-exposure matrix was developed and an exposure level for each individual worker, for each year, was determined based on his job category, interpolating from earlier and later years to fill in missing data. Two analyses were done: First, a categorical analysis in which person-years in the cohort were divided into four exposure categories by cumulative exposure. Expected leukemia deaths were estimated from U.S. white male rates for the same 5-year age and calender period. Standard mortality ratios were calculated by dividing observed by expected leukemia deaths and multiplying by 100. From these, a clear, and highly nonlinear dose–response relationship emerged (Fig. 11-1).

The second analysis was a nested case-control design. A control was selected from the cohort for each case, matched by year of birth and first year of exposure. These were analyzed with conditional logistic regression. Cumulative exposure, exposure duration, and average exposure rate were fit to the model individually and together; only cumulative exposure was found to contribute materially to the model in predicting the risk of leukemia deaths. The equation best predicting the odds ratio for leukemia was

$$OR = e^{(0.0126 \times \text{ppm-years})}$$

$$\text{chi-square} = 6.4, \qquad p = 0.011$$

This odds ratio is relative to an unexposed worker and estimates the relative risk at the given cumulative exposure level. It does not consider

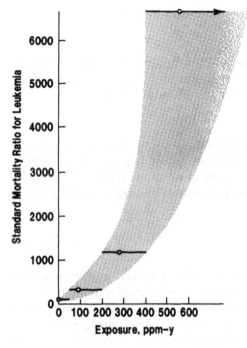

FIGURE 11-1 Dose–response relationship exposure from epidemiological study of Rinky et al. (1987). Number of deaths given in parentheses.

Exposure (ppm-y)	Standard Mortality Ratio for Leukemia
0.001–40	109 (2)
40–200	322 (2)
200–400	1186 (2)
> 400	6637 (3)

any latent period between exposure and death. To account for the latent period between exposure and clinical manifestation of the cancer, another analysis was run in which benzene exposures within 5-years of death were not considered as part of the cumulative exposure; this resulted in:

$$OR = e^{(0.0169 \times \text{ppm-years})}$$

$$\text{chi-square} = 6.7, \qquad p = 0.010$$

Based on the latter equation, and omitting the last 5-years exposure, a worker with 40 years exposure at 1 ppm would have an increased relative risk of dying from leukemia (based on the odds ratio) of

$$e^{(0.0169 \times 1 \times 35)} = 1.8$$

Assuming the same dose–response function applied to lifetime average exposures, then a lifetime exposure to 1 ppm for 70 years would produce an increased relative risk (again based on the odds ratio) of

$$e^{(0.0169 \times 1 \times 65)} = 3.0$$

Multiplying by the same lifetime probability of dying of leukemia used by CAG in 1979 yields an increase in the leukemia rate due to a lifetime exposure of 1 ppm of 0.02, actually quite close to the 0.015 estimated by CAG almost 10 years earlier with much less data and the grossest possible assumptions.

Polycyclic Organic Matter

Polycyclic organic matter (POM) has probably received greater attention in terms of quantitative dose–response function development than any "chemical." POM includes the polycyclic hydrocarbons and other heterocyclic organic compounds which often contain oxygen, nitrogen, or sulfur as well as hydrogen and carbon. Such an organic mix of pollutants results from the combustion of fossil fuels, although the total pollution mix from combustion also contains inorganic compounds such as sulfur dioxide which may also enter into the dose–response relationship. It is a good example of the problems of developing and using dose–response curves for chronic exposure to a complex mixture or a class of chemical pollutants using an exposure index. Essentially all of the commonly used POM dose–response functions are based on one of three studies. Some of these were introduced earlier in this chapter.

The first was an ecological study which regressed age-, sex-, and race-specific lung cancer mortality rates by state against per-capita cigarette sales and benzo[a]pyrene (BaP) concentrations in air (NAS, 1972a; Carnow and Meier, 1973). This study concluded that an increase in urban pollution corresponding to an increase in average BaP of 1 ng/m³ (almost a doubling of average BaP concentration in ambient air) may result in a 5% increase in the lung cancer death rate. The results were carefully phrased to make explicit that the exposure was to the total air pollution mix, and not simply to BaP. Although the resulting dose–response function, especially as it was part of a National Academy of Sciences (NAS) report, was widely used, the study suffered from the common problems of an ecological study: (1) cancer rates were statewide, thus it was implicitly assumed that BaP measurements from a few points in the state were representative of statewide exposure. Yet, BaP is extremely variable across an area as large as a state. (2) BaP measurements were of outdoor air. Even to the extent they reflect statewide averages (which is doubtful) they did not reflect the exposure actually received by the population. (3) Lung cancer rates were compared with BaP levels for roughly the same time period, yet it was the air pollution levels of 20 or more years before which would have been related to the observed lung cancers. These earlier air pollution levels were unknown, but were probably higher due to greater use of coal. Nisbet et al. (1983) attempted to estimate exposure levels for the period 1935-1945, which they felt to be the effective population exposure for cancers developing in the 1960s, by using dustfall rates as a surrogate index of likely BaP levels. They concluded these effective levels were twice those measured in the 1960s and used in the ecological studies. This has the effect of doubling the NAS dose–response function. The difficulty with such speculative analysis can be seen by the fact that a different set of analysts made the opposite assumption and halved the NAS estimate (Wilson et al., 1980). Most important is that there is no reason to believe that the raw statistical results originally reported (NAS, 1972a) are more valid than those based on speculative assumptions. (4) Smoking was based on per capita cigarette sales, yet these data are incomplete, suffer from "smuggling" of cigarettes across state lines (which can be substantial in border areas when large tax differences exist), and, because of urban–rural smoking differences, may vary geographically within the state in a way related to BaP levels in the air, introducing problems of collinearity.

The second study was of British gas retort workers whose work exposure to BaP was about 2 $\mu g/m^3$, more than 1,000 times ambient exposures (Lawther et al., 1965). These workers were shown in a prospective epidemiological cohort study to have an elevated lung cancer mortality rate compared with unexposed workers (Doll et al., 1972). A quantitative dose–response function was not derived by the authors of the original study, but separately by others using the gas retort worker data (Pike et al., 1975). The calculation was simple:

> The [gas retort workers] were exposed to an estimated 2000 ng/m^3 BaP for about 22 percent of the year (assuming a 40-hour week, 2 weeks paid leave, 1 week sick leave); very roughly, the men were exposed to the equivalent of 440 (2000×0.22) ng/m^3 BaP general air pollution. This exposure caused an extra 160/105 lung cancer cases, so that we may estimate, assuming a proportional effect, that each ng/m^3 BaP causes 0.4/105 (160/105/440) extra lung cancer cases per year." (Pike et al., 1975)

With an average background lung cancer rate in the United States of about $40/10^5$, this would be a 1% increase in the lung cancer death rate, about an order of magnitude lower than the earlier estimate from an ecological study. No adjustment was made to account for the fact that the gas retort workers were not followed through their entire lives. Assuming a relative risk approach, this could lead to a factor of 3 underestimate of dose–response (Nisbet et al., 1983). A subsequent case-control study on this population is discussed at the end of this section, however, which suggests that, contrary to underestimating dose–response, the Pike estimate, and by extension, all of the POM dose–response functions discussed here, substantially overestimate dose–response for exposure to the general population at current ambient levels.

Third was a long-term prospective study of coke-oven and coke by product workers done as part of the Pittsburgh Steelworkers Study (Lloyd, 1971; Redmond et al., 1972, 1976). Initial studies compared men who worked on top of the coke ovens where the exposure was highest, with those who worked on the side of the coke oven, to workers in other parts of the steel mill. Although there was no quantitative measurement of exposure, a clear dose–response relationship emerged. Relative risks for lung cancer in workers at the three different qualitatively defined exposure levels in Allegheny County (Pittsburgh) coke ovens were 6.9, 1.9, and 1.1, and for coke ovens outside Allegheny County 3.5, 2.3, and 2.1. By the time the importance of quantitative exposure data was apparent, regulatory action had already taken place and exposures were curtailed. Limited older data were coupled to the existing epidemiology results by job category (Mazumdar et al., 1975). Exposures ranged from 0.88 to 3.15 mg/m^3 coal tar pitch volatiles (CTPV), a measure of the benzene soluble fraction of total particles. Measurements at other coke ovens suggest a ratio of CTPV to BaP of about 140 (Jackson et al., 1974), suggesting coke-oven worker exposures were equivalent to about 6 to 20 ug/m^3 in terms of BaP, even higher than the British gas retort workers. Despite the shortcomings of the exposure measurements, these data proved to be the strongest epidemiological data available. EPA conducted a quantitative risk analysis with these data using the Weibull and multistage models and considering four different "lag times." That is, estimates were generated assuming that an exposure-related cancer would not appear before 0, 5, 10, or 15 years after the exposure. Cancers appearing within this interval are assumed to be unrelated to the exposure. A number of similar analyses based on the coke-oven worker data are compared in Table 11-2. Different approaches and assumptions lead to variation in the risk estimates, even though all are based on the same data set. All used a model linear at low doses, except Brown (1981), who used a model

TABLE 11-2 Various Estimates of Increased Lifetime Lung Cancer Risk Per Million Person-$\mu g/m^3$ Exposure to CTPV

871	Land (1976)
925	CAG (1981)
225	Morris and Thode (1981)
9	Brown (1982)
360	EPA (1984)

All are derived from the coke-oven worker study (Mazumdar et al., 1975).

in which age-specific mortality rates varied exponentially with exposure. The risk estimate shown in the table is for low doses, as much as four orders of magnitude below the coke-oven workers' exposure. The exponential dose–response function form explains why Brown's estimate is so much lower than the others.

A similar listing of dose–response estimates for organic pollutant mixtures using BaP as an index is given in Table 11-3. Several authors estimated ranges of 0 to 40 annual lung cancer deaths per million person-ng/m^3 BaP lifetime exposure.

The problems associated with use of BaP as an index chemical were discussed in Chapter 4. Uncertainties associated with the CTPV index stem from (a) shortcomings of the coke-oven worker epidemiologic study itself, (b) uncertainties introduced in analysis of the data to produce a more generalized dose–response function, and (c) uncertainties introduced in the application of the results to a general population exposed to a different mix of pollutants at much lower concentrations.

TABLE 11-3 Dose–Response Estimates for Polycyclic Organic Matter Exposure Based on Benzo[a]pyrene index

17	NAS (1972a)[a]
4	Pike et al., (1975)
14–40	Cuddihy et al. (1980) from urban pollution and smoking
0.8	Cuddihy et al. (1980) from coke-oven workers
10–40	Myers et al. (1982)
11	Nisbet et al. (1983)

[a]Originally reported as 5% increase in lung cancer death rate per ng BaP/m^3. Using the 1970 lung cancer death rate of 34/10^5, 5 is 1.7/10^5 or 17/10^6.
All are expressed here as annual increased fatal lung cancers per million people per ng BaP/m^3.

Uncertainties stemming from the original study include the limited exposure data, lack of smoking data, and possible interactions associated with race. Exposures were characterized by 319 samples taken at 10 different plants in a one-year period. This is insufficient to fully understand the variability among different workers in the same job and over time. Most coke-oven jobs are outside and thus more variable then indoor exposures not subject to weather. No information beyond CTPV is available from this sampling so the character of the complete mix indexed by CTPV is unknown. No information on smoking habits of the coke-oven workers was available. The dose–response was sufficiently large to rule out the possibility it was an artifact of smoking, but different levels of smoking within groups at different exposure could affect the quantitative dose–response estimate. Even the quantitative effect is probably not large, however, because the BaP exposures from coke-ovens were roughly 100-times that of heavy smokers (Cuddihy et al., 1980). Potential racial interactions could affect interpretation. Fifty-eight percent of the coke-oven cohort was nonwhite, but the ratio varied by exposure level. In the highest quartile of exposure, nonwhites were 87% of the population. Differences were observed in cancer rates between white and nonwhite workers. The influence of race has never been determined. If blacks and whites are equally susceptable to lung cancer from coke-oven gas exposure, there is no problem. Although it seems unlikely, if blacks were more susceptible than whites, then part of the effect attributable to coke-oven exposure would be due to this increased susceptability.

The coke-oven worker exposures were on the same order as those given laboratory animals in toxicology experiments so that all the cautions of high-dose to low-dose extrapolation discussed in Chapter 9 apply. The effect of using a different shape dose–response curve was seen in the work of Brown (1982) in Table 11-2. The coke-oven worker data are truncated; that is, the population has not been followed over its full lifetime. Since most background lung cancers appear at older ages (roughly half after age 65), how the continued influence of coke-oven exposures in the workers is treated when constructing a dose–response function can significantly affect the results. Yet, if the dose–response function is to reflect the total impact of the exposure, such an extrapolation must be made since it is doubtful that all the cancers associated with the exposure had been seen at the time the cohort was "truncated." If a relative risk model is used, in which it is assumed the effect of the exposure is to increase the cancer rate in proportion to the background rate at the age the cancer is manifested, then exposure-related cancers will continue to increase as background cancer rates increase, and a large number of additional cancers in older age groups will be predicted. If an absolute risk model is used, in which it is assumed the effect of exposure is to add an absolute increase to the background cancer rate, without regard to its size, the additional number of cancers predicted will be lower. If it is assumed that whatever increase is imposed by the exposure decreases after the exposure stops (as is seen in ex-smokers), then the additional number of cancers in older age groups of workers who are retired and no longer exposed will be predicted to be much lower. Only time and further follow-up of the cohort (which is happening) will resolve which is the right approach. The coke-oven worker study provides an excellent opportunity to add considerably to knowledge of chemical carcinogenesis in this regard.

Finally, there are two principal considerations in applying the results: exposure and the character of the population. Because combustion-related air pollution is a common problem which appears in many circumstances, dose–response functions derived from coke-oven workers or gas-retort workers find many applications. In addition to being at much lower concentrations, the air pollution mix in each case is qualitatively different. Sometimes these differences can be of great importance. Samples taken at modern coal gasification plants have had few or none of the 4-and 5-ring polycyclic compounds in the CTPV samples which were believed to be the active agents in the coke-oven case. In diesel exhaust, the nitro-aromatic compounds seem likely to be the more important agents. Both of these situations might well result in poor predictions of cancer risk when estimated directly from coke-oven worker dose–response functions. Even when applied to the "same" situation there can be problems. Because of the pollution controls and other safeguards in place at coke ovens today, the exposure to coke-oven workers is not only lower than before, but undoubtedly different qualitatively. Even in applying the ecological study results of BaP and air pollution, one finds that in the past 20 years BaP levels have decreased considerably although some other components of the organic mix have not (Nisbet et al., 1983). A method of "tailoring" the epidemiologically derived dose–response functions using results of short-term bioassays is described in Chapter 12.

Regarding the character of the population, when applying dose–response functions derived from occupational studies to the general population for many environmentally induced diseases, it is important to recognize that healthy, and often highly selected workers have lower sensitivity to disease than the general public. This is not as true with cancer for which the commonly found "healthy worker effect" is not as strong. In the future, as screening methods and biotesting in the workplace improve, this may change. The general population still differs considerably in age distribution, however, from an occupational group. In particular, the effect due to childhood exposures introduces an unknown quantity to worker-to-general population extrapolations.

An example of how an extrapolated dose–response function can give an inaccurate prediction of cancer risk and how epidemiology can resolve the discrepancy was mentioned earlier. Pike et al. (1975) applied their dose–response function extrapolated from gas retort workers to explain an increase in lung cancer found in an ecological study in areas of Los Angeles with high BaP levels. In a subsequent case-control study, the same group was able to account for essentially all of excess cancer risk by considering occupational exposure in the petrochemical industry which was producing the high ambient levels (Pike et al., 1979). Although the authors concluded that this could not completely eliminate the possibility that air pollution caused some increased lung cancer, the environmental exposure could no longer be considered the principal cause of the excess cancers. One possibility is that the different qualitative mix in the Los Angeles air produced a different, and much lower, relationship with the BaP index; another is that the linear extrapolation used is not correct and that the effect is less per unit dose at lower dose rates. The findings cast doubt on the validity of all of the POM dose–response fuctions discussed above when applied to ambient exposure levels. Additional validation studies of this kind are needed to confirm the findings of this single study.

SUMMARY

Epidemiology is an important source of dose–response information for risk assessment. Since the data are derived directly from human populations, the interspecies extrapolation associated with animal studies is avoided. High-dose to low-dose extrapolation is still often necessary and differences between the character of the original study population and that of the population to which the derived dose–response function is to be applied must be considered. An example using epidemiologically derived dose–response functions for assessing risks of ambient air exposure to polycylic organic matter illustrates methods of dose–response assessment and some of the pitfalls in extrapolation.

REFERENCES

Aksoy, M., S. Erdem, and G. DinCol. 1974. Leukemia in shoe-workers exposed chronically to benzene. *Blood* 44:837–841.
Bartman, T.R. 1982. Regulating benzene, Chapter 4 in L.B. Lave (ed.), *Quantitative Risk Assessment in Regulation*. Brookings Institution, Washington, D.C., pp. 99–134.

Blot, W.J. and J.R. Fraumeni, Jr. 1976. Geographic patterns of lung cancer: industrial correlations. *Am. J Epidemiol.* 103:539–550.

Blot, W.J., J.F. Fraumeni, Jr., T.J. Mason, and R.N. Hoover. 1979. Developing clues to environmental cancer: a stepwise approach with the use of cancer mortality data. *Environ. Health Perspect.* 32:53–58.

Brown, C.D. 1982. Analysis of the level of health risk posed by emission of volatile organic compounds released during continuous operation of a commercial scale coal gasification facility. In K.M. Novak, W.H. Medeiros, and E.A. Coveney (eds.), *Health and Environmental Risk Analysis Program Workshop: Potential Health Impacts of Airborne Organic Combustion Products* (BNL 51542). Brookhaven National Laboratory, Upton, NY, pp. 96–117.

Brown, S.M. 1980. The use of epidemiologic data in the assessment of cancer risk. *J. Environ. Pathol. and Toxicol.* 4-2,3:573–580.

CAG. 1978. Carcinogen Assessment Group's preliminary report on POM exposures. U.S. Environmental Protection Agency, Washington, D.C.

Carnow, B. and P. Meier. 1973. Air pollution and pulmonary cancer. *Arch. Environ. Health* 27:207–218.

Coleman, M., J. Bell, and R.Skeet. 1983. Leukaemia incidence in electrical workers. *Lancet* 1:982–983.

Cuddihy, R.G., F.A. Seiler, W.C. Griffith, B.R. Scott, and R.O. McClellan. 1980. Potential health and environmental effects of diesel light duty vehicles (LMF-82). Inhalation Toxicology Research Institute, Lovelace Biomedical and Environmental Research Institute, Albuquerque, NM.

Cuddihy, R.G., W.C. Griffith, C.R. Clark, and R.O. McClellan. 1981. Potential health and environmental effects of light duty diesel vehicles II (LMF-89). Inhalation Toxicology Research Institute, Lovelace Biomedical and Environmental Research Institute, Albuquerque, NM.

Cuddihy, R.G. 1982. Potential health impacts of light duty diesel vehicles. in K.M. Novak, W.H. Medeiros, and E.A. Coveney (eds.), *Health and Environmental Risk Analysis Program Workshop: Potential Health Impacts of Airborne Organic Combustion Products* (BNL 51542), Brookhaven National Laboratory, Upton, NY, pp. 26–36.

Cuddihy, R.G., W.C. Griffith, and R.O. McClellan. 1984. Health risks from light-duty diesel vehicles. *Environ. Sci. Technol.* 18:14A-21A.

Doll, R., M.P. Vessey, R.W.R. Beasley, A.R. Buckley, E.C. Fear, R.E.W. Fisher, E.J. Gammon, W. Gunn, G.O. Hughes, K. Lee, and B. Norman-Smith. 1972. Mortality of gasworkers—final report of a prospective study. *Br. J. Ind. Med.* 29:394–406.

Enterline, P.E. 1983. Population selection criteria: do they introduce bias. In L. Chiazze, Jr., F.R. Lundin, and D. Watkins (eds.), *Methods and Issues in Occupational and Environmental Epidemiology.* Ann Arbor Science Publishers, Ann Arbor, pp. 143–146.

Grimshaw, C.A. 1987. Computer code user manual and documentation for (1) manipulation of mortality and population data files and (2) calculation of mortality rates. Brookhaven National Laboratory, Upton, NY.

Hamilton, L.D. 1983. Alternative interpretations of statistics on health effects of low-level radiation. *Am. Stat. 37*:442–451.

Higgins, I.T.T. 1983. Cross-sectional studies. In L. Chiazze, Jr., F.R. Lundin, and D. Watkins (eds.), *Methods and Issues in Occupational and Environmental Epidemiology*. Ann Arbor Science Publishers, Ann Arbor, pp. 37–49.

Infante, P.F., R.A. Rinsky, J.K. Wagoner, and R.J. Young. 1977. Leukaemia in benzene workers. *Lancet 2*:76–78.

Infante, P.F. and M.C. White. 1985. Projections of leukemia risk associated with occupational exposure to benzene. *Am. J. of Ind. Med. 7*:403–413.

Jackson, J.O., P.O. Warner, and T.F. Mooney, Jr. 1974. Profiles of benzo(a)pyrene and coal tar pitch volatiles at and in the immediate vicinity of a coke oven battery. *Am. Ind. Hygiene Assoc. J. 35*:276–281.

Kleinbaum, D.G., L.L. Kupper, and H. Morgenstern. 1982. *Epidemiologic Research, Principles and Quantitative Methods*. Lifetime Learning Publications, Belmont, CA.

Land, C.E. 1976. Presentation for OSHA hearings on coke oven standards.

Lave, L.B. and E.P. Seskin. 1977. *Air Pollution and Human Health*. Johns Hopkins University Press, Baltimore.

Lawther, P.J., B.T. Commins, and R.E. Waller. 1965. A study of the concentrations of polycyclic aromatic hydrocarbons in gasworkers retort houses. *Br. J. Ind. Med. 22*:13–20.

Lipfert, F.W. 1985. Mortality and air pollution: is there a meaningful connection? *Environ. Sci. Technol. 19*:764–770.

Lloyd, J.W. 1971. Long-term mortality study of steelworkers. V. Respiratory cancer in coke plant workers. *J. Occup. Med. 13*:53–68.

Lloyd, J.W. 1983. Cohort or longitudinal studies? In L. Chiazze, Jr., F.R. Lundin, and D. Watkins (eds.), *Methods and Issues in Occupational and Environmental Epidemiology*. Ann Arbor Science Publishers, Ann Arbor, pp. 11–25.

Lyon, J.L., M.E. Klauber, J.W. Gardner, and K.S. Udall. 1979. Childhood leukemia associated with fallout from nuclear testing. *N. Engl. J. Med. 300*:397–402.

Marsh, G.M. and R.J. Caplan. 1986. The feasibility of conducting epidemiologic studies of populations residing near hazardous waste disposal sites. In F.C. Kopfler and G.F. Craun, *Environmental Epidemiology: The Importance of Exposure Assessment* (EPA/600/9–86/030). Environmental Protection Agency, Cincinnati, pp. 64–85.

Maclure, M. 1985. Popperian refutation in epidemiology. *Am. J. Epidemiol. 121*:343–350.

McDowall, M.E. 1983. Leukaemia mortality in electrical workers in England and Wales. *Lancet 1*:246.

Mason, T.J. and F.W. McKay. 1974. *U.S. Cancer Mortality by County: 1950–1969* (DHEW Pub. No. NIH 74-615). National Cancer Institute, Bethesda, MD.

Mason, T.J., F.W. McKay, R. Hoover, W.J. Blot, and J.F. Fraumeni, Jr. 1975. *Atlas of Cancer Mortality for U.S. Counties: 1950–1969* (DHEW Pub. No. NIH 75-780), National Institutes of Health, Bethesda, MD.

Mazumdar, S., C. Redmond, W. Sollecito, and N. Sussman. 1975. An epidemiological study of exposure to coal tar pitch volatiles among coke oven workers. *J. Air Pollution Control Assoc.* *25*:382–389.

Mazumdar, S. and C.K. Redmond. 1982. Evaluating dose-response relationships using epidemiological data on occupational subgroups. In N.E. Breslow and A.S. Whittemore (eds.), *Energy and Health.* SIAM, Philadelphia, pp. 265–282.

Meuck, H.R., J.T. Casagrande and B.E. Henderson. 1974. Industrial air pollution: possible effects on lung cancer. *Science 183*:210–212.

Milham, S., Jr. 1982. Mortality from leukemia in workers exposed to electrical and magnetic fields. *N. Engl. J. of Med. 307*:249.

Monson, R.R. 1980. *Occupational Epidemiology.* CRC Press, Boca Raton, FL.

Morris, S.C. and H.C. Thode, Jr. 1982. Estimating the risk of chronic occupational disease per person-year worked. In J. Van Ryzin and D. Barleta (eds.), *Proceedings of the 1981 DOE Statistical Symposium* (BNL 51535). Brookhaven National Laboratory, Upton, NY.

Morris, S.C., J.O. Jackson and M. A. Haxhiu. 1987. Kosova coal gasification plant health effects study. Brookhaven National Laboratory, Upon, NY.

Myers, D.K., N.E. Gentner, J.R. Johnson, and R.E.J. Mitchel. 1982. Carcinogenic potential of various energy sources (IAEA-SM-254/2). In *Health Impacts of Different Sources of Energy.* International Atomic Energy Agency, Vienna, pp. 539–552.

Najarian, T. and T. Colton. 1978. Mortality from leukaemia and cancer in shipyard nuclear workers. *Lancet 2*:1018–1020.

NAS. 1972a. Particulate Polycyclic Organic Matter. Committee on Biologic Effects of Atmospheric Pollutants, National Research Council, National Academy of Sciences, Washington, DC.

NAS. 1972b. *The Effects on Populations of Exposure to Low Levels of Ionizing Radiation.* Report of the Advisory Committee on the Biological Effects of Ionizing Radiations. National Research Council, National Academy of Sciences, Washington, DC.

NAS. 1985. *Epidemiology and Air Pollution.* Committee on the Epidemiology of Air Pollutants, National Research Council. National Academy Press, Washington, DC.

NCHS. 1987. Annual summary of births, marriages, divorces, and deaths: United States, 1986. *Monthly Vital Statistics Report 35*:no. 13.

NCRP. 1984. Evaluation of occupational and environmental exposures to radon and radon daughters in the United States (NCRP 78). National Council on Radiation Protection and Measurements, Bethesda, MD.

NIH. 1984. SEER Program: Cancer Incidence and Mortality in the United States 1973–81 (NIH Pub. No. 85-1837). National Cancer Institute, Bethesda, MD.

Nisbet, I.C.T., M.A. Schneiderman, N.J. Karch, and D.M. Siegel. 1983. Review and evaluation of the evidence for cancer associated with air pollution (EPA-450/5–83–006). Clemet Associates, Inc., Arlington, VA.

O'Berg, M.T. 1983. Study of active employees. In L. Chiazze, Jr., F.R. Lundin, and D. Watkins (eds.), *Methods and Issues in Occupational and Environmental Epidemiology*. Ann Arbor Science Publishers, Ann Arbor, pp. 93–96.

Ott, M.G., J.C. Townsend, W.A. Fishbeck, and R.A. Langner. 1978. Mortality among individuals occupationally exposed to benzene. *Arch. of Environ. Health 33:*3–10.

Percy, C., E. Stanek, and L. Gloeckler. 1981. Accuracy of cancer death certificates and its effect on cancer mortality statistics. *Am. J. Public Health 71:*242–250.

Pike, M.C., R.J. Gordon, B.E. Henderson, H.R. Menck, and J. SooHoo. 1975. Air pollution. In J.F. Fraumeni, Jr. (ed.), *Persons at High Risk of Cancer, An Approach to Cancer Etiology and Control*. Academic Press, New York, pp. 225–238.

Pike, M.C., J.S. Jing, I.P. Rosario, B.E. Henderson, and H.R. Menck. 1979. Occupation: "explanation" of an apparent air pollution related localized excess of lung cancer in Los Angeles County. In N.E. Breslow and A.S. Whittemore (eds.), *Energy and Health*. SIAM, Philadelphia, pp. 3–16.

Preston, D.L., H. Kato, K.J. Kopecky, and S. Fujita. 1987. Studies of the mortality of A-bomb survivors, 8. Cancer mortality, 1950–1982. *Rad. Res. 111:*151–178.

Redmond, C.K., A. Ciocco, J.W. Lloyd, and H.W. Rush. 1972. Long-term mortality study of steelworkers. VI. Mortality from malignant neoplasms among coke oven workers. *J. Occup. Med. 14:* 621–629.

Redmond, C.K., B.R. Strobino, and R.H. Cypress. 1976. Cancer experience among coke by-product workers. *Ann. NY Acad. Sci. 271:*102–115.

Rinsky, R.A., R.D. Zumwalde, R.J. Waxweiler, W.E. Murray, Jr., P.J. Bierbaum, P.J. Landrigan, M.Terpilak, and C. Cox. 1981. Cancer mortality at a naval nuclear shipyard. *Lancet 1:*231–235.

Rinsky, R.A., A.B. Smith, R. Hornung, T.G. Filloon, R.J. Young, A.H. Okun, and P.J. Landrigan. 1987. Benzene and leukemia, an epidemiologic risk assessment. *N. Engl. J. Med. 316:*1044–1050.

Sartwell, P.E. 1983. Case-control studies. In L. Chiazze, Jr., F.R. Lundin, and D. Watkins (eds.), *Methods and Issues in Occupational and Environmental Epidemiology*. Ann Arbor Science Publishers, Ann Arbor, pp. 27–35.

Shear, C.L., D.B. Seale, and M.S. Gottlieb. 1980. Evidence for space-time clustering of lung cancer deaths. *Arch Environ. Health 35:*335–43.

Slesin, L. 1987. Power lines and cancer: the evidence grows. *Technol. Rev.* October 1987, pp. 53–59.

Smith, A.H. 1983. Factors in the selection of control groups. In L. Chiazze, Jr., F.R. Lundin, and D. Watkins (eds.), *Methods and Issues in Occupational and Environmental Epidemiology*. Ann Arbor Science Publishers, Ann Arbor, pp. 107–115.

Snow, J. 1855. On the mode of communication of cholera. As reprinted in *Snow on Cholera*. Hafner Publishing Co., New York (1965).

Susser, M. 1986. the logic of Sir Karl Popper and the practice of epidemiology. *Am. J. Epidemiol. 124:*711–718.

Wald, N.J. and R. Doll (eds.). 1985. Interpretation of Negative Epidemiological

Evidence for Carcinogenicity. International Agency for Research on Cancer, Lyon.

Weed, D.L. 1986. On the logic of causal inference. *Am. J. Epidemiol. 123*:965–979.

Weiss, N.S. 1981. Inferring causal relationships, elaboration of the criterion of dose-response. *Am. J. Epidemiol. 113*:487–490.

Wilson, R., S.D. Colome, J.D. Spengler, and D.G. Wilson. 1980. *Health Effects of Fossil Fuel Burning*. Ballinger Publishing Company, Cambridge, MA.

Wong, O. and P. Decoufle. 1982. Methodological issues involving the standardized mortality ratio and proportionate mortality ratio in occupational studies. *J. Occup. Med. 24*:299–304.

World Health Organization. 1975. *Manual of the International Statistical Classification of Diseases, Injuries, and Causes of Death*. World Health Organization, Geneva.

Wertheimer, N. and E. Leeper. 1979. Electrical wiring configurations and childhood cancer, *Am. J. Epidemiol. 109*:273–284.

Wright, W.E., J.M. Peters, and T.M. Mack. 1982. Leukaemia in workers exposed to electrical and magnetic fields, *Lancet 2*:1160–1161.

12

Combined Approaches to Dose–Response: Putting It All Together

Dose–response assessment must draw on all available data sources to assure the best picture of dose–response emerges. This picture should ideally include an understanding of (1) the concept of dose in the particular application; (2) the mechanism of dose–response; (3) the form of the dose–response function; (4) quantification of the dose–response function; (5) the role of other factors which affect dose–response; and (6) quantified estimates of uncertainty. Such a full understanding cannot come from one study or one discipline alone; it must draw on everything available. But this is an ideal. In a real situation, data are generally so sparse that the need to draw on all available sources of information is dictated by the need to achieve the barest minimum understanding to allow an assessment. Dose–response assessment is generally the weakest and most uncertain part of a risk assessment.

Consistency in results among different kinds of studies has always been a source of assurance that a causative effect exists and that there is a dose–response function. Quantification of dose–response for purposes of risk assessment is a relatively new trend, however. Despite the pressing need, there are no generally accepted methods for combining quantitative results of different disciplines or even different studies within the same discipline. Statistical methods do exist for combining data collected under similar designs, but these are not applicable to data which are qualitatively different. The most common approach has been to draw on a wide variety of sources to achieve a broad qualitative understanding of the dose–response picture, then to select one or more specific studies for quantitative analysis. There are usually only one or a very few studies available which can support a quantitative analysis. If the methods were available, fragmentary information from other studies or other sources might be brought into play, but these methods have generally been ad hoc. If sufficient human data are available, they are generally used preferentially, even though they may be weaker than available animal data. That is, weak human studies tend to displace strong animal studies because they are more directly applicable. The stronger animal data are used merely as qualitative reassurance that there is a causative relationship. Ideally, the strength of the animal data would be used in developing the quantitative dose–response function. The ability to do this properly depends on improved understanding of the quantitative relationship between cancer in animal test species and human cancer. We forget that, if the human data were not there, we are generally quite willing to jump right to the animal data and extrapolate human risk from them. Why be so hesitant to use them in combination with weak human data?

The first approach, which requires no methodological advance, is to estimate risk independently from both animal and human data and compare the results. Rowe and Springer (1986) do this for asbestos. They conclude that animal extrapolations based on cumulative exposure lie well within the range of results from human studies. On a concentration per day basis, risks estimated by animal extrapolation are lower, but within an order of magnitude of those for nonsmoking asbestos workers (an order of magnitude is closer than should be expected from such comparisons). In another comparison, Hearne et al. (1987) report an epidemiological study of an occupational cohort exposed to methylene chloride numbering approximately 1000. Over half the cohort had more than 30 years exposure and exposure was well defined quantitatively. Two analyses were done: (1) Expected deaths by cause were estimated from state mortality records by age, sex, and race. These were then compared against observed deaths in the cohort. No significant differences were found for any cancer deaths and no evidence of dose–response either by length of exposure, cumulative exposure, or both. (2) Expected deaths for lung and liver cancer were calculated based on an upper 95 percentile unit risk estimator extrapolated from long-term animal bioassay (EPA, 1985). These were also compared with observed deaths and found to exceed the observations at every dose level. Overall, 36.3 deaths from lung and liver cancer were predicted by the animal model, 21.8 predicted from the state mortality data, and only 14 observed (Table 12-1).

Comparisons such as this provide additional information to the risk analyst since they add comparison values for which exposures are well characterized and other experimental conditions maintained. When complete data sets are available from both animal and human studies, comparisons also helps to further establish the correlations between the two and the limitations of each. This leads to better understanding of animal extrapolations in cases where human data are lacking and might help to indicate ways data from both sources can be used jointly.

TABLE 12-1   Comparison of Epidemiologic Findings and Predictions from Animal Models

Mean exposure	Observed	Expected[a]	Predicted[b] (ppm-y)
153	4	4.2	4.9
531	5	8.1	11.8
1212	5	9.5	19.6
Total	14	21.8	36.3

[a]Based on New York State mortality rates.
[b]Predicted from upper 95 percentile estimate of animal model.
Source: From Hearne et al., 1987.

Combining data in quantitative dose–response curve development is not limited to animal and human data. Appropriate methods for combining the much broader range of biological data, especially data from the various short-term bioassays, is needed. Combining different types of data, however, is chancy. It is akin to going out on a scientific limb. Critics can always point out the lack of valid biological evidence and statistical method to support joint analysis. It is one of the areas in risk analysis with the greatest need for methodological development. An early example was in the acute effects of radiation (UNSCEAR, 1962). Limited human data were available, but several good animal studies had been reported. The shape of the dose–response function and its slope were drawn from data derived from dogs and the human data used to "calibrate" the curve. Creative thinking applied to dose–response assessment might unearth opportunities for this kind of combination, in which each kind of data has its own particular role to play in the whole. Combining data sets in situations where each plays the same role, where the combination simply expands the amount of data available, surprisingly, is more difficult. Such synthesis is called meta analysis. Increasing the amount of data has the potential to increase statistical power, reduce bias, and produce more robust results. To realize this potential, however, a study design must surmount many difficulties. The method of selection of the population of studies is important. Has the full universe of studies been sampled, or only a biased subsection surveyed? A more difficult test for the population to meet is, is the sample representative of the universe of possible studies? That is, are there biases in the kinds of studies that are done or that are reported in the literature that would slant the sample of studies selected? Similarly, are different studies truly independent? Wachter (1988) argues that the cumulative properties of science and networks of shared beliefs make even studies by different research teams less than independent. It would appear almost impossible to pass these tests rigorously, yet in a practical world, the statistical requirements for most kinds of analysis are seldom rigorously enforced. Wachter (1988) suggests this should be interpreted constructively, as a call for more flexible and robust statistical procedures. How does one judge the balance between the advantages to be gained from combining several studies against the danger that the results may be biased and misleading? Meta analysis is an area of growing interest, but has yet to achieve the full acceptance needed. Further references include Hunter et al. (1984), Hedges and Olkin (1985), and Wolf (1986).

Three different concepts are discussed in this Chapter: (1) combining similar data from different studies of animals or people using the improved Mantel-Bryan procedure to increase the size of the data set, thus improving the random error estimate; (2) using decision aiding techniques to apply scientific judgment to combine results for several dose–response models in a consistent manner; (3) the relative potency approach to combining different kinds of data from different sources to use toxicological results to adjust dose–response estimates developed from human data.

IMPROVED MANTEL-BRYAN PROCEDURE

The improved Mantel-Bryan procedure (Mantel et al., 1975) was mentioned briefly in Chap. 9 in discussing high- to low-dose extrapolation methods to interpret animal bioassay results. One attribute of this procedure is that it provides a method for determining risk (in this case expressed as the "safe" dose) from the data of several experiments. The basic assumption of the approach is that the agent is equally potent in the different experiments, the carcinogenic response differing only in the background cancer rates. When combining data of different sex, species, or other physiological characteristic, or data from different experimental protocols, these differences must be taken into account before combining the results. Crump (1986) reviews some approaches used to do this and gives examples. He also suggests alternative approaches that would allow relaxing the assumption of equal potency in different species.

Maximum likelihood estimates are determined iteratively. Some experiments are more "informative" than others because of differences of uncertainty inherent in the design or the results. The calculation is more influenced by informative experiments than uninformative experiments. In the case of a more informative experiment with a high "safe" dose combined with a less informative experiment with a low "safe" dose, the resulting "safe" dose would be higher than would be the case if all the data were simply combined and analyzed as a single experiment. The approach requires imposition of a single, preselected shape for the dose–response curve. Mantel et al. (1975) use a lognormal model, but the approach could be applied to any of the commonly used mathematical dose–response models. Crump (1981, 1986) applies it to the multistage model.

Crump (1986) works several examples, showing that maximum likelihood results usually lie between those computed from the two data sets being combined, while the upper confidence limits from the combined data frequently are less than any of the corresponding limits from the separate data sets, noting that this simply reflects the narrower confidence bounds resulting from the use of more data. Since the approach assumes the agent is equally potent in both data sets, care must be taken in interpreting the results when the individual data sets show significantly different slopes. Nonetheless, Crump (1986) concludes that combining data seems to be more scientifically acceptable than simply using the data set that shows the greatest effect and offers a more balanced approach than simply choosing one data set over another.

DECISION ANALYSIS

The improved Mantel-Bryan procedure allows the combination of data from different sources, but retains the limitation that the analysis revolves around a single extrapolation model. That is, the results, including all uncertainty estimates, are based on the assumption that the dose–response model used in the analysis is correct. While different authors or agencies support one or another model, most allow that current knowledge is insufficient to be certain of any one model. While Mantel-Bryan may solve the problem of how to handle multiple data sets, it does not solve the problem of what to do with multiple dose–response models. Many studies simply report the results of analysis with several different models. At the present, this is without doubt the best thing to do; it gives the reader a notion of the potential variability of the results due to uncertainty in the correct dose–response model without the interjection of any bias on the part of the author. A difficulty is that dose–response estimates are seldom the ultimate objective of an analysis. These must in turn be combined with exposure estimates, and possibly other factors, to produce effects. Carrying several lines of analysis through multiple calculations not only increases the effort required in the analysis, but ultimately leaves one with numerous answers that may differ widely. How does one choose among different possible answers that reflect different assumptions about dose–response? The standard response has been to chose the simplest model, the model that gives the most conservative results, or the model one believes best represents the truth. Without sufficient information, it is a matter of judgment or choice. Decision analysis (see further discussion in Chap. 16) provides a way to combine the results of multiple dose–response models by weighting each by the degree of belief it is true. It provides no greater scientific validity to the result, but it can prove a useful way to integrate the quantitative uncertainty associated with the several different models. Morris et al. (1984) analyzed three animal studies of benzo[a]pyrene using six dose–response models (1-hit, multihit, multistage, probit, logit, and weibull). They gave equal weight to the statistical, hit, and stage models, combining the six models into three groups. These results were treated as data in a probabilistic analysis to produce a combined distribution of dose–response results, producing an 80% "confidence range" from 10^{-23} to $10^{-2.2}$ with a median of $10^{-4.3}$. This range includes interstudy and intermodel sources of uncertainty. Since the contribution of the former source of uncertainty could be determined independently, the intermodel uncertainty, representative of incomplete knowledge of the carcinogenic process, could be determined; it was found to the largest source of uncertainty in the overall estimate of dose–response. It is, of course, not possible to know the amount of uncertainty associated with incomplete knowledge; to do so would be a contradiction. Estimates must be based on analysis of what is available. Today, growing confidence with physiologically based models may improve our ability to estimate the effect of this source of uncertainty, as well as offer new ways to do so.

Decision techniques provide a means to make use of scientific judgment to combine results from different models in a consistent way. They are widely used for similar purposes in other applications, but have not been generally accepted for combining cancer potency estimates.

RELATIVE POTENCY

One approach that uses human and toxicological data in combination is "relative potency." This method is based on an assumption that the relative potency between two carcinogens (C_1 and C_2) in one bioassay is directly proportional to their relative potency in another bioassay (Lewtas et al., 1983). This can be stated as:

$$\frac{P_{1,1}}{P_{1,2}} = k \frac{P_{2,1}}{P_{2,2}} \tag{1}$$

where $P_{i,j}$ is the potency of carcinogen i in bioassay system j. Given this assumption and a value of k, one can estimate the unknown potency of a *particular test chemical* (T) in one bioassay system from the potency of a reference chemical (R) in the test system and the potency ratio of the test chemical to the reference chemical in a second bioassay system. Using the same format as above:

$$P_{T.1} = k\, P_{R.1}\, \frac{P_{T.2}}{P_{R.2}} \qquad (2)$$

If "bioassay system 1" is the effect in the exposed human population and "bioassay system 2" a quick test, the usefulness of the method is readily apparent. The potency in the human population is taken from well established epidemiological findings. This approach can, therefore, be used to base extrapolations from animal or in vitro bioassays to risk estimates in human populations using actual epidemiological results for a reference chemical as a kind of catalyst which sweeps aside all the considerations of interspecies extrapolation discussed in Chap. 9 by assuming their action on the test chemical is the same as on the reference chemical. For example, the ratio of bioavailability of the test chemical in the bioassay to its bioavailability in human populations is assumed to be the same as the parallel ratio for the reference chemical. The same might be said for other interspecies and interorgan differences such as distribution of particulate exposure, extractability of particulate-bound organics, target site of action, metabolism, and genetic repair mechanisms. This is, at best, an approximation, and, depending on the reference chemical and test system chosen, could be far from accurate. Once the assumption is accepted, the reference chemical and the reference bioassay system from which the relative potency will be determined must be selected and the potencies of the test and reference chemical in the test bioassay and of the reference chemical in the human population calculated.

The most extensive application and discussion of the relative potency method has been in the risk assessment of diesel particulate emissions. Following the oil crisis in 1974, a shift to diesel engines in automobiles and light trucks in the United States was predicted to grow to 20-30% of the entire fleet. Diesel engines emit more particles into the air than gasoline engines. These particles have a higher concentration of extractable organic matter than particles from gasoline engines and not surprisingly proved to be mutagenic in early in-vitro bacterial bioassays. The specter of a technological change with a potentially large and rapidly growing exposure of the population to mutagenic particles led to the initiation of a large and intensive research and assessment program. The only available epidemiological estimates directly applicable to diesel exposure was a study of London Transport Authority (LTA) diesel bus garage workers which did not show an effect (Waller, 1979). The study had many limitations: genetic, socioeconomic, and smoking were not considered and there was no follow-up of workers after retirement or leaving for other reasons. It was thus not sufficiently powerful to exclude an effect. In a reanalysis, bus garage engineers were compared to other LTA workers; 95% confidence bounds on the relative risk of lung cancer in the garage engineers were calculated to be 0.7 to 1.6, considering uncertainties in exposure and smoking habits (Harris, 1981, 1983a). Expressed as a dose–response coefficient, this translated to 12 lung cancers per ng particles per m^3-person-year with 95% confidence range of 24 to 49.

Extensive short-term bioassays were conducted on extracts of particles collected from the exhausts of several diesel engine types and, as possible reference chemicals, on extracts of coke oven emissions, roofing tar, and cigarette smoke condensate for which human epidemiological estimates were available (see discussion in Chap. 11). Assuming relative potencies are constant across human and nonhuman biological systems (i.e., $k = 1$), Harris (1981, 1983a) substituted data on four different bioassays for particulate samples from each of three different light-duty diesel engines into equation (2) using coke oven and roofing tar exposures as the reference chemical. There were thus eight results on each of three engines or 24 results total. These relative risk estimates ranged from 0.1 to 28 per ng particles per m^3-person-year. If each result was regarded as an equally likely measure of the true value, the overall mean estimate would be 3.5 per ng particles per m^3-person-year with 95% confidence range of 18–25.

The differences between the relative and absolute risk models for extrapolation of epidemiological results were discussed in Chap. 11. The relative potency method is applicable to both. Harris (1981, 1983a) applied relative potency to relative risk estimates while Albert et al. (1983) applied much the same procedure to absolute risk estimates. Dose–response assessment was done in two steps in the latter study. The assumption of direct proportionality of relative potency was examined for three complex organic mixtures known to be human carcinogens. Mouse skin tumor initiation relative potencies were directly proportional to the relative potency estimated from lung cancer epidemiological data to within a factor of two. The in vitro bioassays, however, were not fully consistent. In addition, the mouse skin bioassay was a whole-animal, mammalian test, qualitative correspondence had been shown between the tumorigenic response of the skin and the lung in rodents and humans, and the mouse skin initiation bioassay was linear over the entire range of tested doses for the three reference chemicals and the Nissan diesel which corresponded to the assumption made in analysis of the epidemiological data. For these reasons, Albert et al. (1983) chose this bioassay as their test system for calculating relative potency. The mouse skin initiation bioassay responded

TABLE 12-2 Unit Lung Cancer Estimates for the Nissan Diesel Particulate Emissions, Based on Relative Potency in the Mouse Skin tumor Initiation Assay

Source	Nissan unit risk estimate[a]
Coke-oven topside	2.6
Roofing tar	5.2
Cigarette smoke condensate	5.4
Average	4.4

[a]Lifetime risk per 10,000 per microgram organics/m^3.
Source: From Albert et al., 1983.

poorly, however, to the diesel particle extracts which were weaker carcinogens than the reference chemicals. Thus, as a first step, unit lung cancer estimates were calculated for one diesel type (Nissan) using the relative potency method based on the skin initiation bioassay and the three different reference chemicals (Table 12-2). The results were surprisingly close and an average of the three was calculated. This average was then used as the reference base for relative potency estimates of the human risk of each of the other diesel types in the study with the combined results from the Ames, SCE, and mouse lymphoma biossays as the test system (Table 12-3). This is a typical judgment that must frequently be made in risk analysis: to use all the data, or to evaluate all the data and select those data which appear to be the most applicable to the task. Harris (1983b) argues that complete reliance on mouse skin initiation bioassay would not exploit the full informative power of the database. When possible, it is worthwhile to do it both ways; differences in the results can yield further insights into what is really happening. In this case, it was shown that the results would not greatly differ if the study had been done as a single stage and the mouse skin initiation bioassay results been used directly as the base for all the individual diesel types (Cuddihy and McClellan, 1983).

It is instructive to compare results from different sources (Table 12-4). Since the different dose–response functions are of different form, the simplest comparison is to apply each to a hypothetical situation. A U.S. population of 230 million with a lifespan of 70 years and annual lung cancer deaths of 100,000 will be used as the base (McClellan, 1986).

The large range of possible effects predicted from the LTA workers study is not surprising given the inherent weaknesses in that work. Other epidemiology studies still in progress may allow more precise estimates. Given this large range which includes no effect (or even a protective effect, although that is a statistical phenomenon rather than a biologically

TABLE 12-3 Unit Risk Estimates of Various Diesel and Gasoline Particulate Emissions Based on Combined Data from Three Assays in Relation to the Nissan

Emission sources	Unit-risk estimates[a]
Nissan (Diesel)	35.0
Volkswagen Rabbit (Diesel)	23.0
Oldsmobile (Diesel)	20.0
Caterpillar (Diesel)	1.8
Mustang II (Gasoline)	60.0

[a]Lifetime risk per million per microgram/m^3.
Source: From Albert et al., 1983).

justifiable possibility), it is also not surprising that the relative potency estimates also fall within the range. Since all the relative potency estimates are based on the same data, not overmuch emphasis should be given to the fact that they are all quite similar.

The relative potency method is a reasonable approach to estimate human cancer risk of exposure to a material when neither direct epidemiology nor long-term animal bioassay results are available. It offers a useful comparison approach even when these other data are available. In the diesel example, consistencies were shown among different selection of bioassay systems and among three different reference materials. Nonetheless, even these comparisons were done within a selected set of bioassays and the relative ranking of the results may depend on the sensitivity of specific bioassays to individual chemicals within the test mixture. Cuddihy and McClellan (1983) point out that the focus of further assessment should be on other factors such as whether or not the mutagenic organics dissociate from the particles after inhalation or ingestion and whether or not they are detoxified before reaching target cells. Relative potency estimates now have their primary use at the stage before such knowledge is available. The time to obtain the detailed information they suggest is

TABLE 12-4 Comparing Relative Potency Results from Different Sources

(1) LTA workers (95% confidence range): decrease of 1700 cancers/year to increase of 3500 cancers/year
(2) Relative potency–relative risk: 250 lung cancers/year
(3) Relative potency–absolute risk: 100 lung cancers/year
(4) Relative potency–absolute risk: 230 lung cancers/year

Sources: 1 and 2 are from Harris, 1981 and 1983a; 3 is from Albert et al., 1983; 4 is from Cuddihy et al., 1984.

on the same order as for long-term animal bioassays and that information would also be useful in the direct extrapolation of animal bioassays to human risk. Still, relative potency offers a different approach to extrapolation which can draw directly on short-term bioassay as well as long-term whole animal bioassay. As data become available, further exploration into developing modifiers to the relative potency calculation (i.e., multiple k values) may prove valuable.

Application of the relative potency method also depends on methods of calculating potency itself (see Chap. 8), on quantification of results of short-term bioassays (Chap. 10), and on methods of quantifying dose--response functions from epidemiology (Chap. 11). Although the Harris (1981, 1983a) and Albert et al. (1983) studies drew on the same studies, the basic potency estimates calculated in each differed due to different mathematical techniques in analyzing the original data (Cuddihy and McClellan, 1983). Beyond the estimates themselves, full characterization of uncertainty in these contributing tasks is difficult, and shortcomings in this may be magnified in the results of the relative potency analysis.

SUMMARY

There is never sufficient information to develop and quantify a dose--response function to the level desired so it is important that all data from all available sources be used to their fullest. While this need is generally recognized, it is seldom followed in a quantitative sense. Methods are available to combine data sets within the context of a single dose--response model, to include alternative dose--response models, and to use various kinds of data in different ways to quantify dose--response. They should be applied more widely to take advantage of data that would otherwise provide only qualitative support but could be used to reduce quantitative error terms and improve quantitative estimates. The development and further refining of methods in this area is an important area of potential advance in quantitative cancer risk analysis.

REFERENCES

Albert, R.E., J. Lewtas, S. Nesnow, T.W. Thorslund, and E. Anderson. 1983. Comparative potency method for cancer risk assessment: application to diesel particulate emissions. *Risk Analysis* 3:101-117.

Crump, K.S. 1981. Statistical aspects of linear extrapolation, in C.R. Richmond, P.J. Walsh, and E.D. Copenhaver (eds.). *Health Risk Analysis*, The Franklin Institute Press, Philadelphia, pp. 381-392.

Crump, K.S. 1986. Investigation of methodologies for estimating human carcinogenic risk using nonhuman data (EPRI EA-4973). Electric Power Research Institute, Palo Alto, CA.

Cuddihy, R.G. and R.O. McClellan. 1983. Evaluating lung cancer risks from exposures to diesel engine exhaust. *Risk Analysis* 3:119-124.

Cuddihy, R.G., W.C. Griffith, and R.O. McClellan. 1984. Health risks from light-duty diesel vehicles. *Environ. Sci. Technol.* 18:14A-21A.

EPA. 1985. Addendum to the Health Assessment Document for Dichloromethane (Methylene Chloride), Final Report (EPA-600/8-82-004FF. Office of Health and Environmental Assessment, U.S. Environmental Protection Agency, Washington, DC.

Harris, J.E. 1981. Potential risk of lung cancer from diesel engine emissions. National Academy Press, Washington, DC.

Harris, J.E. 1983a. Diesel emissions and lung cancer. *Risk Analysis* 3:83-100.

Harris, J.E. 1983b. Diesel emissions and lung cancer revisited. *Risk Analysis* 3:139-146.

Hearne, F.T., F. Grose, J.W. Pifer, B.R. Friedlander, and R.L. Raleigh. 1987. Methylene chloride mortality study: dose–response characterization and animal model comparison. *J. Occup. Med.* 29:217-228.

Hedges, L.V. and I. Olkin. 1985. *Statistical Methods for Meta-Analysis*. Academic Press, NY.

Hunter, J.E., F.L. Schmidt, and G.B. Jackson. 1984. *Meta-Analysis: Cumulating Research Findings Across Studies*. Sage, Beverly Hills, CA.

Lewtas, J., S. Nesnow, and R.E. Albert. 1983. A comparative potency method for cancer risk assessment: clarification of the rationale, theoretical basis, and application to diesel particulate emissions. *Risk Analysis* 3:133-137.

McClellan, R.O. 1986. Health effects of diesel exhaust: a case study in risk assessment. *Am. Ind. Hygiene Assoc. J*:1-12.

Mantel, N., N.R. Bohidar, C.C. Brown, J.L. Ciminera, and J.W. Tukey. 1975. An improved Mantel-Bryan procedure for "safety" testing of carcinogens. *Cancer Res.* 35:865-872.

Morris, S.C., H. Fischer, L.D. Hamilton, P.D. Moskowitz, K. Rybicka, H.C. Thode, Jr., and A.A. Moghissi. 1984. Why we can't accurately predict chemical cancer risks, presented at the annual meeting, Society for Risk Analysis, Knoxville, TN.

Rowe, J.N. and J.A. Springer. 1986. Asbestos lung cancer risks: comparison of animal and human extrapolations. *Risk Analysis* 6:171-180.

UNSCEAR. 1962. Report of the United Nations Scientific Committee on Effects of Atomic Radiation to the General Assembley, United Nations, New York.

Wachter, K.W. 1988. Disturbed by meta-analysis? *Science* 242:1407-1408.

Waller, R. 1979. Trends in lung cancer in London in relation to exposure to diesel fumes. In *Health Effects of Diesel Engine Emissions: Proceedings of an International Symposium*, Volume 2 (EPA-600/9-80-057b). U.S. Environmental Protection Agency Health Effects Research Laboratory, Cincinnati, OH, pp. 1085-1097.

Wolf, F.M. 1986. *Meta-Analysis: Quantitative Methods for Research Synthesis*. Sage, Beverly Hills, CA.

PART IV

RISK CHARACTERIZATION AND IMPLICATIONS

This concluding section begins with uncertainty. Uncertainty is a vital, perhaps the most important aspect, of quantitative risk analysis. Specific aspects of uncertainty were discussed with each of the topics covered earlier; Chapter 13 presents some general principles of uncertainty in risk analysis. Risk characterization, the final phase of quantitative risk analysis in which exposure and dose–response are combined, is discussed in Chapter 14. Risk perception and risk communication, two new and quickly developing fields that are of direct importance in risk characterization are included in that chapter.

Quality assurance and its role in risk assessment is discussed in Chapter 15, along with validation and peer review. Credibility is essential to effective risk analysis. All the effort spent in characterizing a risk is useless if no one believes in the result.

This book is about risk assessment, not risk management, but the risk analyst must be aware of how the results will be used. Like risk perception concepts, risks cannot be effectively characterized without an understanding of how the characterization will be used. Chapter 16 describes some of the techniques used in risk management and the formats or contexts in which they are used.

Lastly, Chapter 17 examines opportunities and research needs in some of the most rapidly advancing areas of quantitative risk analysis.

13

Characterization of Uncertainty

ROLE OF UNCERTAINTY IN RISK ASSESSMENT

A recent critical review of problems in risk assessment concluded that " . . . risk assessors must do a better job of identifying and assessing uncertainties and communicating them to policymakers and the public" (Hattis and Kennedy, 1986). Given the uncertainties in all of the sciences upon which risk assessments are based, identifying and assessing the uncertainties of estimated risks is the most important, although sometimes the most neglected, aspect of risk assessment. Consider an example in financial risk. You have the option of two investments. One offers 8% return on your money, the other 25%. No sensible person would make a choice without knowing the "risk" involved; that is, what is the chance of losing the principal. In this context, the word risk itself can be understood to mean uncertainty. Cancer risk assessment is no different. It would be folly to institute a regulatory policy based on an analysis that one option would result in ten times the number of cancers as another when equally likely, or only slightly less likely, assumptions could lead to the opposite result. Uncertainty is inherent in cancer risk assessment. Both exposure and dose–response contain uncertainties. We cannot even look back on a past event and determine precisely what a population's exposure was and how many cancers resulted. It has been said that the difference between risk assessment and a five-year weather forecast is that at least with the weather forecast, if you wait five years you find out whether you were right. Exposure usually involves too many chemicals to measure each one, and differences among individuals are so great that individual exposures and responses vary widely. In the usual case of a potential or future exposure, additional uncertainties are introduced. Often, the uncertainty is so large that a point estimate is simply not useful. An understanding of the size of the uncertainty associated with various risks can be the prime objective of an assessment.

How to deal with uncertainty is also a key element of cancer risk management. Risk managers, however, can do no better in dealing with uncertainty than the information provided them on uncertainty in risk assessments. Risk assessments which do not include consideration of uncertainty are a disservice to risk management. An analysis indicating that a given technology, industrial process, or food causes some number of cancers can have a disrupting effect on society. Resulting market, political, and regulatory actions can involve large economic cost and further social disruption. While there is a responsibility to avoid or limit environmental cancer, starting the process in motion without an adequate examination of the uncertainties associated with the results is irresponsible. Further reasons for trying to develop estimates of uncertainty in risk assessments are listed in Table 13-1.

Ideally, cancer risk assessments would include complete consideration of all sources of uncertainty, leading to a full characterization of uncertainty in the final estimates. Consideration of uncertainty, however, is frequently complicated. In some cases a full consideration of uncertainty seems impossible. One approach commonly used to keep the analysis simple is the use of so called "conservative" estimates. The general philosophy in the field of public health is, when in doubt, one should err on the side of public health. The health effects are more important than the economic costs which are often involved on the other side of the equation. Following this, models in health risk assessment frequently have conservative assumptions "built in." For example, emission estimates are selected from the high end of the range and assumptions in environmental transport and exposure models are selected to assure overestimates rather

TABLE 13-1 Reasons for Explicit Estimates of Uncertainty in Risk Analysis

1. To avoid misunderstanding that often results from using a single point estimate
2. To focus on those uncertainty contributions which are the largest, to determine if further research can reduce them
3. To give regulatory decisionmakers a range of options consistent with the state of scientific knowledge
4. To show that a risk estimate, while not exact, is not so uncertain as to be useless
5. To respond to objections that the estimates are based on so many assumptions as to be useless by carefully estimating the uncertainty introduced by each assumption
6. To prevent the loss of partial and not totally scientifically-based information which still can be of value

Source: From Cothern et al., 1986.

than underestimates. The result is to produce point estimates which presumably overestimate the cancer risk, but by an unknown amount. In its extreme, this approach is sometimes called "worst-case analysis." It avoids treating uncertainty by looking only at the worst case, so that all the uncertainty is on the side of lower effects than those estimated. Worst-case analysis can be a useful screening tool, but has a number of unfortunate results which are discussed in Chapter 16. Explicit characterization of uncertainty is an essential aspect of risk assessment and should be considered the most important part of the analysis, even if available knowledge or resources limit the work to crude or even qualitative treatment of the subject.

Uncertainty is such a pervasive subject in cancer risk analysis that it is included to some degree in almost every chapter in this book. Methods and applications of uncertainty analysis are integrated into the presentations of exposure modeling, dose–response function development, and risk characterization. This chapter provides an overview of uncertainty and its role in risk assessment and examples of techniques for explicitly quantifying uncertainty in cancer risk assessment.

WHAT IS UNCERTAIN?

Exactly what are these uncertainties that are so important? They can be classified in several broad categories, only some of which are classically considered uncertainty. All involve the fact that different answers can be obtained under different assumptions or conditions, or even in different trials of the same experiment under the same conditions. Different kinds of uncertainty are appropriately handled in different ways in an analysis, of course. The kinds of uncertainties to be discussed are policy uncertainties, natural variability, and knowledge uncertainties.

Policy Uncertainty

First are policy uncertainties. Risk assessments often aim at predicting effects following developments currently being considered. For example, what will be the expected impact on the cancer rate in the surrounding population of a new industrial development? The answer to this question obviously depends on many decisions yet to be made. Exactly where will the development be located? How large will it be? What pollutants will be emitted? What pollution controls will be included? What routes of exposure are available? These questions are themselves part of, or a result of, the decision to be made or related public or private decisions that will be made as planning and implementation progresses. The risk analyst should not expect all the answers to be available. The risk assessment should be started early enough in the process so that many of these policy questions are still open. In fact, final decisions on many of these policy questions may not come until much later in the process. For example, final decisions on pollution control technology are reasonably delayed until after process technology is fully developed and at times not until after construction is underway. This allows the maximum amount of information to be brought to bear on the question. The risk assessment itself will provide some of this information and may be a key factor in subsequent decisions. Some policy uncertainties might be on a continuous scale, e.g., pollution control requirements might range from 50% to 90%, but many will be discrete, e.g., three different possible locations may be under consideration or one of two different chemical processes might be used. In the policy arena, specific, discrete options tend to evolve, even for variables that are naturally continuous.

Analysis of policy options is often called "policy analysis" (e.g., Quade, 1975). It can be a link between risk assessment and risk management. The implications of each policy option are explored, including the associated uncertainty. But often policy options must be considered even if they are not the focus of the analysis. An example is "generic" risk assessments done to investigate the risks of new technologies. The Department of Energy conducted several "generic" risk assessments for new energy technologies to help decide which were worth further development and to identify potential sources of risk which could be reduced or eliminated as part of the overall technological development (e.g., Cuddihy et al., 1981; Moskowitz et al., 1983). Other generic assessments have been done as part of environmental impact statements on new technologies (AEC, 1974) or for general comparisons such as coal vs. nuclear as fuel for electric power production (Hamilton, 1984). These generic assessments often ignore technological, operational, and locational differences among individual plants of the same type. They are often based on a typical "reference facility" at a real or fictitious "reference location." An example of how a policy uncertainty can be explicitly included in a generic analysis is given by Rowe (1980, 1981) for the case of location. An air pollution dispersion model was run repeatedly to produce a matrix containing the cumulative population exposure nationwide due to a unit emission source in each U.S. county. A probability distribution could then be developed to express the range of population exposure which could result from a reference plant at an unknown location. The range of effects, depending on where the plant was located, could then explicitly be factored into the analysis. This provides a base for later policy analyses which might compare the implications of different emission control levels with different plant locations.

The best way to handle policy uncertainties depends on the objectives of the analysis. The key in all cases is to examine differences in the final effects estimated from different assumptions about how policy questions will be resolved, and to separate the implications of the policy uncertainties from those of the more basic scientific uncertainties.

Natural Variability

Natural variability stems from random or otherwise varying behavior in the quantity being measured or estimated. All scientific information is subject to what is usually called random error. Any experiment in which some quantity is measured is likely, upon the measurements being repeated, to yield a different value for the quantity measured. How closely grouped repeated measurements are depends on the underlying variability of the process, the design of the experiment, and the precision of the instrument used to make the measurement. Animal experiments from which cancer dose–response functions are derived are an example. The precision, or repeatability, of these experiments is a function of the number of dose levels used and the number of animals in each dose level. Larger experiments and more experiments will reduce the random error in the results. Similar error is introduced in risk assessments from experiments to determine "spreading" coefficients in atmospheric dispersion models or deposition rates of various airborne material. The less random error in the input data, the less uncertainty in the risk estimates. Practical limits are soon reached, however, in the amount of gain that can be expected in uncertainty from this source.

While it may initially seem different than random error in experiments, a similar phenomenon is the day-to-day, minute-to-minute variability in weather or the movement of people. Exposures leading to possible cancers following an industrial accident, for example, will depend on the direction of the wind and the stability of the atmosphere at the time of the accident. This could never be predicted in advance, but we know from past experience what fraction of the time the wind blows in each direction at a given location. Variability in these factors can be reduced in a probabilistic sense by learning more about the likelihood of the accident happening at different times of day or seasons of the year and correlations of time with wind direction and population movement. Probabilities can then be weighted by these correlations.

Uncertainties in overall risk cannot be fully quantified without the inclusion of natural variability. In addition, because many aspects of natural variability are more easily appreciated than scientific uncertainty, it provides some perspective against which the importance of other contributions to uncertainty can be judged. Natural variability is often the smallest of the uncertainties found in a risk assessment.

Knowledge Uncertainty

Finally, the kind of uncertainty which forms the real substance of uncertainty analysis in cancer risk assessment is uncertainty due to lack of knowledge. This includes vagueness or indefiniteness in an analysis, a stated conclusion, or stated value (Vesely and Rasmuson, 1984), and is termed knowledge uncertainty. Considering the advanced state of science today, the number of things we still do not know sometimes seems almost incredible. The deeper one looks into almost any question, the more knowledge gaps one finds, gaps which prevent us from pinpointing the answer, forcing it to be expressed as within some range. In cancer risk assessment, the range is frequently large. Scientific uncertainties can be reduced through further research. Research also raises new questions, opening up new, previously unsuspected, uncertainties. Thus, research may seem to increase uncertainty rather than reduce it. But it only seems so. In fact, in such a case research moves us from the dangerous situation of thinking we know more than we do, to recognition of some of the things we do not know. In decisionmaking, ignorance is not bliss.

While natural variability is usually associated with the input parameters in an assessment, knowledge uncertainties may be associated with either parameters or models. When the values of parameters can be estimated from large statistical databases fully applicable to the case under study, the dominant parameter uncertainty is from natural variability. This is seldom the case in risk assessment, however. Parameter values may be drawn from small samples or from situations different from the case at hand. Examples of the latter include high-dose to low-dose extrapolation, assumptions that the chemical of interest has the same environmental transport characteristics as a better understood chemical, application of regional or national characteristics to the exposed population, or application of specific characteristics of the current population to populations that may be exposed in the future. Methods to characterize uncertainty in model parameters when sufficient data are available are well established and described in texts on statistical error analysis (e.g., Taylor, 1982). Even when data available are insufficient for standard statistical techniques, alternative methods, such as subjective probability analysis, are available (Morgan et al., 1985).

Uncertainty in whether or not the correct model has been selected is the hardest to treat quantitatively. Numerous models are used in cancer risk assessments. These include source term models, environmental transport models, population projection models, population activity models, exposure models, dose–response models, and metabolic models. Vesely and Rasmuson (1984) divide model uncertainty into (1) indefiniteness in the model's comprehensiveness, and (2) indefiniteness in the model's characterization. The former is the uncertainty of whether the model accounts for all the variables which can significantly affect the results. For example, most models of air transport of sulfur oxides and associated chemical transformation assume uniform, linear chemical transformation of sulfur dioxide to sulfates. They do not include cloud chemistry, a process now believed to be important, which leads not only to nonuniform but virtually noncontinuous transformation. All models, of course, are simplifications of reality and exclude consideration of unimportant factors. Incompleteness may result from a lack of knowledge of a factor or from a misunderstanding of the importance of a factor. Some factors may be important for certain purposes, but not for others. The analyst must beware of selecting a model without careful study to assure it is appropriate for the aims of the assessment. For example, "conservative" air transport models designed for estimating inhalation exposure often ignore ground deposition. Such a model would be inappropriate for a case in which ingestion through drinking water via deposition from air to ground with subsequent runoff to surface water was a potentially important exposure route.

The second form of model uncertainty, indefiniteness in characterization, refers to the processes or relationships expressed in the model. Even if all the significant factors are included in the model, the model may represent an inaccurate understanding of how the world operates. Many of the models used in risk assessments are empirical and either are not fully validated or do not have an adequate basis in theory. The most obvious example is the variety of different high-dose to low-dose extrapolation models used in developing cancer dose–response coefficients. The model uncertainty in these, expressed as the differences in results when using different models, can be many orders of magnitude.

Wong (1984) explored the question of using the dose extrapolation model to design the experiment so as to provide more precise results. The uncertainty in the final risk estimate is composed of model uncertainties and sampling uncertainties. The sampling uncertainty can be reduced by using more animals in each dose group in the bioassay, while the model uncertainty can be reduced by using more experimental doses. If the bioassay is done with the aim of supplying data to an extrapolation model and finally to estimate the risk at low dose, these design aspects should be examined jointly. An important factor is the length of extrapolation necessary. Uncertainty generally increases the further one extrapolates from the experimental data. Larger samples reduce uncertainty associated with shorter extrapolations, but their effect decreases with distance; long extrapolations may be insensitive to larger sample sizes. Model uncertainty remains a limit, however. As sample size increases, total uncertainty approaches model uncertainty. The rate of convergence depends on the design. If convergence is fast, a large increase in sample size may have little effect, the limit being essentially reached with a small increase in sample size.

The experimental dose range is roughly fixed by the preliminary studies to fix the maximum tolerated dose. If the aim of the assessment is to determine the risk associated with a given dose, the length of extrapolation is known. If the aim of the assessment is to set an exposure standard at an acceptable level of risk, one can fix the desired risk level by policy (say a lifetime cancer risk of one in a million), but the associated dose level is, of course, the object of the study and is unknown ahead of time. The shape of the (unknown) true dose–response function is also important. An increase in sample size may not be efficient in reducing uncertainty in extrapolation if the true uncertainty is highly nonlinear.

QUANTITATIVE VS. QUALITATIVE

Some uncertainties are easily quantified. Most can be quantified in principle, but prove difficult in practice due to lack of sufficient information. Some involve discrete options so that their implications are categorically quantified. That is, the results can be quantified for each case. For some uncertainties there is no theoretically rigorous or approved method of analysis. An idea of the variability or range may be had through applying various models or assumptions, but these results are not a full quantitative characterization. Some uncertainties defy quantification completely and must be handled qualitatively. All uncertainties should be described qualitatively. For those quantified in an analysis, the basis of quantification should be explained, including qualitative factors which might affect the quantitative results. Usually quantification involves some assumptions; these, and their implications, should be understood.

All uncertainties which can reasonably be quantified should be. One must, however, not lose sight of the potential importance of those uncertainties which cannot be quantified. As with estimates themselves, ignoring uncertainties which cannot be quantified is burying one's head in the sand. Hattis (1984) has noted that the tendency is to quantify uncertainties that can be quantified and not to deal with those that cannot be quantified. He proposed a law that the uncertainties that can be quantified are always (1) the least interesting kinds of uncertainties, such as statistical variability, and (2) nearly always a small fraction of the overall uncertainties.

There is an argument that quantification, particularly via computer models, makes the results seem unjustifiably accurate. The fact that risk assessments invariably have many assumptions and scientific judgments built-in, which can be hidden in a seemingly sophisticated analysis makes this danger more acute. Providing a full and explicit quantification of the associated uncertainties can remove much of the impact of this concern, but it is important to keep it in mind. Quantifying uncertainties often requires even more assumptions and scientific judgments than quantifying the estimates themselves. These may be as simple as assuming a given parameter is distributed lognormally, when in fact the distribution may be quite different at the extremes, or they may involve a total judgmental extrapolation of the implications in man of tumors in animal tissues which do not exist in man. These assumptions must be explicitly stated; the uncertainties they introduce must be considered and, if possible, investigated.

Quantitative assessment is to aid in decisionmaking. If its results are misleading, it does not achieve this end. Quantitative conclusions cannot stand on their own. They should be interpreted only in light of the assumptions and methods used. Analysts have little control over how their results may be misused, but do have an obligation to make the presentation of their work and their conclusions as clear and explicit as possible.

An important gain from quantifying both the risk estimates and their associated uncertainty is that it imposes a more rigorous process on the analyst. Thinking about how one might quantify uncertainty helps in understanding uncertainty, even if the information available is too scant to allow any meaningful quantification.

HOW BIG ARE UNCERTAINTIES?

Size of uncertainties vary, of course, by the situation. As an example, however, Table 13-2 provides estimates of uncertainty ranges for various components of an Environmental Protection Agency risk analysis done as the basis of a possible standard for volatile organic compounds (VOC) in drinking water. These estimates are mostly subjective, without any explanation of the process involved in their development and are described by their authors as ". . . a rough measure of the subject degree of uncertainty faced by the assessor and regulator" (Cothern et al., 1986).

METHODS OF QUANTITATIVELY CHARACTERIZING UNCERTAINTY

Uncertainty implies that an estimate is not pinpointed, but might take on one of many values. Uncertainty can be characterized in a discrete case

TABLE 13-2 Estimated Level of Uncertainty in Different Components of a Risk Analysis for Volatile Organic Compounds in Drinking Water

---

Factor of 20-50%
   Pollutant level in consumed water
   Selection of dose levels in animal study
Factor of 2:
   Generation of monitoring data
   Assumptions on oral exposure rates
   Variations in animal chow formulation
   time-to-tumor in animal studies
   Inclusion of benign tumors in animal results
   Statistical noise in animal study
Factor of 3:
   Respiratory exposure rates
   Inclusion of pre-cancerous lesions in animal results
Factor of 10:
   Selection of body weight vs. surface vs. concentration as basis of dose–response extrapolation
   Assumption of human effect when animal tumor occurs in animal tissue for which there is no corresponding human tissue
Factor of 10 *to* 100:
   Purity of test compound in animal studies
   Toxicological synergisms or antagonisms
Factor of 1000:
   Distribution of animals among dose levels and number used
Factor of 100,000:
   Extrapolation of animal data from high to low dose

Source: From Cothern et al., 1986.

by listing all of the possible values and in a continuous case, by the range of possible values or the range of values within which the true value falls with a given probability. The frequently used 95% confidence interval is an example of the latter. A more complete characterization accounts for some values having a greater likelihood than others of being the true value. Specific probabilities (summing to 1) might be assigned to each of several discrete points or a range be further characterized with a statistical probability density function.

Similar techniques are used (although sometimes in different ways) to determine ranges and distributions. The simplest way of defining a range is the limits of physical possibility. The range of temperatures within which water exists as a liquid at normal pressure is 0 to 100 °C. Worst-case analysis can be thought of as consistently using the upper boundary of a range, without explicitly stating the range. In many cases, there is no easily definable physical limitation. A more common problem with this approach to defining the limits of a range is that the physical limits include absurdly high or low values, thus unnecessarily expanding the range and overstating uncertainty. Following the example of water temperatures, if we are characterizing the temperature of a lake measured at 25 °C, we might reasonably expect it to hit the lower physical limit in the winter, but would not expect it to even come near the upper physical limit. The difficulty is that there is no particular upper cut-off; even the highest recorded water temperature might be exceeded at a future date. Different approaches have been developed in different contexts to define an arbitrary upper cut-off. Terms like "maximum credible," for example, have been used. The result is always a judgment call; seldom can any rational argument be presented to justify the selected number as opposed to one just slightly higher. Yet, something like this is necessary, particularly in cases where there is insufficient statistical data to shift to an alternative approach. How does an expert determine the point where something is no longer "credible," while still unwilling to classify it as impossible? In the absence of anything else, an expert's "gut feeling" and nothing more may be the only straw to grasp, but for a judgment to be credible, the rationale behind it must be understood. Such a rationale involves physical or biological characteristics, but should also have a probability as a guideline.

The classical approach to defining ranges (or confidence limits) is statistical analysis. Harking back again to our lake, if we measured the temperature every day for a year, and found the daily temperature had a mean of 25 and a standard deviation of 5, we could calculate the 95% confidence range of the mean as

$$25 \pm \frac{(1.96)(5)}{\sqrt{365}} = 25 \pm 0.5 \tag{1}$$

or 24.5 to 25.5. Seldom are the necessary data available to rely solely on this classical analysis. In the example, we assume the measurements have been taken in a place representative of the lake as a whole. Consider, however, whether the year was representative, or was it unusually hot or cold? Suppose that some data were missing; was it on icy, cold days that no one went out to measure the water temperature? The calculation above assumes normally distributed data, probably reasonable here, but not necessarily reasonable in all cases. In cancer risk analysis, classical statistical procedures should be used when appropriate. Their use when not appropriate is a misuse of statistics and usually leads to an underestimate of the range of uncertainty. Statistical methods should not be ignored or forgotten, however. They represent a disciplined approach to uncertainty analysis that can provide the framework for a necessarily less rigorous approach in situations where statistics cannot be used directly. The same can be said for the extension of uncertainty characterization to probability density functions. An understanding of the distribution of a parameter enables one to properly propagate errors through a series of calculations or a model.

Uncertainty analysis is the determination of the variation or imprecision in quantitative conclusion of a risk assessment model (e.g., the predicted exposure or effects) that results from the collective variation associated with the variables in the model (Iman and Helton, 1988). Methods used for uncertainty analysis in computerized risk assessment models, as described by Iman and Helton (1988) include:

1. Response surface replacement, wherein the model is evaluated at many selected sets of input-parameter values and the results fitted in a general linear model which is then used as a replacement for the computer model. The time or cost involved in the large number of computer runs required to obtain sufficient data to fit the linear model limit the applicability of this technique
2. Modified Monte Carlo or latin hypercube sampling, wherein the range of each variable is divided into nonoverlapping intervals with equal probability and one value is selected at random from each interval. From these values, sets of input parameters are selected randomly to form the Latin Hypercube sample that is then used for the uncertainty analysis
3. Differential analysis, wherein a Taylor series approximation is used in conjunction with Monte Carlo analysis to estimate distribution functions

The numerous assumptions, simplifications, and extrapolations that must be made in risk analyses introduce uncertainties beyond those seen in experimental science and narrow conclusions. For this reason, 95% or 99% confidence intervals, commonly used in science, are usually inappropriate for risk analysis. One may calculate a 99% confidence interval, but seldom are the parameters sufficiently understood that one can have any assurance in stating that there is only a 1% or 5% chance the true value lies outside stated bounds. It is much better, and probably more honest, to give 80% confidence bounds. These are easily calculated for normal and log-normal distributions. Factors for estimating confidence limits for Poisson distributed parameters are given in Tables 13–3 to 13–5.

Expert judgment is often called upon to quantify uncertainty in risk

TABLE 13-3 Confidence Limits on the Poisson Distribution

Probability	Upper bound number of counts (h)
Upper bound (h) on the expected number of counts in a Poisson distribution when the observed number of counts was zero[a]	
0.025	3.69
0.05	3.00
0.10	2.30
0.15	1.90
0.1587	1.84
0.20	1.61
0.25	1.39
0.30	1.20
0.3174	1.15

[a]Probability the expected number of cases is greater than h. For h = upper limit of confidence interval (1-α), enter table with value of α. For upper bounds consistent with upper bounds of confidence intervals based on positive counts (i.e., with α/2 probability in the upper tail), enter the table with α/2 instead of α. Note that α = 0.1587 results in an upper bound analogous to one standard deviation above the mean.

assessment. If probability is accepted as a means of representing a statement of degree of belief, then probability distributions can be used as a means to characterize the views of experts on how well or how poorly a given value is known (Morgan et al., 1985). Unlike public opinion polling, risk assessment requires careful, critically considered, professional judgments.

The decisions which risk analysis support are made by people, people whose judgment in weighing the different facets of such decisions is trusted. These decisionmakers do not have the knowledge to make the detailed scientific judgments necessary in the assessment. Where such scientific judgments are necessary, they should be made by competent scientific experts. The worth of uncertainty estimates based on expert judgment depends on the degree of judgmental extrapolation from "solid" data that is necessary. One does not ask an expert to judge the degree of uncertainty in the number of lung cancers in the United States attributable to polycyclic hydrocarbon emissions from coke ovens. The purpose of analysis is to break down such questions into discrete parts, each within the competence of different experts. One can provide judgments on *the uncertainty in* source terms, another on specific uncertainties in air

TABLE 13-4 Confidence Limits on the Poisson Distribution—Poisson Confidence Limit Factors Based on Chi-Square

N	95%		90%		80%		68%	
	L	U	L	U	L	U	L	U
1	0.03	5.55	0.05	4.75	0.11	3.89	0.39	2.36
2	0.12	3.60	0.18	3.15	0.26	2.65	0.58	1.76
2	0.21	2.92	0.27	2.58	0.37	2.23	0.66	1.55
4	0.27	2.56	0.34	2.29	0.44	2.00	0.71	1.44
5	0.33	2.33	0.39	2.10	0.49	1.85	0.75	1.37
6	0.37	2.18	0.44	1.98	0.53	1.76	0.77	1.33
7	0.40	2.06	0.47	1.88	0.56	1.68	0.79	1.29
8	0.43	1.97	0.50	1.81	0.58	1.63	0.81	1.27
9	0.46	1.90	0.52	1.74	0.61	1.58	0.82	1.25
10	0.48	1.84	0.54	1.70	0.62	1.54	0.83	1.23
11	0.50	1.79	0.56	1.20	0.64	1.51	0.84	1.21
12	0.52	1.75	0.58	1.62	0.65	1.48	0.85	1.20
13	0.53	1.71	0.59	1.59	0.67	1.46	0.85	1.19
14	0.55	1.68	0.60	1.56	0.67	1.44	0.86	1.18

Upper bound (h) on the expected number of counts in a Poisson distribution when the observed number of counts was greater than zero.
Source: Based on a relationship described by Johnson and Kotz (1969) for counts of 1 through 14, and on a normal approximation for count 15 and over

transport, another on uncertainties in the dose–response function, and so forth.

Elicitation of expert opinion for risk assessment requires advance planning and careful protocol design, a good understanding of the subject by the elicitation team, and significant investment of time on the part of the experts. The elicitation protocol must be designed to avoid, to the extent possible, cognitive biases recognized in the psychological literature such as anchoring and adjustment (Kahneman et al., 1982; Morgan et al., 1980). It is often necessary to challenge the expert to assure the full extent of uncertainty has been considered. In one protocol for example (Morgan et al., 1980), limits to the range of consideration were obtained by first asking experts how large a given parameter might possibly be. They then were asked to imagine they left the field for a period of several years and came back to find that someone had definitively demonstrated the actual value was somewhat higher than what they had just stated. Could they think of any explanation that would account for such a finding? The experts then recognized that, if they could find a rationale for the higher value, the limits of the possible range must be expanded to include that value. This elicitation team also challenged the experts by pointing

TABLE 13-5 Upper Bound Poisson Limit Factors Based on Normal—Lower Bound Factor Is Reciprocal of the Upper Bound Factor

N	95%	90%	80%	68%
15	1.65	1.52	1.39	1.29
16	1.62	1.50	1.38	1.28
17	1.60	1.48	1.36	1.27
18	1.58	1.47	1.35	1.27
19	1.56	1.45	1.34	1.26
20	1.54	1.44	1.33	1.25
21	1.53	1.43	1.32	1.24
22	1.51	1.42	1.31	1.24
23	1.50	1.41	1.30	1.23
24	1.49	1.40	1.30	1.23
25	1.48	1.39	1.29	1.22
26	1.47	1.38	1.28	1.22
27	1.45	1.37	1.28	1.21
28	1.45	1.36	1.27	1.21
29	1.44	1.35	1.27	1.20
30	1.43	1.35	1.26	1.20
35	1.39	1.32	1.24	1.18
40	1.36	1.30	1.22	1.17
50	1.32	1.26	1.20	1.15
60	1.29	1.24	1.18	1.14
70	1.26	1.22	1.17	1.13
80	1.24	1.20	1.15	1.12
90	1.23	1.19	1.14	1.11
100	1.22	1.18	1.14	1.11
200	1.15	1.12	1.09	1.07
300	1.12	1.10	1.08	1.06
400	1.10	1.09	1.07	1.05
500	1.09	1.08	1.06	1.05
600	1.08	1.07	1.05	1.04
700	1.08	1.06	1.05	1.04
800	1.07	1.06	1.05	1.04
900	1.07	1.06	1.04	1.03
1000	1.06	1.05	1.04	1.03

out values in the literature which were near or higher than the limits they set.

It is important not to lose sight of the fact that, although expert judgments can be appropriately and usefully applied in risk assessments, they are no substitute for research. Not only must the research necessary to narrow the estimated uncertainty be considered, but the need for research to verify the judgment must be considered. Judgment provides an interim result needed now, research provides a better answer later. Few questions of cancer risk are answered definitively and forever; they return again and are reconsidered as knowledge increases.

PROPAGATION OF UNCERTAINITY

Cancer risk analysis usually involves a number of steps, for example: emissions, environmental transport, exposure, dose, dose–response. Each step has an associated uncertainty and the final result includes the combined uncertainty from all steps. Propagation of uncertainty through several steps in an analysis is often the weakest aspect in risk analyses, although the theory of error propagation is well developed. If the formula for calculating the risk is a simple multiplication of the estimate from each step, the estimates are all independent, and the uncertainty associated with each is characterized as a probability density function (pdf), then the propagation of uncertainty through the analysis is the convolution of all the pdfs. This can be thought of as the product of all possible combinations of the values of all the pdfs with appropriate probability assigned to each. For example, take the sequence of events from a pollutant emission to air, through dispersion and transport, leading to population exposure and ultimately a health impact. The emission rate can be estimated but, because of imperfections in measurement techniques and some variability in the release rate over time, is not known precisely. It is estimated as a pdf rather than a single point value. The result of transport and dispersion (involving complex processes) can, for simplicity, be reduced to a linear relationship represented by a single expression normally called χ/Q. This is the quotient of the concentration to which people are exposed (χ) divided by the emission rate (Q). This value, usually obtained by computer models, may also be expressed as a pdf representing uncertainties involved in the process. To complete our simple analysis, we assume a linear dose–response relationship parameterized as a coefficient, E, lifetime effects per unit exposure. This is also expressed as a pdf. As discussed in earlier chapters, while the emission rate and dispersion relationship is specific to the case being studied, the dose–response coefficient is usually derived from the literature. In preliminary or scoping studies, χ/Q may be drawn from literature sources also.

Were each component a point value, the risk (R) in this simple assessment would be calculated:

$$R = Q \ (\chi/Q) \ E \tag{2}$$

Each parameter is, however, expressed as a pdf and can assume any value within its range. It might be that the true value of Q is at the low end of its pdf, the true value of X/Q at the middle of its pdf, and the true value of E at the upper end of its pdf. Any combination is possible. The uncertainty in the calculated risk must reflect all of these possibilities. To do this, the product of every possible combination of the three parameters must be combined with the appropriate probability associated with that combination and accumulated in a frequency distribution to obtain the pdf of risk. This is most easily seen in Monte Carlo analysis, a computer simulation technique which performs this analysis. Each pdf is expressed in its cumulative form. A random number is selected and used to enter the probability side of the function (vertical axis), and the value of the parameter determined from the horizontal axis (Fig. 13–1). This is done for each distribution. The results are one possible set of estimates for each of the contributing parts of the risk formula, called a "realization." The parameter values selected in this realization are all multiplied to yield the risk estimate for that realization. The probability of that realization occurring is calculated as the product of all the individual probabilities. This is done many (perhaps 1000) times and a new cumulative distribution constructed from all the results. Repeatability can be checked by running another 1000 realizations and comparing the cumulatives resulting from the two. If they are not the same, a larger number of realizations are

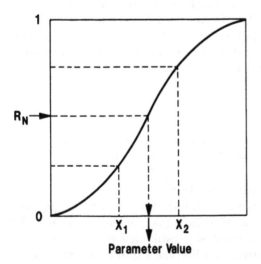

FIGURE 13-1   Monte Carlo selection of parameter value. Random number is enterd on y axis, determining parameter value on x axis. Shape of curve determines distribution of parameter values. In this example, randomly selected numbers on y axis will concentrate parameter values between x_1 and x_2.

necessary. Computer environments have been developed to simplify this process (e.g., Henrion and Morgan, 1985).

This assumes that all the parameters are independent. If the parameters are correlated in some way, say that at high emission rates different dispersion processes come into play, then this must be built into the Monte Carlo analysis. If two parameters are perfectly correlated, that is, if one is from the high end of its pdf, than the other will be from the high end of its pdf to exactly the same degree, then the same random number is used to select the values for each.

In specific circumstances, this analysis can be done analytically without the need for computer simulation. One common case is a multiplicative model such as the example above in which all the pdfs are lognormal. In this case, the overall estimate of uncertainty is determined by the following relationship (Layton and Anspaugh, 1981):

$$\text{Var}(\ln R) = \text{Var}(\ln Q) + \text{Var}[\ln (\chi/Q)] + \text{Var}(\ln E) \tag{3}$$

where, for example,

$$\text{Var}(\ln E) = \ln^2 Sg(E) \text{ and} \tag{4}$$

$Sg(E)$ = geometric standard deviation of R.

Since many parameters used in risk analysis are approximately lognormal, this approach is often useful for a first order estimate of uncertainty.

The following example is taken from an analysis of health effects of geothermal energy production (Layton et al., 1981). The risk of leukemia in the general public exposed at a distance of 10 km to benzene emissions from a 100 MWe geothermal plant was estimated as

$$R = C E (\chi/Q) P \tag{5}$$

where:

R = an individual's lifetime probability of developing leukemia resulting from benzene exposure from the geothermal plant

C = Benzene concentration in geothermal fluid

E = The extraction rate of geothermal fluid

χ/Q = The annual average ambient concentration of benzene per unit emission rate averaged over all sectors (i.e., 360 degrees) at 10 km from the plant. Since the plant was estimated to have only a 30 year life, this was converted to a lifetime exposure by multiplying by 30/70, the ratio of plant life to average human life expectancy

P = life time probability of leukemia per average lifetime exposure to atmospheric benzene, as derived from epidemiological studies of Turkish shoe workers (Aksoy et al., 1974) and U.S. rubber workers (Infante et al., 1977)

TABLE 13-6 Parameters Used in Estimating Leukemia Risk to Benzene Emissions

Parameter	Geometric mean	Geometric SD	ln 2 Sg
C	4 x 10-5 g/kg	8	4.32
E	1.9E3 kg/s	1.5	0.164
χ/Q	0.08 μg s/m^3 g	2.5	0.840
P	7.6E-6 per μg/m^3	1.8	0.346

Sg = Geometric standard deviation.
Source: From Layton et al., 1981.

The lognormal parameters used in the analysis are shown in Table 13-6. The mean value is:

$R = 2 \times 10^{-8}$

$Var(\ln R) = 4.32 + 0.164 + 0.840 + 0.346 = 5.67$

$Sg(R) = 11$

95% confident limits (mean/1.96Sg to mean × 1.96Sg) are thus:

2×10^{-10} to 2×10^{-6}

This approach is much quicker and simpler than Monte Carlo analysis, but only applies in narrow circumstances. In addition, correlations are much more complicated in analytical solutions. An important consideration is spatial correlation. In the example, air dispersion results were restricted to a single distance and averaged over the 360 degrees of the compass. In a more detailed analysis, one might wish to multiply the individual risk by the number of people in each sector. In such an analysis, however, the concentrations in each sector (and thus the χ/Q for each sector) are spatially correlated. That is, if the concentration is high in one sector it is probably high in adjoining sectors. This kind of correlation is difficult to handle analytically. In Monte Carlo analysis, on the other hand, each realization is like an experimental data set and can be treated directly as such.

For regulatory purposes, it is generally thought that only the upper confidence bound is useful. A regulatory authority aims to protect public health and generally tries to take a conservative approach to doing so. Effects are overestimated resulting in regulatory action that is overly stringent, presumably assuring a "margin of safety" to account for any uncertainty. According to this philosophy, an approach that is sometimes proposed as a way to deal with propagation of uncertainty is to replace each parameter in the calculation with its upper 95% confidence limit. This is mathematically an incorrect way to propagate error distributions, but it does assure that the resulting risk estimate overestimates the actual risk. The difficulty is that the degree of overestimation is unknown and

TABLE 13-7 Upper Confidence
Bounds of Each Parameter in Table
13-6, Calculated from Geometric
Means and Standard Deviations

Parameter	95% Upper bounds
C	2.36×10^{-3}
E	4.21×10^{3}
χ/Q	4.82
P	2.41×10^{-5}

may be absurdly high. Upper 95% confidence bounds of each parameter in the previous example, as calculated from the geometric means and standard deviations, are give in Table 13–7. Substituting these values in Eq. (5) yields a risk of 1.1×10^{-3}, nearly three orders of magnitude higher than the upper bound calculated from the proper method of error propagation (2×10^{-6}). Looking at this another way, we can calculate how far out on the distribution of risk 1.1×10^{-3} is. The upper bound is the mean times $Z \times Sg$. Setting this equal to 1.1×10^{-3} and solving for Z gives 4.57. Entering this in a cumulative normal table, we find that 1.1×10^{-3} is the 99.9995% upper bound of the risk; there is less than a 2.5 in a million chance that the true value exceeds this estimate. The problem in terms of interpreting the risk estimates is that, if one is thinking in terms of 95% confidence bounds, the estimated risk far exceeds that, and the misperception can lead to gross overregulation. Moreover, since the amount by which the calculated value exceeds a 95% confidence bound on risk is unknown and varies by the number of parameters in the formula, risk estimates for different hazards will be based on different "margins of safety."

It can be argued that proper methods of error propagation, whether analytic or Monte Carlo, require knowledge of the shape of the error distribution for each parameter, something which is generally not known. This is true, but reasonable assumptions about shape can be made and the sensitivity of the results to these assumptions examined. Moreover, this argument is somewhat disingenious since calculation of 95% confidence bounds on the parameters themselves implies some knowledge or assumption on the shape of the error distribution.

A practical example illustrates how the use of even moderately "conservative" estimates (i.e., those which would overestimate effects) can lead to absurd results when several such estimates are propagated through an analysis. This example is drawn from an analysis criticizing supporting

TABLE 13-8 Assessment Overestimates at Boundary of Uranium Mill-Tailings Pile

Factor	Overestimate	
	Range	Mean
Area of the tailings pile	0.8–2.3	1.2
Radon flux per unit radium-226 concentration in pile	1.1–5.5	1.8
Transport and diffusion	2–10	5
Equilibrium factor	1.4–2.3	1.7
Exposure-dose relationship		0.5
Risk coefficient	1.7–11	6
Overall product		55

Source: From Hamilton and Nagy, 1984.

calculations for proposed EPA standards on radon-222 emissions from inactive uranium mill tailings sites (Hamilton and Nagy, 1984).

Six parameters were involved in the calculation of risk from mill tailing sites. EPA's conservative estimates for each of these parameters averaged about a factor of 2 higher than what Hamilton and Nagy (1984) judged the "best" estimate based on an extensive review. Yet the EPA risk estimate, the product of the six parameters, exceeded the risk calculated from the product of the best estimates by a factor of 55 (Table 13–8).

Propagation of uncertainty is not limited to combining the results from the different subparts of a risk analysis. It must originate with the data and models at the most preliminary calculations of the analysis. For example, uncertainties in emission rate, stack height, and atmospheric parameters that serve as input to an air dispersion model used to estimate exposure should be propagated through to the exposure estimates. Most air dispersion models do not provide for this analysis, but the need for uncertainty analysis in risk assessments is forcing their development. A recent example of this kind of effort is given by Freeman et al. (1986).

Despite the importance of propagation of uncertainty, too frequently it is ignored and the uncertainties represented in the final risk estimates allowed to reflect only one aspect of the process. Even in complex probabilistic analysis of nuclear power plants in which highly sophisticated methods are used to propagate uncertainties through fault trees used to develop the probability of major accidents, little or no attempt has been made to propagate uncertainties in the consequence modeling.

BENEFITS OF REDUCING UNCERTAINITY

Most risk analyses include many built-in assumptions that lead to overestimates of risk. This reflects the preference of regulatory agencies to err on the side of protecting public health. The degree of overestimation needed, however, can be reduced by replacing uncertainty by knowledge. Dupuis and Lipfert (1986) state: "Reliance upon modeling as the basis of regulatory policy dictates an examination of model improvement needs and the economic benefits that could result from the use of improved models." Model improvements have the potential to eventually result in large savings in pollution control costs. A quantitative technique of decision theory, the analysis of value of future information, can help to determine how much effort could profitably be put into improving the models basic to risk assessments. Computer programs are available to carry out this type of analysis (Finkel and Evans, 1987).

SENSITIVITY ANALYSIS

Sensitivity is different from uncertainty. In its simplest form, sensitivity analysis varies each parameter in an analysis in turn and determines the effect on the final risk estimate of a given (say 10%) change in each. In an analysis which involves many different models, each with multiple parameters, the design of a sensitivity analysis can be complex and its conduct time-consuming and computer intensive. The sensitivity of each parameter can be analyzed independently or several parameters changed simultaneously to evaluate interactions. In addition, the effect of small changes to parameters and large changes, possibly using bounding values, may be assessed separately. These are termed local and global sensitivity analyses (Vesely and Rasmuson, 1984).

Sensitivity analysis is conceptually straightforward and an easier task than uncertainty analysis. While it is an important and a useful task, it is sometimes used misleadingly as a substitute for uncertainty. Sensitivity analysis gives no indication of how much each parameter might vary. An arbitrary change of 10% in an input parameter in a sensitivity analysis gives one an understanding of how a change in that parameter affects the final risk estimate, but it does not suggest whether a 10% change is the size of variation to be routinely expected or whether this would represent a large and unexpected change. Without full explanation the reader of the analysis might wrongly assume that a 10% change represents an uncertainty range. Uncertainty analysis goes beyond sensitivity analysis by developing these uncertainty ranges.

IMPLICATIONS OF UNCERTAINITY FOR POLICY APPLICATIONS

Policymakers simply cannot make a reasonable decision if they do not know the uncertainty associated with the "facts" they are getting. Sometimes, policymakers may get frustrated with scientists who give fuzzy answers. There is a story of a senator who, after hearing the testimony of several experts phrased in the form of "Well, on the one hand . . . but then, on the other hand . . .," said that what he needed was some one-handed scientists. To the policy questions which arise on cancer risk, scientists can seldom give one-handed answers. The state of knowledge simply does not allow it. Yet, scientific and technical input to policy decisions in this area is essential. The answer lies in methods of making public decisions under uncertainty. First, a scientist can give fuzzy answers without "waffling." It is done by describing uncertainties scientifically and, to the extent possible, quantitatively. Second, while everyone would like to have needed policy decisions on cancer based on better information than is available, today's decisions must be made with today's knowledge. That does not make cancer risk unusual; few public decisions are made with a full understanding of their consequences. Building the groundwork for a policy decision from the existing body of scientific knowledge requires some leaps, some assumptions, some guesswork, some philosophical basis. Some of this is scientific and should be done by scientists, although where the facts stop and the assumptions begin must be clear to the policymaker. How one leaps over uncertainties, however, involves attitudes toward risk that are more in the political realm than the scientific. Here the risk assessment should layout the science in a way that helps the policy maker reach these decisions.

The uncertainty in the results of an analysis may actually vary according to the policy use. Uncertainties discussed in this chapter are based on estimating absolute risk levels; that is, the risk of a given technology or exposure has a particular value, and there is a quantitative level of uncertainty associated with that value. Many policy applications, however, involve comparisons of risks. Many of the same kinds of knowledge uncertainty apply to all options being compared, and thus are canceled out. For example, many of the uncertainties in the transport of polycyclic organic particles through the atmosphere will cancel when comparing the risk of exposures from coal and oil power plants. Thus the total uncertainty associated with a single risk value may make the significance of the difference or the ratio of two risk values appear to be greater than it actually is. Determining what can be canceled out can be challenging, however. Properties such as particle size which affect the transport of polycyclic organics may be similar for coal and oil power plants, but may be sufficiently different for emissions from home furnaces and power plants as to limit the amount of canceling that can be done.

An important role of risk assessment is to identify the contribution of scientific uncertainties to the final risk estimates so that the value of reducing each source of scientific uncertainty by a given amount can be measured in terms of its effect on the final risk estimates and their contribution to a specific decision. For example, the cancer risk to the public from formaldehyde off-gassing from household construction materials and furnishings depends in part on the level of exposure from this source. The information available on exposure in early risk assessments was from a relatively small number of homes which were not at all representative of the overall distribution of housing types. This is a gap in knowledge which could be improved by more research studying larger numbers of homes over longer periods of time using better measurement techniques. Quantitatively characterizing the uncertainty in the exposure estimates and determining how much this source contributes to the overall uncertainty in the final cancer risk estimates provides the base for a policy analysis which would combine this information with the value placed on the possible cancers to be avoided, the cost of various options to reduce exposure, and the cost of the more extensive surveys to help decide if more research is worthwhile and if regulatory action or other mitigative measures should proceed or should await the results of additional research. Just because a given source of uncertainty is a large contributor to overall uncertainty does not mean that source should have highest priority for additional research. Setting that priority also depends upon the cost of the research, the length of time before the research would produce the result, and the likelihood that the research would actually reduce the uncertainty to the extent expected. The cost, delay, and the expected reduction in uncertainty of the survey of formaldehyde exposure in more homes can easily be estimated. The contribution of uncertainty in risk due to uncertainty in dose–response information can also be estimated in a risk assessment (although perhaps not with as much confidence), but best experiments to reduce that uncertainty, the amount of expected reduction in uncertainty in dose–response resulting from those experiments, and the likelihood that a given reduction in uncertainty will be achieved at a given cost would be much harder to judge.

While discussing the contribution of risk assessment to setting priorities for research to reduce uncertainties in risk, it is important to take note of the need for a balance in the size of the different sources of uncertainty. If one source contributes a large uncertainty to the overall risk estimate, it is of little use to reduce the contribution of smaller sources, since their reduction will have little effect on the overall uncertainty in risk. While this truth must be remembered, there are yet reasons why one may choose to attack small contributors to uncertainty. For example, if the reduced uncertainty can be easily accomplished, it may add to the credibility of the work.

SUMMARY

Estimating uncertainty can be the most important aspect of quantitative risk analysis. Providing decisionmakers estimates of environmental cancer risks without corresponding estimates of the associated uncertainty is irresponsible. This chapter reviewed policy uncertainties, knowledge uncertainties, and natural variability. Examples of the characterization and propagation of uncertainty were given, illustrating the effect of improper uncertainty propagation. Sensitivity analysis was introduced The role of uncertainty in policy applications was discussed.

REFERENCES

AEC. 1974. Proposed final environmental impact statement, liquid metal fast breeder reactor program (WASH 1525). U.S. Atomic Energy Commission, Washington, DC.

Aksoy, M., S. Erdem, and G. Dincol. 1974. Leukemia in shoe-workers exposed chronically to benzene. *Blood* 44:837-841.

Cothern, C.R., W.A. Coniglio, and W.L. Marcus. 1986. Development of quantitative estimates of uncertainty in environmental risk assessments when the scientific data base is inadequate. *Environ. Int.* 12:643-647.

Cuddihy, R.G., W.C. Griffith, C.R. Clark, and R.O. McClellan. 1981. Potential health and environmental effects of light duty diesel vehicles (LMF-89). Lovelace Biomedical and Environmental Research Institute, Albuquerque, NM.

Dupuis, L.R. and F.W. Lipfert. 1986. Estimating the cost of uncertainty in air quality modeling (EA-4707). Electric Power Research Institute, Palo Alto, CA.

Finkel, A.M. and J.S. Evans. 1987. Evaluating the benefits of uncertainty reduction in environmental health risk management. *J. Air Pollut. Control Assoc.* 37:1164-1171.

Freeman, D.L., R.T. Egami, N.F. Robinson, and J.G. Watson. 1986. A method for propagating measurement uncertainties through dispersion models. *J. Air Pollut. Control Assoc.* 36:246-253.

Hamilton, L.D. 1984. Health and environmental risks of energy systems (IAEA-SM-273/51). In *Risks and Benefits of Energy Systems*. International Atomic Energy Agency, Vienna, pp. 21-57.

Hamilton, L.D. and J. Nagy. 1984. Management of uranium mill tailings: a critique of standards (BNL 37750), Brookhaven National Laboratory, Upton, NY.

Hattis, D. 1984. Mechanisms of carcinogenesis: implications for expectations about dose–response relationships. In Workshop on Problem Areas Associated with Developing Carcinogen Guidelines (BNL 51779). Brookhaven National Laboratory, Upton, NY, p. IV-9.

Hattis, D. and D. Kennedy. 1986. Assessing risks from health hazards: an imperfect science. *Technol. Rev.* 89 (4):60-71.

Henrion, M. and M.G. Morgan. 1985. A computer aid for risk and other policy analyses. *Risk Analysis* 5:195-208.

Iman, R.L. and J.C. Helton. 1988. An investigation of uncertainty and sensitivity analysis techniques for computer models. *Risk Analysis* 8:71-90.

Infante, P.F., J.K. Wagoner, R.A. Rinsky, and R.F. Young. 1977. Leukaemia in benzene workers. *Lancet* 2:76.

Johnson, N.L. and S. Kotz. 1969. *Discrete Distributions*. John Wiley & Sons, New York.

Kahneman, D., P. Slovic, and A. Tversky (eds.). 1982. *Judgment Under Uncertainty: Heuristics and Biases*. Cambridge Univ. Press, New York.

Layton, D.W. and L.R. Anspaugh. 1982. Health impacts of geothermal energy (IAEASM-254/38). In *Health Impacts of Different Sources of Energy*. International Atomic Energy Agency, Vienna, pp. 581-594.

Layton, D.W., L.R. Anspaugh, and K.D. O'Banion. 1981. Health and environmental effects document on geothermal energy—1981 (UCRL-53232). Lawrence Livermore National Laboratory, Livermore, CA.

Morgan, M.G., M. Henrion, and S.C. Morris. 1980. Expert judgments for policy analysis (BNL 51358). Brookhaven National Laboratory, Upton, NY.

Morgan, M.G., M. Henrion, S.C. Morris, and D.A.L. Amaral. 1985. Uncertainty in risk assessment. *Environ. Sci. and Technol.* 19:662-667.

Moskowitz, P.D., E.A. Coveney, M.A. Crowther, L.D. Hamilton, S.C. Morris, K.M. Novak, P.E. Perry, S. Rabinowitz, M.D. Rowe, W.A. Sevian, J.E. Smith, and I. Wilenitz. 1983. Health and environmental effects document for photovoltaic energy systems—1983 (BNL 51676), Brookhaven National Laboratory, Upton, NY.

Quade, E.S. 1975. *Analysis for Public Decisions*. American Elsevier, New York.

Rowe, M.D. 1980. Human exposure to sulfates from coal-fired power plants. *J. Air Pollut. Control Assoc.* 30:682-4.

Rowe, M.D. 1981. Human exposure to particulate emissions from power plants (BNL 51305). Brookhaven National Laboratory, Upton, NY.

Taylor, J.R. 1982. *An Introduction to Error Analysis*. University Science Books, Mill Valley, CA.

Vesely, W.E. and D. M. Rasmuson. 1984. Uncertainties in nuclear probabilistic risk analysis. *Risk Analysis* 4:313-322.

Wong, S.C.Y. 1984. Model uncertainty: implications for animal low-dose cancer risk assessment experiments. Presented at the annual meeting, Society for Risk Analysis, Knoxville, TN.

14

Risk Characterization, Communication, and Perception

INTRODUCTION

Risk characterization is the fourth and final step in risk assessment. Exposure and dose–response information developed earlier in the process are combined to estimate cancer risk. This crucial step brings everything together in a way that makes sense to decisionmakers and the public. It should give an understandable accounting of known scientific and technical information in a way that allows that knowledge to be brought to bear on the problem. It must also describe what is not known, in a way that gaps in knowledge and uncertainties can also be fully taken into account in addressing the problem. The risk analyst must realize that the risk characterization is not the end, it is merely one of many inputs to a decision. The analyst should understand the elements of that decision and something about the other factors that contribute to it to assure that health risk is characterized in a way that will be useful in decisionmaking.

Because it must be tooled to focus on each specific problem, it should not be surprising that risk characterization is the least formalized, the least well-defined step in quantitative risk assessment. The National Academy of Sciences' report, *Risk Assessment in the Federal Government*, that established the steps of a risk assessment, has little instruction or advice on risk characterization compared to the earlier stages of analysis (NAS, 1983). Its discussion of risk characterization focuses on characterization of uncertainty, selection of dose–response and exposure models to be used, and on selection of the population at risk that provides the most meaningful expression of the health risk.

Risk characterization is, in one sense, the final product of assessment. It is the place for interpretation of the results and it provides the link between the analysis and later policy or risk management work. A careful and objective analysis can be spoiled by a poorly done or biased character-

331

ization stage. The selection of what parts of the analysis are to be emphasized or even included can obviously introduce personal or policy bias into the characterization. Even decisions on how to aggregate results to simplify and clarify presentation, especially those on how to treat highly uncertain or improbable results, sometimes made without much thought beyond the need to reduce a complex set of analyses to an understandable presentation, can have significant downstream implications. The format of the characterization may make some policy choices easier to understand or to manipulate than others, for example.

A decade ago, a discussion of risk characterization would have focused only on the ways of bringing together exposure and dose–response information to quantitatively estimate risk. Today, the subject of risk characterization is sterile without including two new and important fields: risk communication and risk perception. The purpose of characterizing risk goes beyond the simple desire to understand risks; it intrinsically includes the need to communicate that understanding to others. Because of their background and training, scientists, engineers, economists, and other quantitatively oriented people who do risk analysis tend to address problems differently than much of the public. Moreover, it is easy for them to fall into the trap of focusing on increasingly narrow, quantitative aspects of risk. It is clear that the public perceives risk differently than the "experts." The solution to this problem once was thought to be public education, we now realize that two-way communication is needed. Those involved in risk assessment must make a better effort to communicate their findings to others and to understand and address the concerns of others. To do this, they must have a better understanding of concepts and methods of risk communication and of the way the public perceives risk but, they must also be open to change the way they characterize risk to meet the needs and desires of the public. This chapter, thus, includes sections on both areas, in addition to more traditional concepts of risk characterization.

RISK CHARACTERIZATION: COMBINING EXPOSURE AND DOSE–RESPONSE TO ESTIMATE CANCER RISK

While the original National Academy of Sciences report provided little guidance on the risk characterization phase of quantitative risk assessment, more informative general guidance is found in a U.S. Department of Health and Human Services task force report on health risk assessment (DHHS, 1986). The task force defines the role of risk characterization as synthesizing information developed in the earlier stages of assessment. Recognizing that synthesis is not as straightforward a process as might appear initially, it suggests methods that might be used: (1) consensus development conferences, (2) criteria documents, (3) state-of-the-art conferences. These, of course, are the processes to build a risk characterization, not the content of the characterization itself. This work can be done "by a single staff analyst, . . . by an assembly of eminent scientists with diverse but relevant technical backgrounds, or by researchers with any intermediate combination of numbers, breadth of expertise, and professional standing." Part of the synthesis process is described as weighing all of the evidence in terms of experimental design, reproducibility, and concordance across several species. This is parallel to the process used by EPA in its "weight-of-evidence" approach to determine if a substance is a carcinogen (see Chap. 3). The principal application of the "weight-of-evidence" approach would seem to be more appropriate in the earlier stages of the risk assessment, but the notion of synthesis clearly belongs with   characterization.

As in the earlier NAS report, the task force stressed the importance of uncertainty in the assessment. When key information in the assessment is missing or subject to excessive uncertainty, a decision must be made on how to proceed. Possibilities suggested by the task force include:

1.   Make a best guess about the missing information
2.   Do another kind of analysis to side-step the gap
3.   Bracket the uncertainty by two or more estimates
4.   Establish and follow some policy on the matter

These decisions require judgment, either on the part of the risk assessment team directly or, through application of agency policy, on the part of policy-level officials. Such judgments are necessary to get on with the assessment, but have often been the focus of concern for critics of risk assessment. It is important that these judgments be explicitly described to assure the absence of policy bias or to make any biases explicit. Otherwise, the credibility of the assessment suffers.

The task force distinguishes between risk assessments made for regulatory and nonregulatory purposes. These differences include "the nature and specificity of legal and regulatory mandates, the deliberateness with which the analyses are structured, the degree of openness of the process, review and clearance procedures, and the type and specificity of reports issued." It notes, however, that these distinctions begin to blur in the risk characterization phase and finds substantial unity in the roots of regulatory and nonregulatory risk characterization.

The following paragraphs of this section touch briefly on various aspects of risk characterization and considerations that go into development of the characterization part of a quantitative assessment.

Qualitative Overview

The numbers in a quantitative risk assessment strengthen it, make the information it conveys more precise, and put greater meaning to caveats and expressions of uncertainty. But, numbers need to be packaged in words to describe the problem addressed, point out important factors that affect the risk, tell which factors can be expressed well in numbers, which cannot, and explain how the latter influence the results of the analysis.

The risk characterization should briefly restate the purpose and motivation for the work. It should describe the scope of the dose–response and exposure assessments and summarize limitations or assumptions made there that might limit or otherwise affect the conclusions to be drawn from the characterization. While the characterization may determine that a certain approach or way of viewing the problem is better for the purposes of the assessment, it should discuss alternative approaches, their relative merits and the implications their application would have on the conclusions. A reader of the characterization should not find any disturbing surprises upon looking back into the more detailed dose–response and exposure assessment.

Risk assessment, and its characterization phase especially, is likely to influence public opinion or policy directly, or to form the basis of later policy analyses or news stories that will do so. While the line between risk analysis and policy analysis is often fuzzy, the risk analyst must be aware of policy questions and options. It is not the role of risk characterization to answer, address, or even necessarily to mention these questions, but it must present the scientific analysis in a way that these questions can be addressed. Too often the design or presentation of a scientific study precludes its direct application to policy questions; this is directly contrary to the function of risk analysis and must be avoided.

Qualitative discussion provides the framework for the quantitative analysis, but it goes beyond that. It must state the limitations of the quantitative analysis, clearly setting forth underlying assumptions and simplifications and noting key factors affecting risk or its valuation that cannot be quantified.

Body Counts or Alternative Measures?

The easiest and most commonly used quantitative measure of risk is the number of "excess cancers" resulting from some exposure source or action. For example, one risk analysis estimated that exhaust from diesel-powered vehicles would cause less than 200 lung cancers per year in the U.S. population (Cuddihy et al., 1984). Another risk assessment estimated that about 0.45 leukemia cases per year result from fugitive benzene emissions in the U.S. (EPA, 1984).

Another way to characterize risk is in terms of increased lifetime individual risk, often to a maximally exposed individual (MEI). For example, the MEI lifetime risk associated with surface water concentrations for 12 hazardous waste sites in one study averaged 6×10^{-5} (Whitmyre et al., 1987). That is, the maximally exposed individual would have 6 chances in 100,000 of developing cancer due to this exposure. Individual risk depends on a great many personal factors, e.g., age, sex, smoking and dietary habits, and occupation. While the variables may be too great to make a prediction for a particular person, the average individual risk can be estimated for a defined population. Often the effect of these various individual risk cofactors, while acknowledged in principle, are in fact unknown and are ignored in a risk calculation.

The individual risk estimate requires exposure information for only the individual or population subgroup of interest, often the fictitious maximally exposed individual. The population risk is the cumulative effect in the population expressed as the number of extra cancers expected in a population as a result of a given exposure. While individual risk can be expected to vary by age, sex, race, occupation, and other factors, the effect over numerous population subgroups is summed to estimate the overall population risk. Population risk estimates thus require a more detailed assessment of population exposure over the entire population than do estimates of individual risk. Statements of population risk often appear to have the characteristics of body counts and are felt by many not to be informative, especially for low-level exposures. Even a small individual risk spread over a large population or a large time period can lead to a seemingly substantial number of cancers. There is a need to place such results in perspective, a topic treated in more detail in a later section.

A supplementary piece of information beyond the risk of cancer or the number of cancers expected is years of life lost due to cancer. Simply giving the number of cancers does not distinguish between an exposure that produces cancers in people 35–50 years old and those 75–90 years old, yet most people would agree there is a difference. This is not holding the lives of older people cheap. Risk assessments seldom consider cancers that have occurred; instead, they estimate future cancers expected to occur in a population. To a 20 year old, it makes a difference whether a current exposure threatens to inflict him with cancer in 15 or 50 years time. For some diseases, distributing environmentally induced cases by age is difficult due to a severe lack of knowledge. Cancers are easier to deal with in this regard since more information is available and only two or three alternative models need be considered. Taking lung cancer from radon *exposure as an example*, a widely accepted model (NCRP, 1984) assumes radiation-induced lung cancers are produced at a rate that is a fraction of the background rate, that size of that fraction being a function of dose modified by a lag time followed by an exponential decline in risk over time. Given a dose regimen, the "excess" lung cancers are calculated in a life-table model. The same model could be used to calculate years of life lost to radon-induced lung cancer; no additional assumptions are necessary.

Explicit Treatment of Uncertainty

As discussed at length in the previous chapter, uncertainty is the dominating factor in risk analysis. Adequate characterization of uncertainty is the hallmark of a superior characterization of risk. The National Academy of Science's report on risk assessment places emphasis on the importance of uncertainty in risk characterization (NAS, 1983).

A minor, but important, point in risk characterization is careful attention to significant figures. Quantitative risk assessments involve computer analysis leading to results stated in 10 or more digits. Risk analysts too frequently forget that it makes no sense to give a result as "174.3697 expected cancers per year" when the probable range is from zero to 300. Seldom do assessments justify the use of more than two significant digits.

Time and Space Considerations

Risk must be defined in terms of time and a population. In the case of individual risk, is it increased annual risk or lifetime risk? For population risk, are the numbers given increased cancers per year, increased cancers accumulated over a specific number of years, or total cancers over all time associated with a specific source? Moreover, population risk estimates must explicitly designate the population at risk and indicate if projected population growth has been included in the analysis. The population may be the entire world, the U.S. population, the population within a given radius of a facility or of a number of facilities. Populations need not be defined geographically; for example, the population at risk may be all those who eat a particular food, or all cigarette smokers. The need to state time and space parameters clearly may seem obvious, but sometimes these factors are so obvious to the analyst that they are not included in the report. One then finds they are not so obvious to those trying to use the results of the assessment. It is always wise for someone not directly involved in the work to review the risk characterization for omissions of this kind.

While it is necessary to be explicit about whatever parameters are used, some time and space units are more appropriate than others. The selection should be based on the underlying science and the policy needs.

Selecting the units based on model capabilities should be avoided. There is little scientific basis for calculating the risk to those within 80 km of a facility simply because that is the range of the available air dispersion model. There is no discontinuity at that distance to make a risk calculation at 70 km valid while one at 90 km is not. Uncertainty increases with distance and it may be appropriate to stop the analysis at some quasi-arbitrary distance, but this should be based on sensitivity analysis or other calculations and the implications discussed. A similar situation arises with time; uncertainty increases as the distance estimates are extrapolated into the future increases. Uranium mill-tailings piles, without protective cover, will continue to emit radon gas into the almost unlimited future. Uncertain low-dose dose–response estimates may be combined with uncertain long-range transport models and the effects cumulated over the uncertain events of a hundred thousand years or more to estimate large numbers of cancers, but these estimates are so uncertain and have such little practical meaning as to be useless. The method generally adapted by regulatory agencies is to cut off estimates after some arbitrary number of years (e.g., 100 or 10,000). An alternative approach would be to estimate the lifetime incremental risk of each future generation.

Synergisms, Confounding Factors, Multiple Sources of Risk, and Complex Mixtures

Synergisms, confounding factors, multiple sources of risk, and complex mixtures are those nagging problems that there is never sufficient information to deal with satisfactorily, but that must be addressed and recognized as potential problems. Most decisions on these issues must be made in earlier phases of the analysis, and have been treated in earlier chapters. There are implications, however, that only appear in synthesis. Potential synergisms in dose–response take on importance only to the extent that people may be exposed to the right mixture of substances, for example. Frankly, because of the inability to do anything beyond speculation, most risk assessments do not go beyond mentioning these problems as caveats, and many do not even to that. Sometimes, useful bounding analyses can be done. These may be "back of the envelope" calculations, or may be simple probabilistic analyses combining exposure and dose–response information. The latter are usually based on input distributions derived from little more than "back of the envelope" calculations. A judgment must be made as to whether synergisms, complex mixtures, and other confounding factors are likely to make a meaningful difference in the risk characterization and bounding calculations can be helpful in that decision. If they may be important, the likelihood and potential consequences of their effect should be discussed and analyzed to the extent possible.

Perspective

Risk characterization is more than simply combining exposure and dose–response estimates. It requires expressing the resulting risk in a way that can be understood by the recipient. The results of risk assessments are often small incremental risks. The risk analyst becomes accustomed to dealing with risks like 10^{-5} or 10^{-6} as a shorthand index. Government or corporate policymakers and the public, however, have little grasp of the meaning of such small incremental risks; indeed, neither may the risk analyst in any practical, real-life way. One way to provide meaning to the numbers is to compare them with common risks that are generally understood. Although seemingly an obvious aid, such comparisons are often not well accepted. The public or the workforce often does not believe the risk to be acceptable, simply does not believe that the exposure of interest has as small a risk as estimated by the analysis, and is not interested in comparisons with familiar acceptable risks such as drinking three cans of diet soda or eating a peanut butter sandwich. Often the public's concern transcends the increased cancer risk and speaks from outrage over the imposition of an unwanted risk with no direct benefit. The comparisons are often voluntary activities or natural risks such as hurricanes or falling meteorites and are different in character from an environmental pollutant or a food additive. Comparisons must be phrased carefully so that it is clear they are used to provide perspective on the size of the risk, and are not meant to imply the risk analyzed is equally acceptable as those used as comparisons. Another approach to providing some perspective is to express the risk relative to the background cancer rate. Not a risk of 10^{-6}, but an increase from a background cancer rate of 35% to one of 35.0001%. Perspective is important to the understanding of risk, but it must be done thoughtfully to avoid being patronizing or losing credibility.

Putting Cancer Risk in Economic Terms

Characterizing cancer risk in monetary terms is often a difficult calculation to explain. How can one set a monetary value on human life? Is not life infinitely precious? Is not any attempt to set such a value bound to be a mechanical exercise in mathematics devoid, not only of feeling, but of any sense of reality? But, look at this question in a different way. Is not life filled with risks, known and unknown? How many people, even if they could afford it, would go to the extremes to avoid risk that Howard Hughes did in the last part of his life? It would mean giving up a part of life itself. Do we do our utmost, expend all our resources to avoid risks? Interstate highways are much safer than secondary roads; but we do not insist that secondary roads be built to the same standards as interstates. The reason is that the cost would be too great, not only in dollars, but in land use, social disruption, and, indeed, the decreased usefulness of the road system itself.

Value-of-life questions take on different meanings under different circumstances: whether it is known who will die; the probability of death; the certainty of death; the timing of death. A coal miner is trapped in a cave-in, sure to die unless rescued within days. Society will expend almost unbounded effort and resources to rescue him. Yet, the event is not a big surprise; everyone knows these things happen in coal mines. Why were the resources not spent ahead of time in prevention? The answer is, of course, that there were considerable resources spent in prevention, but no amount would be enough to eliminate the risk; more would just reduce the probability. When it comes to actually putting up the cash, society is unwilling, indeed is unable, to spend infinite amounts to avoid something that might happen to someone who cannot as yet be identified. A similar situation exists in the regulation of exposure to potential carcinogens, except there are more qualifiers: there is usually considerable uncertainty over whether the exposure actually will produce any increase in cancer; the effect, if it did occur, would not be expected for two or more decades in the future; and, even if it did, it may never be known since the cancer produced is unlikely to be connected directly to the previous exposure. The impact of expenditures to reduce environmental cancer is thus less quantifiable, or even verifiable, than that, say, to provide improved emergency medical service.

The value of a particular life, at immediate risk of death now, is quite different than the value of a small change in the risk of cancer decades in the future. Yet, the former, never the case in cancer risk assessment, is what often comes to mind when the question arises of "putting a price on life." Howard (1980) proposes a method to extrapolate what he calls the small-risk life value from indifference curves constructed by asking questions about alternate life incomes and life expectancies. Various points of view on valuing life may be found in Rhoads (1978), Singer (1978), Etzioni (1979), and Hapgood (1979).

Graphic Presentation

A graph can be worth a thousand numbers. Graphical presentation of the results of a risk analysis can serve to make the findings clearer. Graphs can cut through pages of complex text to bring understanding. The graphics must be, of course, well thought out; bad graphics may confuse *rather than elucidate* and at worst may mislead. Special care must be taken to assure that the graphs do indeed display the findings and do not mislead. The analyst or the analysis team should develop the graphics, possibly using a graphics consultant. This should be done as part of the synthesis process of risk characterization. The need to produce a graph serves to focus the mind and can help to clarify the thoughts to be expressed in the text as well.

Seldom are graphics meant to replace text; they are supplements only. By helping the reader to quickly grasp the key points, they make the text easier to understand. Recommendations on how to handle the mechanics of graphics to improve their usefulness include: (1) assign each figure a number so it can be clearly referenced in the text; (2) provide a main title for the figure as well as a sufficient caption; (3) label all axes, columns, and rows; (4) specify the units; (5) define all special symbols and abbreviations (Rathbone, 1972).

Risk analyses frequently must present information expressed as probability distributions. These curves can be difficult for the untrained eye to interpret. Cumulative plots can be especially misleading. While the median is evident, the mean value cannot be determined from a plot of a cumulative distribution function. It is recommended that a cumulative distribution function be plotted in alignment with a probability density function using the same horizontal scale, and that the mean be clearly marked on both curves (Ibrekk and Morgan, 1987).

RISK PERCEPTION

Until recently, the risk assessment community adhered to a belief that physical actions (emission of a toxic pollutant, exposure to a radioactive substance, etc.) posed a risk to people that could be completely described in terms of their physical, chemical, or biological characteristics. There was disagreement within the community on how well these risks could be quantified and even the extent to which they should be quantified, but there was little question that scientifically based study and analysis was the only way to understand these risks and the only justifiable basis for regulating risks. After two or three decades of increasingly widespread development of quantitative risk estimates, however, it became apparent that something was wrong. This scientifically based approach was not leading to a rational policy for regulating risks. Regulation is a political process highly influenced by the public's perception of risk. Gradually, research by a small group of psychologists began to show that public perception of the risk of hazardous activities, substances, and technologies is shaped by factors quite different from the scientifically based risk estimates developed by risk analysts (Slovic et al., 1980; Slovic, 1987).

People's perceptions of environmental and occupational risk is shaped to some degree by personal observations, but perhaps more broadly by the news media. Calamity and risk are news; safety is not. Rarity is news, the commonplace is not. Yet, with our worldwide news coverage, we are deluged with rarity on a regular basis; we come to believe rarity to be common, the common to be rare. Asked to estimate the frequency of fatalities from different causes, people overestimate the effect of the rarities botulism and tornados, effects that are newsworthy so that everyone hears about virtually every case, while they underestimate common causes such as stroke, diabetes, and stomach cancer, effects that are not newsworthy and so people only know of a small percentage of all cases (Lichtenstein et al., 1978). Another characteristic of news coverage that biases public perception is that news stories tend to present viewpoints, not truths. Sandman (1988) points out that if all possible positions on an issue are ranked on a scale of 0 to 10, responsible journalists give short shrift to the extremes (0, 1, 9, and 10), but also pay little attention to the middle (4, 5, and 6) that does not provide good copy. Most of the news consists of 2s and 3s and 7s and 8s in alternating paragraphs. The controversy increases the news value, while giving "both sides" of the story maintains objectivity. The middle ground, where most scientific experts might fall much of the time, becomes lost in the controversy between the credible extremes. Although both sides may be given, the "bad" news generally gets better coverage than the "good" news. Moreover, it is easy to read personal or corporate financial interest in those who report low risk, while those who report findings of high risk are more likely to be seen to be acting in the public interest. Even the lack of trust in government commonly seen today has a similar bias: government reports stating that actions of industry or government agencies pose high risk are more readily believed than reports from the same agencies that actions of industry or government pose little or no risk. Interestingly, the same is not true in other circumstances. Government reports that radon gas in homes may present a high cancer risk receive little response in the public, perhaps because there is no outrage, no industry to blame, or perhaps because people cannot accept that their familiar homes pose such a risk (or perhaps because the public has a more sensible attitude toward such risks than regulatory agencies).

The public does misperceive risks because of the biases in their sources of information, but the difference in perception of risk between experts and the public is much deeper than that. It strikes at the very concept of what risk means. Risk analysts generally equate risk to the probability of increased death or disease, although even among experts there is argument on exactly how risk should be expressed. The "body counts" or

TABLE 14-1 Measurement Scales for Perception of Risk

Factors related to dread
  Controllable–uncontrollable
  Dread–Not dread
  Global catastrophic–not global catastrophic
  Not equitable–equitable
  Catastrophic–individual
  High risk to future generations–low risk to future generations
  Not easily reduced–easily reduced
  Risk increasing–risk decreasing
  Involuntary–voluntary
Factors related to unknown
  Not observable–observable
  Unknown to those exposed–known to those exposed
  New risk–old risk
  Risks unknown to science–risks known to science

Source: From Slovic, 1987.

narrow expression of risk in terms of expected fatalities often have little meaning to the public who think in terms of much broader characteristics. Paul Slovic and his colleagues (e.g., Slovic et al., 1980; Slovic, 1987) investigated people's perception of risk using many different scales of measurement (Table 14-1). These scales were reduced to two principal components: measures of dread and measures of the unknown. Simply scanning the table provides some appreciation of the complexity in people's thoughts about risk.

Since the development of this list, three other metrics have been suggested as important in evaluating how people perceive risks. *First* is the signal effect; this is the ability of an event to have impact far beyond its immediate effects by acting as a signal or an alert that other similar events may be in the offing (Slovic, 1987). The extensive social and political impact of the Three Mile Island nuclear power plant accident is an example. Not a single person died, no latent cancers were expected. Some analysts, in fact, proclaimed TMI demonstrated that a major reactor accident would not result in the massive health effects predicted. Yet, TMI apparently was the death knell for nuclear power in the United States; despite its own lack of direct health effects, it served as a signal (or perhaps a symbol) of what might be. The *second* newly described factor is outrage. Although backed primarily by anecdotal evidence, a group at Rutgers University (Hance et al., 1988) suggest there is an "outrage" dimension in addition to a "hazard" dimension to risk. Some of the factors contributing to outrage (Table 14-2) are the same or similar

Table 14-2   Factors Contributing to Outrage

Voluntary risks are accepted more readily than those that are imposed
Risks under individual control are accepted more readily than those under government control
Risks that seem fair are more acceptable than those that seem unfair
Risk information the comes from trustworthy sources is more readily believed than information from untrustworthy sources
Risks that seem ethically objectionable will seem more risky
natural risks seem more acceptable than artificial risks
Exotic risks seem more risky than familiar risks

Source: From Hance et al., 1988.

to Slovic's "dread" and "unknown" factors, but their implication is slightly different. It literally reflects a sense of community or personal outrage that a particular risk should be foisted on "us." The *third* factor is stigma. In some cases, environmental contamination can stigmatize an area, its products, or even its people, in the sense, for example, that the public will refuse to buy food produced in a region where contamination has been publicized. There is little scientific information on this effect, and no evidence that the effect is long-lasting, but there is no doubt that the perception that such effects could occur affects people's thinking about risk. Some people who express no fear of direct health effects from a nuclear power plant in their community, for example, have expressed the fear that in the event of an accident new industry and new people would refuse to move into the area leading to economic stagnation.

To summarize, the public often has misperceptions about risks that have proved difficult for risk experts to understand. But, the public also has a much broader concept of risk than is included in formal scientifically based risk assessments. What is generally seen by risk analysts as the key conclusions of a risk assessment, namely the increased cancer incidence or fatality rate associated with a substance or an action, may be seen by the public as only a small, and possibly insignificant measure of the risk. To some degree it is the role and responsibility of government, industry, and professionals to carry out the analyses that assure excessive health impacts will not occur, regardless of the importance placed upon this by the public. Nonetheless, recent research results in this area should give pause. Regulatory agencies and the risk analysis profession should consider whether overmuch reliance is being placed on esoteric calculations of extremely small effects on cancer rates to the almost total exclusion of consideration of many of the reasonable and practical considerations that *the public appears to consider important.*

Risk Communication

Risk communication is a natural extension of risk characterization. We characterize risks because we wish to communicate their meaning to policy makers and the public. Usually, the principal focus has been on the policy makers; the public were secondary. Stallen and Coppock (1987) give four reasons for communicating risk to the public:

1. People at risk ought to be informed so they can avoid harm
2. People have a right to be informed
3. People want to be informed
4. People need information to check whether government is doing its regulatory job adequately

Until recently, there was little emphasis on risk communication to the public. Risk analysis was simply a matter of estimating the risk and presenting the findings. When the public seemed not to accept the results, education was the recommended solution. Research findings on public perception now help to explain *why* the public did not accept many of the results. These findings also provided the basis for a new and growing field. Government and industry officials responsible for explaining risks to the public have an expanding kit of tools to use.

Keeney and von Winterfeldt (1986) offer six objectives for this new field of risk communication

1. Educate the public about risks, risk analysis and risk management
2. Inform the public about specific risks and actions taken to reduce them
3. Encourage personal risk reduction
4. Improve understanding of public values and concern
5. Increase mutual trust and credibility
6. Resolve conflicts and controversy

When a new niche is formed, government and corporate bureaucracies expand to accommodate it: federal and state agencies and industry are hiring risk communicators. That provides recognition of the importance of risk communication, but opens the dangerous possibility that a gulf will open between risk assessment and risk communication. The opposite effect is needed. Risk analysis, risk communication, and management at the policy level should be brought closer together. That is because effective risk communication must be two-way communication. To the extent that the problem is not so much that people disbelieve the risk estimates as it is that the numbers being generated in the analyses simply do not address people's concerns, communication must seek to find out what those concerns are and to incorporate them in the assessment.

TABLE 14-3   Seven Cardinal Rules of Risk Communication

1. Accept and involve the public as a legitimate partner
2. Plan carefully and evaluate performance
3. Listen to your audience
4. Be honest, frank, and open
5. Coordinate and collaborate with other credible sources
6. Meet the needs of the media
7. Speak clearly and with compassion

Risks associated with memorable events are considered more risky
Risks that are undetectable create more fear than detectable risks

Source: From Covello and Allen, 1988.

While research results on risk perception provide a solid foundation, exactly how to apply these results effectively involves guidelines and rules of thumb more than any specific scientific method. As in any interpersonal interactions, although there are techniques that can be learned, much depends on the individuals involved. An EPA publication lists "seven cardinal rules" for effective risk communications (Table 14-3). In addition, two highly useful guides are available that are filled with guidelines and suggestions, one designed for industrial plant managers (Covello et al., 1988), and one designed for government regulatory agency personnel (Hance et al., 1988). The former focuses more on the technical information to be presented, providing guidelines for explaining risk-related numbers and risk comparisons, and includes numerous concrete examples. The latter focuses more on the methods of communication itself, covering topics such as how to overcome outrage, how to earn trust and credibility, how to communicate with different audiences, and how to deal with values and feelings. Both address the problem of communicating to the public in a local geographic area on risk issues of local concern, e.g., local concerns for risks at a chemical plant or hazardous waste site. Both provide useful guidance beyond their narrow original scope and anyone anticipating interacting with the public on risk issues is well advised to obtain copies of both.

When thinking about communicating risks to the public, analysts should not forget about policy makers. They, after all, are part of the public, too, and are likely to share many of the same characteristics that separate the rest of the public from the experts. It may be that by improving communication with the public, risk analysts will improve their communication of risk to policymakers also.

SUMMARY

Risk characterization, the final step in quantitative risk assessment, synthesizes information developed in the earlier hazard identification, dose–response assessment, and exposure assessment phases. Risk characterization's purpose is to communicate the risk to policy makers or the public. Recent findings in risk perception demonstrate biases in public perception of risks that must be overcome to communicate the scientific information in the assessment. This research also indicates, however, that the public perceives risk in a much broader context than the narrow "body counts" on which quantitative risk assessments have focused. This calls for increased two-way communication and greater consideration of broader aspects of risk in analysis.

REFERENCES

Covello, V. and F. Allen. 1988. *Seven Cardinal Rules of Risk Communication*. U.S. Environmental Protection Agency, Washington, DC.

Covello, V.T., P.M. Sandman, and P.Slovic. 1988. *Risk Communication, Risk Statistics, and Risk Comparisons: A Manual for Plant Managers*. Chemical Manufacturers Association, Washington, DC.

Cuddihy, R.G./, W.C. Griffith, R.O. McClellan. 1984. Health risks from light-duty diesel vehicles. *Environ. Sci. Technol.* 18:14A-21A.

Davies, J.C., V.T. Covello, and F.W. Allen (eds). 1987. *Risk Communication*. The Conservation Foundation, Washington, DC.

DHHS. 1986. *Determining Risks to Health, Federal Policy and Practice*. U.S. Department of Health and Human Services, Auburn House Publishing Company, Dover, MA.

EPA. 1984. National emission standards for hazardous air pollutants; benzene equipment leaks. *Fed. Reg.* 49:23498-23520.

Etzioni, A. How much is a life worth? *Social Policy* 9(5):4-8.

Hance, B.J., C. Chess, and P.M. Sandman. 1988. *Improving Dialogue with Communities: A Risk Communication Manual for Government* Environmental Communication Research Program, Rutgers University, New Brunswick, NJ.

Hapgood, F. 1979. Risk-benefit analysis, putting a price on life. *The Atlantic* (January) 33-38.

Howard, R.A. 1980. On making life and death decisions. In R.C. Schwing and W.A. Albers, Jr. (eds), *Societal Risk Assessment, How Safe is Safe Enough?* Plenum Press, New York, pp. 89-106.

Ibrekk, H. and M.G.Morgan. 1987. Graphical communication of uncertain quantities to nontechnical people. *Risk Analysis* 7:519-529.

Keeney, R.L. and D. von Winterfeldt. 1986. Improving risk communication. *Risk Analysis* 6:417-424.

Lichtenstein, S., P. Slovic, B. Fischoff, M. Layman, and B. Combs. 1978. Judged frequency of lethal events. *J. Exp. Psychol.: Human Learning Memory* 4:551-578.

NAS. 1983. *Risk Assessment in the Federal Government: Managing the Process*. Committee on the Institutional Means for Assessment of Risks to Public Health, National Research Council, National Academy Press, Washington, DC.

NCRP. 1984. *Evaluation of Occupational and Environmental Exposures to Radon and Radon Daughters in the United States* (NCRP Report No. 78). National Council on radiation Protection and Measurements, Bethesda, MD.

Rathbone, R.R. 1972. *Communicating Technical Information*. Addison-Wesley, Reading, MA.

Rhoades, S.E. 1978. How much should we spend to save a life? *Public Interest* 51:74-92 (Spring).

Sandman, P. 1988. Telling reports about risk. *Civil Eng.* August, pp. 36-38.

Singer, M. 1978. How to reduce risks rationally. *Public Interest* 51:93-112 (Spring).

Slovic, P., B. Fischoff, and S. Lichtenstein. 1980. Facts and fears: understanding perceived risk. In R.C. Schwing and W.A. Albers, Jr. (eds.), *Societal Risk Assessment, How Safe is Safe Enough?* Plenum Press, New York, pp. 181-214.

Slovic, P. 1987. Perception of risk. *Science* 236:280-285.

Stallen, P.J. and R. Coppock. 1987. About risk communication and risky communication, *Risk Analysis* 7:413-414.

Whitmyre, G.K., J.J. Konz, M.L. Mercer, H.L. Schultz, and S. Caldwell. 1987. The human health risks of recreational exposure to surface waters near NPL sites: a scoping level assessment. *Superfund '87, Proceedings of the 8th National Conference*. The Hazardous Material Control Research Institute, Silver Spring, MD, pp. 143-148.

15

Quality Assurance, Validation, and Peer Review

If something is worth doing, it is worth doing well! Quality assurance is how one makes sure the job is being done well, while validation and peer review are how one finds out afterward if it was done well. Risk assessments often become the basis of regulatory action or policy, even if not conducted for that purpose. They can thus affect both lives and fortunes and it is most important that they be done well. Policies or regulations are more readily accepted if it is felt that the assessments they are based on are solid, objective, and trustworthy. Unlike most scientific endeavors, however, there is so much uncertainty in quantitative cancer risk assessment, so many assumptions which must be made, so many different fields that must contribute, that errors in judgment, mistakes, and bias can easily, and unwittingly, creep in. The uncertainty cannot be avoided; the mistakes can. Moreover, the uncertainty can be identified and in most cases quantified. The user cannot expect the risk assessment to do more than the state of knowledge allows, but should expect the risk assessment to describe the limits of the state of knowledge and the resulting uncertainties in the assessment.

QUALITY ASSURANCE

Quality assurance (QA) is a planning and management process which assures the assessment is of a specified quality. Quality assurance comes from production systems where the product was a piece of hardware and QA involved production quality control, acceptance testing, and product inspection. Quality is no less important in risk assessment, however, where it helps to assure confidence in the validity and integrity of the reported data, analyses, computer codes, procedures, and methods used.

Quality assurance can extend beyond the assessment itself in the form of records management to assure the protection, retrievability, and

348

possibly replicability of the data. Risk assessments which form the basis of government regulations or the basis of decisions made on regulated activities must meet the QA and record keeping requirements of applicable government guidelines and regulations or national consensus organizations (e.g., "Quality assurance criteria for nuclear power plants" in the Code of Federal Regulations, 10 CFR 50 Appendix B; ANSI/ASME, 1983; and DOE, 1985). Evidence from a QA program may be equally useful in environmental or consumer product litigation which may result from decisions based in part on risk assessments.

Quality assurance includes scientific and technical procedures and administrative procedures. For risk assessments, technical QA procedures generally formalize what might otherwise be called "good practice." Examples are documentation and various validity checks of data sources, computer programs, procedures for carefully maintaining calculations in notebooks or other written form, assuring internal consistency in calculations, and similar activities. Administrative procedures include planning, management controls, and quality verification. These might include formal internal reviews and peer reviews which are discussed in more detail below.

VALIDATION

Validation is the process of assuring that something is sound and able to withstand criticism. In computer modeling, an important aspect of QCRA, validation means to compare model predictions with actual laboratory or field experimental results to assure that the model predictions approximate reality within acceptable limits. Validation is part and parcel of model development. Model development and validation require two independent data sets, one on which to develop and calibrate the model, the second on which to test or validate the model. Calibration is like adjusting the dial on the radio to fine tune the station. One adjusts the "dials," or coefficients, in the model to make it fit the data. That is not proof the model is any good, though. A model that has enough "dials" might be made to fit any data set. The "proof of the pudding" is if the model fits the second, independent data set with the same "dial settings," i.e., the same coefficients.

So often there are such scant data available for risk assessment that all of the data must be used for model building, leaving none for validation. This was the case with some structure-activity model building discussed in Chapter 10. There is no satisfactory way around a shortage of data. One possibility is to split what data there are and use part for model building and part for validation. This can result in an unrealistic model and in insufficient data for a proper test. There is no reason, however, not to try this and then recombine all the data and repeat the model-building steps. The final model will be the same as what would have been developed if all the data had been used in the first place. The ability to draw statistical interpretations from the result is impaired because of the earlier manipulation of the data, but this is a small price to pay since statistics must be interpreted cautiously for analyses run with limited data anyway. In addition to a limited validity test, the difference between the two models provides additional insight into the effect of the shortage of data.

The independence of the model-building and validation data sets is important. Calibrating an air pollution model with this year's pollution measurements and validating it with next year's data may not be very rigorous. Next year's data are probably spatially and temporarily correlated with this year's. In its most rigorous form, validation is an experimental process which requires a prior design with prescribed protocols and statistical performance evaluation to measure for the absence of bias, gross error, correlation and goodness of fit between residuals and observed values and correlation between residuals and exogenous variables. A model should be validated for all situations for which it is applicable.

Verification is a related term. It is the process used after encoding a mathematical model in computer language to assure the equations are properly coded. Verification tests can be made by means of hand calculations or comparisons with previously verified results. Verification assures that the computer code reflects what the modeler had in mind. Validation assures that the model as encoded adequately reflects reality.

In many cases, a secondary standard of validation is used. Model results are compared with results of another model which has previously been validated and accepted. Specific test conditions are established to indicate potential errors and highlight the implications of differences between the models.

No model reconstructs the real world to perfection. By their nature, models are simplifications of the real world. So when we talk about validation of a model, we must establish criteria for how close to reality a model must be to be deemed valid. Perhaps surprisingly, there are no general standards for such criteria. This is largely because each model does something different, and the validation criteria must be unique. A model may be valid for one purpose, but not for another. For example, a long-range air pollution transport model is designed to predict the annual average concentration of a carcinogen in each county of the United States. For one purpose, the model may be acceptable if the cumulative population-weighted exposure over the country checks out against measured national average values. For another purpose, it might be important that the population-weighted exposure must check out for each state. For a third purpose, it might be necessary that the predicted concentration in each county is accurate. This is similar to the problem facing weather forecasters. Conditions may enable them to predict with great confidence that it will rain somewhere in the northeast, but the reliability of a prediction that it will rain in New York City specifically is much lower.

Another side of validation should be brought into this discussion. In comparing model results with measurements, one should not necessarily assume that the measurements are right. In the above case, for example, how does one measure the population-weighted exposure level for the nation or even the concentration in a county? Measurement stations are usually few and far between and linear interpolation among them is often not valid, even when sophisticated techniques such as Kriging are used. Indeed, most of the models used in cancer risk assessment cannot be validated in the rigorous way described above. The solid, validated models are inadequate to deal with the questions a cancer risk assessment must address. So models, approaches, and assumptions are used that are pushing the frontier, that are predicting values that cannot be measured. Obviously, we must go ahead and use unvalidated models. So why talk about validation? It is the ideal, the standard against which any judgments about the validity of a model must be based.

Validation and Replication

Validation is generally considered a necessary part of the design of a single study. However, because it so often is not included, it should be recognized that validation can be done in a separate, later study. When inadequate data are initially available for validation, studies to collect more data may be specifically directed at validating the earlier model.

There is always a question of how much data are really needed to develop an adequate model, and how much data are needed to test or validate it. When is it better to lump all the data and develop a new model? Lave and Seskin (1970) used all the (then) available data in a correlation of air pollution and mortality for urban areas to develop a model relating sulfate aerosol to mortality. Later, they "validated" their model with an improved and expanded data set (Lave and Seskin, 1978). Leaving aside the question of the independence of the two data sets, the model was found to "fit" to the second data set, statistically meaning that one could not reject the hypothesis that the second data set came from a world that looked like the model.

Replication is one bulwark of science. Particularly in the physical sciences, publication of an important new discovery leads to a rush in other laboratories to repeat or replicate the experiment. This redundancy and duplication, so often decried by bureaucrats and congressmen, provides credibility and assurances that the original findings were real, and not an artifact of the local experimental set-up or other anomaly. Moreover, the essence of scientific results is that they *can* be replicated if the same circumstances are recreated. In biology, experiments are less frequently replicated, partly due to time and expense. Because of greater random variation in biology, even exact replications cannot be expected to give the same results. Nonetheless, closely related studies with similar findings greatly increase the value of information. One of the reasons that benzo[a]pyrene is so well understood and so frequently cited as an example of chemical carcinogenesis is that there have been many experiments and studies with this one substance. When in vitro tests, animal studies and epidemiology all show a chemical to be a carcinogen, there is little question left.

What replication means specifically in risk assessment is not clear. Presumably, two risk assessment teams doing the same study from start to finish and getting a similar result. This happens frequently. Organizations with different attitudes about how to assess cancer risks conduct separate analyses. For example, several organizations have reported assessments of the risk of radon exposure among the general public (e.g., NCRP, 1984; GAO, 1986; ICRP, 1987). They overlap in the sources they cite and frequently cite each other, but they are in a sense replication. Their conclusions sometimes agree, but not always; replication is not always successful. Searching out the underlying reasons for the differences can be rewarding, often showing that the differences are not real, but simply show that the uncertainty is in fact bigger than estimated in any single assessment.

One must be careful to recognize that, at times, what seems like a separate, new analysis is not that at all, but simply the old analysis in a new wrapper. Risk analysts are known for "borrowing" from one another. There is a case in which two U.S. studies which appeared to be different but with similar (although not exactly the same) results, turned out to be the same. The newer study drew on a European study, which in turn had drawn upon the earlier American study. The slight differences in results were attributable to the double-rounding error in the conversion from English units to metric and back again!

PEER REVIEW

Peer review is the traditional review and validation process in science. A journal article or a grant proposal is submitted to referees for peer review, referees are chosen from a pool of reviewers qualified in the area. Although most scientists have a story to tell of peer reviews which treated them unfairly, almost every scientist is in favor of it. A study suggesting that the peer review process for reviewing grant proposals at the National Science Foundation involved a significant element of chance (Cole and Cole, 1981) flushed out much support of the peer review system (e.g., Clark, 1982). The consensus seems to be that it may not be a perfect system, but it generally works and it is preferred over its alternatives.

In risk assessment, peer review means different things to different people. To some it is a method for assuring greater consistency and identifying areas where scientific uncertainty is so high, additional research is required (Flamm, 1986). To others, it is the means of supervising the integrity of the risk assessment process (Samuels, 1983).

Peer review should be built into the assessment process and into its time schedule. Government agencies usually require this step, and establish requirements and procedures for peer review. Too often, however, the requirements and procedures, although well intentioned, are perfunctory. Everyone expects the job to be done well in the first place and for the peer review report to have only minor criticism at most. Schedules often provide for draft reports to reach the peer review committee a week before the review and for the final report to be completed a month following the review. Such hopeful plans virtually never come to pass. Risk assessments are too complex and offer too many pitfalls. No matter how competent the assessment team, reviewers unearth problems, often substantial ones. Then, either the schedule falls apart or an unsatisfactory report is published. This does not have to be the case. One can assume there will be substantial revisions following peer review and allow time. A better approach, however, is to provide for staged, or continual, review. The plans and design of the assessment can be subjected to peer review, each stage of the work can then be subjected to peer review as it progresses. That avoids a peer review committee being hit with a *fait accompli* at the end where they might find fault with early assumptions, necessitating that much of the later work be redone. The Rasmussen Reactor Safety Study conferred repeatedly with a parallel American Physical Society study which provided some degree of ongoing review. On a smaller scale, the Preliminary Risk Characterization Assessment for the high-level civilian radioactive waste program was specifically designed with continual peer review. The assessment itself was conducted by a team at Battelle Pacific Northwest Laboratories. A review team was established at Brookhaven National Laboratory. A series of reports was scheduled, beginning with the program plan and a report detailing assumptions, approaches, *and models. Each report* was submitted to the Brookhaven group for detailed review, as well as being circulated for review to several program offices within the Department of Energy. In addition, periodic review meetings were held. A review of this sort helps to take advantage of outside advice as part of the study and eliminate surprises at the end. Going even further, an open review, in which preliminary materials are made widely available, including to potential opponents, can assure no aspect important to the assessment, and no way of looking at the problem, is omitted. This can greatly increase the confidence with which results are held. The process, however, involves considerable investment in time and effort.

Scientific Review

Who are the "peers" in peer review? Peer review generally means review by other people working in the same or related areas. Risk assessment models are different from models that researchers who are on the cutting edge of a science build. The latter are built to test hypotheses and to generate new hypotheses. They often delve deeply into narrow areas of science to address specific questions. Models built for risk assessment are generally greatly simplified and much broader in scope. They usually deal with questions in which researchers on the cutting edge have little interest; not because they are not interesting questions or because the answers are known, but because they are questions which cannot be solved directly by experiment. Yet, risk assessment models must maintain as high a degree of scientific credibility as possible. Often, scientists look on risk assessment models with disdain at first acquaintance. After understanding their purpose, however, most will recognize that, for what it is meant to do, the model is sufficiently based in science. Involving scientists on the cutting edge of research in the review of risk assessment models is important. It helps to assure that the models do indeed reflect the science adequately and to the maximum extent consistent with their purpose. It also is a way to bring in new ideas and new hypotheses. Risk assessments must consider the possibilities of several variants in the state of nature, that is the essence of dealing with uncertainty. It is the scientists on the cutting edge who can best see what variants are just appearing on the horizon. Dealing with these scientists takes tact and patience, however, on both sides.

Adversarial Review

Peer review is objective. A peer review committee can be tough and often will play the devil's advocate to avoid missing a problem with the assessment. Their role is to assure the work is good and, where necessary, to point out needed improvements. Adversarial review is tougher. An adversary has a vested interest in finding fault with the assessment. An industry's assessment may face adversarial review in a regulatory agency or by an environmental or public interest organization. A government assessment may face adversarial review by affected industries or by an environmental organization which believes the assessment understates the risk. The tobacco industry painstakingly reviews assessments on cancer and other health effects of smoking. The most searching review can come as part of litigation of issues based on cancer risk assessments. Adversarial reviewers may not always play fair, but they often put a great deal more resources, time, effort, and thought into their reviews than peer reviewers usually can. Because they have more incentive to find faults in the analysis, they are more likely to find faults that exist. They may do more extensive sensitivity analysis, may rerun the analysis with different assumptions or different models.

In some cases, adversarial review can lead to polarization and difficulty in eventually reaching agreement on a course of action. Channeled properly, however, adversarial review can be highly valuable. It can force the assessment to adhere to the highest standards possible. It can provide the most searching review. To the extent that faults in the analysis are minor or can be overcome, it can be an avenue of consensus and of confidence building.

What Fraction of the Total Effort for Review?

A conventional peer review, in which the reviewers serve on a volunteer, consulting, or part-time basis, might involve less than 10% of the total project effort. An ongoing, continual review might involve 20% or more, depending on the depth of independent analysis done by the reviewers. The Nuclear Regulatory Commission's reviews of probabilistic risk assessments for nuclear power plants may involve as much as 40-50% of the total effort. That is, the review may be as extensive as the original analysis itself. While that may sound extreme, it must be remembered that a risk assessment has attributes different from other scientific endeavors. It has many different parts from different fields linked together. It involves many assumptions that can be embedded in layers within the analysis. Simply understanding all the ramifications of what was done can be a time-consuming task. Often, an adequate review may require new and independent analyses to test various aspects of the assessment. In this sense the review can make a genuine contribution to the assessment.

Sometimes, the review can far exceed the original effort. This happens when an assessment which has important regulatory or policy implications is poorly done. Under legislative pressure, budgetary constraints, or simply ignorance of the size of the task, an agency may carry out a "quick and dirty" assessment, pulling a hodgepodge of material from previous assessments and patching them together, or making unwarranted simplifying assumptions as a short-cut. Sometimes such a study is meant to be a quick and dirty study for screening purposes or as preliminary work to get a feel for the problem before designing a more definitive assessment. Such a preliminary study can appear just at a time when there is great pressure to formulate a policy or promulgate a regulation. It then is offered or perceived as the best available basis for action. For example, an exposure analysis, designed to be one leg of a cancer risk assessment for public exposure to exhaust gases from diesel cars was released in the late 1970s, a time when diesel cars were first being introduced and looked like they would quickly become an important part of the U.S. automobile fleet. Whether by design or not, this was no more than a scoping study. Taking advantage of other work just completed in Kansas City, it assumed that the entire United States looked like downtown Kansas City! Several government agencies, industries, and public interest groups had a vital interest in studies which might affect government policy on the growth of the diesel car fleet. Easily 10 or 20 times the effort involved in the original study was spent on reviews and criticisms. While helping to assure that an inadequate piece of work was not used as the basis of an important cancer risk assessment, the resources, effort, and time could have been much better spent doing a more complete exposure assessment. The short-cut approach, taken to save time and money, generally ends up with more time and more money being expended before a decision can be reached. Worse, a decision may eventually be based on a series of corrections to the original study. The appropriate study, which would provide more useful information, and which could have been done with far less time and effort, is never done.

CONFIDENCE BUILDING

Risk assessment models can rarely be adequately verified. They frequently deal with events that will happen only under circumstances which do not yet exist. Even when these events come to pass, it may still be impossible to verify what happened because assessments often focus on effects which are in the "noise" level, that cannot be experimentally measured. Effects of air pollution from coal power plants is an example. There is great controversy over whether current pollution from existing plants causes health effects, and predictions of the effects of a new plant may never be proved right or wrong. Risk management decisions are made under uncertainty. Nonetheless, we want to be as sure as we can of these decisions. Validation and peer review are part of the process to build confidence in risk assessment models. This is not the kind of confidence built through advertising; it is confidence built through testing, comparison, and review. It will never be possible to develop the level of confidence that everyone would desire, but all models and methods should be subjected to as much "confidence building" as is feasible.

SUMMARY

Quantitative cancer risk assessments are generally done amid controversy. Neither public nor corporate decisionmakers or the public will accept policies based on analysis in which they have no confidence. Validation and peer review are part of the process of confidence building. The professional assessment team must convince themselves of the validity of their assessment, they must then convince their scientific peers and the public. In the process, feedback they receive can help to improve and strengthen the assessment.

REFERENCES

ANSI/ASME. 1983. NQA-1 Quality assurance program requirements for nuclear facilities. American National Standards Institute/American Society of Mechanical Engineers.

Clark, A.H. 1982. Luck, merit, and peer review (editorial). *Science* 215 [1Jan]

Cole, J.R. and S. Cole. 1981. Peer Review in the National Science Foundation: Phase Two of a Study. National Academy of Sciences, Committee on Science and Public Policy, Washington, DC.

DOE. 1985. Quality assurance management policies and requirements (DOE/RW-0032). Office of Civilian Radioactive Waste Management, U.S. Department of Energy, Washington, DC.

Flamm, W.G. 1986. Risk assessment policy in the United States. In P. Oftedal and A. Brogger (eds.), *Risk and Reason*, Alan R. Liss, Inc., New York, pp. 141-149.

GAO. 1986. Air pollution, hazards of indoor radon could pose a national health problem (GAO/RCED-86-170). U.S. General Accounting Office, Washington, DC.

ICRP. 1987. Lung cancer from indoor exposures to radon daughters (ICRP 50). Pergamon Press, Oxford.

Lave, L.B. and E.P. Seskin. 1970. Air pollution and human health. *Science* 169:723-733.

Lave, L.B. and E.P. Seskin. 1978. *Air Pollution and Human Health*. Johns Hopkins University Press, Baltimore, MD.

NCRP. 1984. Evaluation of occupational and environmental exposures to radon and radon daughters in the United States (NCRP 78). National Council on Radiation Protection and Measurements, Bethesda, MD.

Samuels, S.W. 1983. Policy of risk assessment of the health effects of hazardous exposures to populations, a report of the subcommittee on environmental carcinogenesis. National Cancer Advisory Board on Quantitative Risk Assessment, National Cancer Institute, Bethesda, MD.

16

Implications for Risk Management

INTRODUCTION

In general terms, risk management is the process by which society and the individuals in it manage or otherwise adjust themselves to the risks they face. Risk assessment, of course, is part of that process. In a more narrow sense, contrasting risk management with risk assessment, risk management involves the political, economic, and social aspects of decisionmaking as apart from the scientific aspects found in risk assessment. Risk assessment unavoidably includes many assumptions that have political, economic, or social implications. The risk analyst, ideally, should not be the one to make these assumptions, they should be established a priori by "management" or should be parameterized so that a choice can be made in the risk management phase. Indeed, the whole purpose of risk assessment is to aid in the process of risk management. The "risk manager" essentially hires the "risk assessor" to provide information. The two must be sufficiently independent to assure objective assessments. The risk assessor is parallel to the accountant who is hired by the manager, but has an independently derived set of professional rules subject to outside audit to assure the financial accounts are not manipulated to suit some private aim of the manager that may be contrary to the interest of the stockholders. The immediate risk manager may be a company president or a regulatory agency official, but the ultimate risk managers are the stockholders or the public. It should be clear that risk management is a broad process encompassing wide societal interests, not a narrow professional field that uses the results of risk analysis to produce decisions. Modern risk management decisions involve complex scientific and technical matters. Just because risk assessment may be independent of risk management does not mean that risk managers need not understand the scientific and technical basis of the problem. Current problems with health and environmental risk at U.S. nuclear weapons plants, for example, have been ascribed to the loss of scientific competence at the management level in the Department of Energy (Butterfield, 1988).

While the risk analyst should be sufficiently independent to avoid being coerced into manipulating the science to meet preconceived ends, he or she must not forget that their aim is to provide information useful to the decision process. To this end, the risk analyst must have an understanding of risk management processes and the kind and form of information that is useful in them. Providing that basic understanding is the aim of this chapter. After discussing risk management philosophies, it looks at risk management in two ways.

First, a number of management techniques are described. One technique may be useful in one situation, an alternative technique in another. They are not all mutually exclusive, however. Two or more techniques may be used together to support a decision. Moreover, a risk management decision need not be a single, one-time decision. Decisions can be, and often are, made in sequence; updating, adjusting, and revising decisions as new information becomes available and unexpected results of earlier decisions appear. The described techniques are not exhaustive and they tend to focus on methods with strong need for quantitative input.

Second, a number of management formats are described. These provide the context within which the techniques are exercised. Individuals are their own risk managers, making choices that affect their level of risk. Part of the responsibility of the risk analyst is to provide information that can help the individual member of the public in doing this. Newspaper headlines giving dire warnings of the "carcinogen of the week" do not provide the public with the coherent information-base necessary for rational decisionmaking about risks. In a complex society, there are many centers of decisionmaking for risk beyond the individual. Industrial firms, government agencies, courts, insurance companies, and others all make decisions affecting cancer risks. Each of these is discussed individually, but it is important to recognize that there is no central person, place, or organization for risk decisionmaking. All of these separate decision-makers act independently or occasionally with limited coordination. Sometimes they act in contradictory ways. No rational decision can be taken without consideration of what others have done or might do.

Compounding this situation, cancer risk management decisions affect other spheres also. They often involve environmental policy, energy policy, nutrition and other aspects of public health, labor-management relations, and industrial or economic development policy. These multiple interests seldom coincide. Even other health issues or environmental concerns may not be best served by a proposed cancer risk management policy. Yet, all of these factors must be taken into account in decisionmaking. To make the decision more burdensome, large amounts of money are at stake; money that could be spent for other worthy purposes—or must be diverted from those purposes—to be spent on uncertain estimates of potential cancer risk.

Risk is a matter of values, knowledge, and circumstances. Primitive cave dwellers 20,000 years ago were exposed to massive doses of carcinogens in the smoke from their cooking fires. Even if they understood the relationship with cancer, it would have been of little concern to them. They had far greater, more important, and more immediate risks to worry about. Today, for most people in the United States, those greater risks are mostly gone. We can afford to be concerned with exposure to carcinogens. Yet, just as scientists may differ over the interpretation of the same data, within the population there are differences of opinion on how safe is safe and how far the government should go to protect the public. In the face of uncertain effects, the more stringent the standard the more certain we can feel we are protected, yet, how certain should we feel? How much should we be willing to pay for additional certainty? These are risk management decisions based on values that vary among the public and change over time. The consensus that is reached, or the social-political-economic compromise that evolves may easily differ from one culture to another and from one political jurisdiction to another.

STABILITY AND FLEXIBILITY

Risk management must be concerned with consistency and stability as well as with the sometimes conflicting need for flexibility and the ability to change as new information becomes available. Risk management is reflected in corporate policy, government regulations, and development decisions. These lead to channeling of people's thinking and to capital investments in new technologies and pollution control measures. The physical implementation of risk management decisions has a time delay of years or decades. Concepts of risk management take time to become established in people's thinking. It is important that risk management decisions receive careful consideration so as not to set implementation steps in motion unnecessarily. Once set in motion, it can be very costly and disruptive to society to change direction in midcourse. Stability is important to the mental, physical, and economic health of a society. Business representatives, for example, are sometimes heard to state their preference for early and decisive regulatory action with some guarantee that it will remain in force for a period of time, rather than a long period of uncertainty even with the expectation that the latter would lead to more favorable rules.

While stability is important, it must be recognized that the scientific basis of risk decisions is constantly improving. Moreover, society itself is changing; with change, come new attitudes toward risk develop. A decision that seems right and sensible today may be viewed differently even 5 years hence. Risk analysis must be updated as new scientific developments emerge. The public, and particularly that section who feel themselves to be at risk, are generally impatient with delays in implementing controls seemingly warranted by new findings, and have little interest in the need for maintaining stability or economic costs, inefficiencies, and loss of credibility that may come from constantly changing the rules. Some laws, such as the Clean Air Act, provide for review and, if necessary, revision of standards on a proscribed basis, e.g., every 5 years. A pressing need in the development of the regulatory process is to find better means of providing both stability and flexibility.

The period between the documentation of a risk in a risk analysis and the promulgation of regulatory standards is often lengthy, and may seem longer since the first announcements of a hazard may precede the conclusions of a formal risk analysis by several years. Every preliminary scientific finding, however, does not turn out to be true. Some degree of verification and assessment is required before regulatory action is taken; the alternative is the chaotic regulatory swings that often appear. Methods used in the analysis and decision processes themselves may be affected by a perceived need for a speedy response. One reason given in favor of a single-step bioassay in preference to the improved knowledge base that could be had with a two-stage bioassay procedure (discussed in Chap. 8) was the anticipation of public perception and public interest group outrage over the delay following a positive first stage result suggesting a substance is a carcinogen or of later having to relax a preliminary standard on the basis of new and different information from the second stage test. Even the built-in periodic re-evaluation of ambient air standards leads to great political trauma for regulatory agencies should a change seem warranted.

RISK MANAGEMENT PHILOSOPHY

Just as there are different philosophies of people management and of money management, there are different philosophies of risk management. A philosophy is, in a sense, the view one takes of life, and so it is not surprising that people's positions in life affects their philosophies. The regulatory official is charged with protection of the public from undue risk. Although perhaps knowledgeable and sympathetic with potentially opposing interests such as manufacturing useful products, protecting food crops from pests, or developing new and beneficial technologies, these are not the responsibility nor the prime interest of the regulator. Industrialists, on the other hand, while not callous to possible risks to occupational or public health, and frequently giving health and safety concerns the highest consideration, must keep other factors in the balance also. Health and safety are not their only concern. This is not a contrast between capitalism and socialism; the American private industrialist shares similar interests and views in this regard with the Soviet Commissar responsible for industrial output or the American government official with operational responsibilities such as energy or defense.

The basis of a philosophy goes beyond individual position, however. It also reflects general societal views. One need only think about the change in societal attitude toward risk that has occurred over the past few decades. This section does not explore different philosophies in detail. It simply discusses some background characteristics that affect management philosophy.

Conservatism

A conservative philosophy in risk analysis and management means overestimating risk in the face of uncertainty to provide some assurance that decisions will protect at least to the degree intended. It would seem hard to fault such a policy. There can be problems with conservatism, however. Concerns include: (a) what degree of conservatism is appropriate? (b) the importance of knowing the degree of conservatism; (c) the problem of propagating conservative values; and (d) the effect of varying degrees of conservatism on comparisons among options.

The appropriate level of conservatism depends on two factors: how well the process is understood and how much risk we are willing to accept. If you drive to work every morning, you know the route and the traffic very well. Perhaps it takes you 20 minutes, seldom varying more than 5 minutes either side of that. Your knowledge is good; you do not need to build in a large "margin of safety" to assure you will get to work on time. Your decision on when to leave for work depends primarily on the consequences of being late, and less on your uncertainty of how much time it will take to get there. If you give yourself 25 minutes, you will almost always be on time; If it is important you not be late, even occasionally, you might give yourself 30–40 minutes and accept that you will be there early most of the time. You probably would never consider leaving an hour ahead of time. On the other hand, if this is not your regular route to work, but an early morning business appointment or job interview, and you are not familiar with the route or the traffic, you might estimate the time required as 15–40 minutes even without considering unusual traffic. Because you know your ability to estimate the time of trip is poor, you will be inclined to add a bigger "margin of safety" above your best estimate to allow for the greater uncertainty. You might easily plan more than an hour to make the trip.

Examine this situation again in more technical terms. In the first case, your estimate is precise, with narrow error bands. Five minutes above the mean may be the upper 90% confidence bound, assuring you are late no more than 5% of the time. In the second case, your knowledge base is smaller and your estimate is naturally less precise; the error distribution around your best estimate is much wider. Making the decision at the 95% upper confidence bound because it is important not to be late, you find yourself at more than 3 times the best estimate. Yet, you are at the same level of confidence that you will be on time as the person who drives the same route daily and allows less time for the trip.

In both cases, the consequences of being late were considered, but in neither was the cost of being early considered. You may not like to get up early or wait around when you arrive early, but these seem small compared to losing your job for being late, and you might find some use of the time you spend waiting. Public health decisions, too, are often made without considering the cost. The costs are there, however. The person with the business meeting "wins" in his decision to leave early if he gets tied up in traffic and the trip does take him an hour. The chances are, however, he ends up arriving in 20 minutes and has to wait for 40 minutes before his meeting begins. Similarly, if the decision is made at the upper 95% confidence level, for every dangerous drug we are "saved" from, we forego the potential health benefit of another 19 that are actually safe are also kept off the market. To do otherwise would either increase the chance of exposing the public to a hazardous product, or would increase the costs by requiring more extensive testing to increase the knowledge base on which the decision is based. Saccharin is an example where the health benefits of weight control and associated decreased risk of heart disease were judged sufficient by Congress in 1977 to outweigh the normally conservative decision process to ban the artificial sweetener as a carcinogen. This led to an extensive study by the National Academy of Sciences of the risks and benefits of saccharin that laid much of the philosophical and technical groundwork for comparisons of this kind (NAS, 1978, 1979). Each risk management decision thus represents an explicit or implicit balancing of risks.

Decisions on the level of conservatism are risk management decisions, and should not be made by the risk analyst. The latter must provide information on the level of knowledge and uncertainty associated with the risk estimates. The risk analyst should also develop information on the costs and consequences of different levels of conservatism. It is unfortunate that much of the conservatism in risk analysis is not explicit, but is built into the models and assumptions made by and used by the analyst. Often conservatisms are so intimately incorporated in the assessment methods that even the scientist-analyst does not know the degree of conservatism involved. Risk management decisions are then made without knowledge of how much conservatism is included, or with a wrong impression of the degree of conservatism. Even when conservatisms built into an analysis are understood, they are often tacked on to a report as caveats that frequently do not find their way into high level briefing documents or public news releases. Thus, when residents of Washington State were asked to choose between loss of jobs by closing smelters or continued increased cancer rates associated with arsenic emissions (Ruckelshous, 1984), it was not clear that the estimated cancer rates were upper 95% confidence levels and not best estimates.

Few people think about how conservative one should be. In high-dose to low-dose extrapolation of chemical cancer potency factors, 95 percentile upper confidence bounds are generally used. This is a clear quantitative policy of the degree of conservatism used, but it applies only to one factor. A cancer risk assessment frequently involves emission rates from a source, environmental transport, and population activity patterns in addition to dose–response. All of these also have conservative estimates associated with them. In many cases, the conservatism is not quantitatively established. Instead, models are used that tend to overestimate exposure to an unknown degree, or it is assumed that the chemical form of a pollutant is the most toxic when the actual form is unknown, or people are assumed to spend an excessive amount of time in a high exposure area. Even the 95 percentile bound on the dose–response curve is not really quantitative since it is the bound on a particular model; the degree to which the choice of model leads to over or underestimating reality is unknown. All of these parts of risk assessment, each estimated conservatively, are combined to estimate risk. An example illustrating how combining several upper bound estimates can lead to highly exaggerated risk estimates is given in Chapter 13.

One clear effect of risk estimates based on unknown conservatisms is in comparative risk assessment. In planning energy policy and developing new energy technologies, for example, it is necessary to compare risk *among existing technologies* and between existing and new technologies.

Yet, inherent conservatisms in the methods, models, and assumptions in assessing risks vary in the different approaches that must be taken to assessing different kinds of risks and different technologies. It is common for risks of one form of energy to have much higher levels of conservatism built-in to its risk estimates than other forms. This distorts the decision process by appearing to make one energy technology "safer" than another, even though the opposite may be the case. This can exclude otherwise useful energy options or cause unnecessary public anxiety if they are pursued.

Closing options has adverse effects, but if conservative regulations focus on only a few areas, society can absorb the increased costs. As the scope of regulation widens to include almost all emissions to air and water, all deposits on land, and all products in the market place, the costs may become unbearable. Wildavsky (1979) puts this concern clearly: "When most substances are assumed safe and only a few are judged harmful, the line may be drawn against risking contact. But when the relationship is reversed, when most substances are suspect and few are safe, refusing risk may become ruinous."

Goals: Acceptability or Zero Risk?

There are basically two philosophies for setting risk goals: acceptable risk levels or zero risk. Zero risk as a societal goal is a false god. It cannot be achieved universally, and striving toward it as a goal distorts rational decisions, cumulatively leading to bad decisions. Moreover, assuming a zero-risk society were possible, would people want to pay the price if they understood what it would be? Wildavsky (1979) claims "No risk is the highest risk of all." Why is this the case? Virtually every human action involves risk. Even actions taken to mitigate risk carry their own risks. Reducing air pollution emissions may reduce risk, but costs increase rapidly as higher percentages of material are removed. Moreover, the material does not disappear; it becomes a solid waste that eventually poses risk to ground water instead of air. If it is especially hazardous, the factory could be closed; alternative products could be found. But alternatives cannot be found for everything within reasonably time or cost. Alternatives have a way of having unexpected risks themselves; risk management in the United States has consisted too frequently of banning a known or suspected risk and turning instead to an unknown risk.

Zero risk thinking is often narrowly restricted. FDA is restricted by the Delaney amendment to allow no food additives that are carcinogenic in animal bioassay, but can ignore natural carcinogens in food that most likely have a much greater role in cancer production than food additives.

IMPLICATIONS FOR RISK MANAGEMENT 367

A recent report (NAS, 1987), examining a new application of the Delaney amendment by EPA to pesticide residues in food, concluded that "certain strategies for implementing the Delaney Clause could increase dietary risk, and vigorous application of the Delaney Clause to tolerances for residues in processed foods may not be the most effective strategy for minimizing dietary exposure to oncogenic pesticides."

Usually, zero risk is stated as a "goal," not a requirement. Thus, EPA established a goal of zero risk for radionuclides in water, but recognizing the impracticality of that, especially in light of naturally occurring radionuclides in waters, established standards at levels higher than zero. But, even as a goal, zero risk can lead to disproportionate effort being put into achieving ever more stringent controls that result in only miniscule reductions in risk.

Another difficulty with a zero risk goal is that standards tend to be based on the ability of chemists to measure the pollutant in the environment. "No risk" translates into goals of "no detectable concentrations," but as the ability to detect chemicals in water moves from milligrams per liter to micrograms per liter to picograms per liter and lower, what may have begun as a practical approach becomes ridiculous. When coupled with the constant reiteration of the zero risk, zero concentration goal, these vanishingly small concentrations take on importance in the mind of the public and of decisionmakers, even though their associated risk may be vanishingly small.

In contrast, the concept of an acceptable level of risk recognizes that risk exists, will always exist, and that there are legitimate trade-offs to be made in balancing among different risks and between risks and benefits. Acceptable risk is obviously not a value that exists waiting to be identified; each individual may have a different idea of what is acceptable. It is a value that must be negotiated through a political process. Moreover, it is not static; levels of acceptability change over time. A truly informed judgment of acceptability, however, requires considerably technical and scientific information and much analysis. Providing the public and nontechnical decisionmakers meaningful and objective information that they can use to guide such decisions is a goal of risk analysis.

Black, White, or Grey?

There is a tendency to view things as either "safe" or "hazardous." "If fluoride is rat poison, we want none in our water, no matter how small the amount." It is difficult to understand that poisons are defined by dose as much as by chemical composition, and still more difficult to grasp the concept that there could be an acceptable level of risk above zero. People like a black and white world. Yet, in some areas, the concept is easily accepted. We recognize the need for a speed limit on the highways and understand that they are not God-given numbers, but are based on fallible human judgment, and are often arbitrary. We accept the findings that reducing the speed limit reduces traffic fatalities, and that driving at speeds above the limit increases the risk of fatalities. Few, however, hesitate to go 5-10 miles per hour above the limit, a level of infraction the police usually ignore, although risks presumably increase incrementally with increased speed. In contrast, we often look at equally arbitrary limits on concentrations of carcinogens to be hard-and-fast, with any exceedence likened to a malicious attempt to poison the population.

Rational or Perceived Risk Basis?

The traditional approach to risk assessment and risk management has been the estimation of risk on a rational, objective, and scientific basis and the institution of risk management on that basis. When people's perception of risks differed from that estimated in scientific studies, the management technique used was education. The distortion in allocation of resources and misdirection of technological development resulting from political decisions stemming from apparent public misperception of risk has been decried by risk experts. Two related develops, however, are leading to a change in this attitude.

First is the body of knowledge generated by psychological researchers on perception of risk (discussed in Chap. 14) demonstrating that people's perception of risks is not at all in line with scientific risk analysis and that risk management attempts to communicate risk information to people does not work because it does not address people's concerns. The result is a lack of understanding, cooperation, and, eventually, loss of trust on the part of the public, who must eventually support any risk management efforts if they are to be successful.

Second is the finding that there exists real effects that are not addressed by most risk assessments and do not easily fall into standard methods. These effects are induced by perception or other secondary factors rather than by the physical source of the hazard directly. Some examples: (1) Evacuation, especially unorganized evacuation, from the scene of a nuclear accident entails its own costs and risks. People may be killed and injured in the crowded rushing to get away; property left unprotected is subject to looting and vandalism. If people perceive a risk and evacuate, these real effects occur even if there is no actual threat of radiation exposure. (2) Studies of the population around Three Mile Island showed psychological impacts resulting from that accident even though there was no significant radiation exposure. People suffered from the shock of what they perceived as a threat independently of the reality of the threat. (3) A region subject to chemical or radiological contamination can be subjected to stigma even if the level of contamination is low. This could effect real estate values, tourism, markets for agricultural products, or attraction of new industry or people into the region.

The body of knowledge on these kinds of effects is small. Research and risk management organizations tend to focus on more tangible effects. The effects discussed may arise only in special circumstances, they may be short lived, and their value may be small compared to more traditionally considered effects. Not enough is known. It is clear, however, that these phenomena also operate at a higher level: even if perception-induced effects do not occur, the perception that they might occur affects risk management decisionmaking. People oppose new development with cancer risk potential because they perceive that accidental contamination of their neighborhood or region will lead to economic stigma as much as because they actually fear the risk of cancer.

Differences between analytically determined risk estimates and publicly perceived risks were discussed in more detail in an earlier chapter; further information can be found in review articles such as Kasperson et al. (1988) and Freudenberg (1988). The key risk management distinction is whether the "manager" bases decisions entirely on analytically determined, "rational" risk estimates from "the experts" or whether risk management decisions remain open to genuine public input and consideration of public perceptions even if they appear "irrational."

MANAGEMENT TECHNIQUES

The management techniques discussed here are not an exhaustive set; others include simply providing information, conducting environmental audits, and negotiation. The techniques discussed were chosen to illustrate the strong linkage between risk assessment and risk management.

Collecting Information

There is an old saying that when you can't decide, you collect more information or form a committee. It is usually invoked disparagingly by people who believe action is preferable to delay. There is a time to act, but sometimes delay is appropriate. If the science is weak, action may not be justified. More scientific data may show the way. Blindly waiting for new data, however, is unjustified, no matter how much money is being poured into research. No one can predict what new data will show or how valuable they will be, but one can make a rational judgment of whether any definitive improvement can be expected in the available information base within a given time. A decision to wait should be based on a rational expectation that this premise is true. Most importantly, a decision to wait for new data should be just that: a decision, made and justified in the same way a decision to take action would be, not simply benign neglect.

It is not only scientific information that is important for risk management; the values and attitudes toward risk of the people involved are of concern. Committees, advisory panels, questionnaires, public hearings are all methods of eliciting values and attitudes of the stake holders in the risk management decision.

Providing Information

Information is power. Perhaps the greatest impact of the National Environmental Policy Act in the early 1970s was that it required information on potential environmental impacts be developed and *placed in the hands of the public*. Although government agencies desiring to develop new projects found many ways to circumvent the Act's requirements, once the public had the necessary information, political and legal forces could be brought to bear to delay, mitigate, and even cancel projects. Opening up the decision process in this way seems philosophically better than leaving it to technocrats. In practice, however, there are risks: complex scientific and technological information is difficult for the public to understand. This allows small activist groups to distort the political process for their own ends. It takes time for the public to learn how to deal with the information and for society to work out a new balance.

New laws requiring disclosure of exposure to carcinogens are now being implemented. California's Proposition 65 came into force in mid-1988. It requires that, "No person in the course of doing business shall knowingly and intentionally expose any individual to a chemical known to the state to cause cancer or reproductive toxicity without first giving clear and reasonable warning to such individual" (Abelson, 1987). New Jersey also requires any facility storing, manufacturing, or handling threshold quantities of listed chemicals to disclose the quantities involved (Levin, 1988). Other states are considering similar requirements. The most massive disclosure program, however, is mandated by the Emergency Planning and Community Right-to-Know Act of 1986, more frequently called SARA Title III, since the act was embedded in Title III of the Superfund Amendments and Reauthorization Act of 1986. This requires any manufacturing facility that meets threshold use levels for hundreds of listed chemicals to report annual releases to air, water, or ground. Levin (1988) states the result clearly: "No plant manager who discovers he has 200,000 pounds annual release of a substance will sit idly by and wait for that figure to be disclosed to his superiors or community. He will immediately start looking for substitute feedstocks, ways to close production loops, and other opportunities for waste minimization in the broadest sense." The impact of mandatory disclosure may ultimately be a much greater force to reduce emissions of carcinogens than any regulations. One report that notes "the potential for public relations problems or serious litigious liabilities resulting [from SARA title III]," recommends a series of comprehensive steps to industries that go far beyond any regulatory requirements (Fisher et al., 1988). These include: "Get companywide commitment to collect all pertinent data . . . Develop computer-based toxic chemical purchasing/usage tracking system . . . Perform a comprehensive survey and documentation of all operating areas . . . Determine ventilation rates and perform sampling on vents/stacks . . . Expand sampling of wastewater being discharged from plant site to an off-site water body . . . Chemically and physically characterize all hazardous wastes . . . inventory all flanges, valves, pumps, vents, pressure relief valves." The director of the EPA program gives an example of a large company in which executives were "taken aback" by the amount of toxic substances they were discharging into the environment once the data were collected in one place for the first time. The company chairman pledged a 90% reduction in air emissions worldwide within 4 years (Elkins, 1988).

De Minimus

It has become the generally accepted practice to assume carcinogens have no threshold of effect, that even the smallest exposure might give some increased risk of cancer. In the absence of information to the contrary, it is, of course, prudent to take due care in the management of even small amounts of carcinogens. The no-threshold viewpoint, taken to extremes, however, can cause unwarranted public concern and lead to wasteful expenditure of regulatory effort over trivial risks. The applicable legal principle is de *minimus non curat lex* (the law is not concerned with trifles). Courts, regulatory agencies, industry, and the public have more important things to do than become embroiled in large controversies over trivial risks. By becoming bogged down with small risks, the regulatory system may give insufficient attention to more important risks. The increasing sensitivity of chemical measurement techniques leads to discovery of *exposure and presumed risk* at lower and lower pollutant concentrations.

The sensitivity with which radioactive materials can be detected is clearly one factor in the degree of concern and regulation of radiation compared to chemical hazards. Strict statutory zero-risk goals can actually impede progress toward risk reduction in some cases since it puts the regulatory agency in an impossible situation (Taylor, 1987).

A *de minimus* risk is one that cannot justify regulatory action. The costs of regulation outweigh the importance of the risk or the incremental risk is so small there is no incentive to modify it. A *de minimus* risk level represents a cutoff below which a regulatory agency could simply ignore alleged hazards (Fiksel, 1985). Essentially it is a standard like an air quality or occupational health standard. If concentrations are below the standard there is no problem; if they are above the standard, regulatory action *may be* necessary to reduce exposures. It is a concept designed to "get around" the problem that standards, the core of the regulatory system, were based on the notion that each pollutant had a threshold level below which there was no effect. Applying threshold-based standards to carcinogens (and to other pollutants that are found to have "effects" at levels below standards) leads to contradictions and other problems. The *de minimus* concept provides an alternative base for a system of standards. An early call for a *de minimus* approach (Comar, 1979) recommended:

1. Eliminate any risk that carries no benefit or is easily avoided
2. Eliminate any large risk that does not carry clearly overriding benefits
3. Temporarily ignore any small risk not already eliminated by the first recommendation
4. Actively study risks falling outside these limits

These criteria provide a concept for setting priorities among different hazards for regulatory decisionmaking. Application of the concept is not as easy as it might seem, however. A number of policy issues must be decided, and it is not clear to what extent they can be decided in an abstract way. The first issue to arise is, at what level should the *de minimus* risk be set. Comar (1979) suggested 10^{-5} per year, although some federal regulatory agencies, while not specifically endorsing a *de minimus* concept, have implicitly used a lower cutoff level of 10^{-6} lifetime risk. For hazardous waste site evaluations, EPA recommended a range of 10^{-7} to 10^{-4} for what appears to be a *de minimus* level of lifetime risk. A uniform *de minimus* risk level applicable to all regulatory agencies would go far toward standardizing risk regulation and avoiding arbitrary differences in the way different kinds of risk are treated. This may be difficult, however, since there is considerable evidence that people perceive similar levels of risk to be of different importance in different situations (Slovic et al., 1980). This is particularly true for voluntary compared to nonvoluntary risks. Most environmental risks are considered nonvoluntary, but the question is sometimes raised as to occupational risks, especially when the circumstances leading to the risk have been part of a negotiated agreement.

When discussion of setting a *de minimus* level gets down to numbers, it soon becomes apparent that the issue is deeper. People disagree on the appropriate way of expressing a *de minimus* level. The numbers suggested above refer to individual risk levels, but it has been argued that the societal risk, i.e., the total number of people affected, and the size of the population at risk, should be taken into consideration. An individual risk level of 10^{-6} annually, for example, implies one individual affected every two years in a city of 500,000, but over 200 people per year if the entire United States were at risk. Should a localized problem be subjected to the same *de minimus* level as a national problem? Mumpower (1986) suggests a dual definition: for example, a risk might be defined as exceeding the *de minimus* threshold if it either (a) exceeded 10^{-6} individual risk *or* (b) was expected to result in more than 100 fatalities annually. This is presented as a question of balancing equity with efficiency, but cannot be addressed in the absence of consideration of uncertainty, of the societal impact of the fatalities rather than simply their number, or of the difference between low-level and high-level risk. First, the risks and the numbers of deaths are uncertain. One hundred deaths annually may seem great, but these are not deaths that are actually counted like the thousands of deaths annually from automobile accidents; these are estimated by modeling national exposure levels and extrapolating dose–response functions from high-dose levels. The uncertainty associated with the number 100 deaths may well range from zero to 1,000. Equally as important is how the uncertainty is incorporated into the decision. EPA, for example, frequently uses 10^{-6} as an implicit *de minimus* level, but when it calculates the risk to compare with this criterion, it uses the upper 95% confidence bound rather than the best estimate. Thus, the *de minimus* level is actually set at the level above which there is only a 2.5% probability of the risk being as high as 10^{-6}. Second, the impact on society of a large number of deaths concentrated in time and space, as in an airplane crash, both seems greater and, to some degree, does have a greater societal impact than the same number of deaths spread out over time and space. One hundred extra deaths in a city of 50,000 is a 20% increase in the death rate; it would probably be noticed and impact the community. One hundred extra cancer deaths distributed throughout the United States would be unnoticed in the over 200,000 background cancer deaths and would not significantly increase societal impact. Finally, it should be recognized that there really is no local–national dichotomy. Low-level risks of concern are national in scope and not limited to any one community. Some communities may be impacted to a greater extent because of emissions from a local facility, but that leads to exceeding the individual risk levels (the example of 100 deaths in a community of 50,000 is a risk level exceeding 10^{-3} and raises no question of *de minimus*).

Another consideration in establishing a *de minimus* level is the possible cumulative effect of many small risks. Mumpower (1986) suggests there may be as many as 40 new carcinogenic chemicals introduced annually and estimates the lifetime effect of such multiple incremental exposures, each at a *de minimus* level. The calculation, however, is made without consideration of background risk. Multiple insults are a consideration, but their effect is limited when they are considered as increments to a background risk and not independent from background.

One further consideration is the applicability of *de minimus* concepts to low probability events as well as low probability consequences. The discussion so far has been in the context of continuous exposures; a population is exposed to a low concentration of a carcinogen that may pose some small risk of cancer. If the risk is negligibly small, it may be ignored. The same concept has been applied to low probability, high consequence accidents, although other considerations also come into play. If the probability is sufficiently low the risk of the accident may be ignored. In this case it seems reasonable that both the event probability and the consequences given the event be considered in establishing the *de minimus* level.

De minimus risk levels are sometimes confused with acceptable risk levels. While all risk levels regarded as insignificant or *de minimus* should be acceptable, other nontrifling risks are often regarded by society as acceptable. Automobile accidents are an example. It has been argued that there are two dividing lines; a *de minimus* level, with all risks below that acceptable, and an unacceptable level, with all risks above that being unacceptable. Between these two limits, benefit/cost tradeoffs decide acceptability. The *de minimus* cutoff represents the boundary below which all risks are acceptable without regard to any consideration of benefits; the very calculation of benefit tradeoffs is not worthwhile for this level of risk.

Finally, the application of the *de minimus* concept depends upon first estimating the level of risk to determine if it is below the *de minimus* level. As has been seen, the analysis and estimation of low-level risk can be a demanding task fraught with difficulties and ending up with great uncertainties. *De minimus* does not limit the scope of quantitative risk analysis to those risks above the *de minimus* limit, it stretches the role of quantitative risk analysis to aid in the *de minimus* determination. The *de minimus* decision may replace in importance the qualitative determination of whether a substance is a carcinogen. That qualitative decision is an important part of risk assessment and often involves quantitative analysis. The *de minimus* decision is more complex: it is clearly quantitative and involves exposure estimates explicitly as well as dose–response considerations. Practical methods must be developed to apply quantitative risk analysis in supporting *de minimus* determinations without requiring too much effort for analysis.

Acceptable Risk

The concept of acceptable risk differs slightly from *de minimus* risk. *De minimus* refers to a risk that is so low it is not only of no regulatory concern, but is beneath any level of concern at all. We can put it out of our minds completely. Acceptable risk, by contrast, need not imply lack of concern. We may accept the risk of driving on a crowded expressway yet still retain a concern for traffic safety. Acceptable risk levels are the result of a balancing process; they may vary depending on the benefits to be gained or other factors. We are undoubtedly willing to accept a higher risk of cancer from food preservatives that protect against other, more immediate, harm than we are willing to accept from food coloring agents that serve a less useful purpose and may even be perceived as deceptive. We may still be concerned, however, about the cancer risk of food preservatives. As a result, we establish programs to find more acceptable substitutes, we limit their use to necessary applications and demand that no more than the necessary concentrations be used. But, until adequate substitutes are found, we accept what seems to be the lesser risk.

Acceptable risk levels might also be considered as targets. The calculation of "safe" exposure levels addressed in Chapter 9 is a quantitative assessment approach designed to aid decisions on this kind of acceptable risk.

Because acceptability involves a balancing process, there is no uniform level of acceptable risk. People tend to be more willing to accept risks they are accustomed to than risks that are new to them; more willing to accept risks they feel some control over than those they have no control over; more willing to accept risks they feel are equitably shared by others, rather than faced by them or their community alone; more willing to accept risks when they are participants in the decision process than when the risks are imposed on them by outside forces. The level of acceptable risk thus depends on the context and character of the risk. It also depends on the character and attitudes of the population. This can be seen in attitudes toward natural risks such as tornados or floods; people in some regions accept natural disasters as fate, others do not and instead take action to avoid or reduce their effects. Some people are "risk adverse"; they are willing to make an extra effort and expend extra resources to avoid risk. Others may be indifferent to risk or may even be "risk seekers." The same person may be adverse to one source of risk and seek out another, a cigarette smoker who actively fights for stricter air pollution control, for example. Finding a common level of risk acceptability is a problem of a political nature.

Acceptability is also a moving target. What is acceptable today, may not be acceptable tomorrow. An increasing standard of living, greater expectations, cleaner and safer new technologies combine to set a new base level of what is acceptable.

The fact that acceptability depends on circumstance could lead to what appears to be a double standard for some pollutants. The circumstances after an accidental environmental exposure are different than before the exposure. Is the level to which contaminated soil must be cleaned up following an accidental spill the same as the level to which uncontaminated soil might be "allowed" to be polluted? Must houses severely contaminated with chloridane be cleaned up to the level that one would like to maintain in a "clean" house? In a court decision on liability, the party that caused the contamination might be made to restore it to its original state, but if the decision were internalized, for example, if the homeowner had caused the contamination, then the decision begins from a new base and one might decide that an exposure level higher than the original state might be acceptable, especially if the cost for the last bit of clean-up were very high.

Uncertainty comes into play in meeting acceptable risk levels. There is uncertainty in estimating risk, and uncertainty in the variation in risk among individuals. To assure that a given level of risk deemed "acceptable" is met, it is necessary that the best estimate of the risk be lower than that acceptable level by some "margin of safety." The size of the margin of safety should depend on the degree of confidence with which one can estimate the risk.

Worst Case

A frequently used screening technique in risk analysis is the upper-bound analysis or worst case. What is the effect on a person who lives 24 hours per day, 365 days per year, for his entire lifetime at the fence-line of an industrial plant, breathes the maximum concentration of toxic air pollutants from the plant and consumes only food grown at the fence-line that contains the maximum amount of toxic agents from the plant likely to get through the food-chain. Also assume all water consumed comes from just below the plant outfall. There is considerable uncertainty in the dose–response relationship of the toxic agents involved; use upper-bound estimates. If the effects under these worst-case conditions are sufficiently low, no further analysis of lesser cases is necessary. This approach has served well in many situations, but under close examination, particularly in situations where low probability—high consequence events are considered, worst-case analysis can be fallacious.

The first problem with worst-case analysis is defining the worst case. The fence-post person may appear to be a physical upper limit, but an imaginative analyst could think of assumptions that would be worse. Perhaps the rate of emissions from the plant vary; then assume they maintain the highest rate ever recorded throughout the fence-post individual's life. Perhaps the greatest dose of the most toxic pollutant comes through concentration in fish; then assume the fence-post individual subsists entirely on fish. And so on and on. These assumptions are not made up to illustrate a point, they are commonly used in assessments. We eventually have an absurd situation, not suited for rational analysis, but was not the fence-post individual an absurd situation to begin with? Attempts to define what is meant by worst case in nuclear reactor accident analysis led to terms such as "worst credible accident." This makes the judgmental nature of the worst case explicit, but does not help to determine what is credible and what is not.

Worst-case analysis may be satisfactory for screening if the worst case shows an acceptable level of risk. It is when the worst case yields an unacceptable level of risk that problems arise. First, a high level of risk in a worst-case screening analysis creates a sensation and sticks in the minds of the public that may not understand the impossible assumptions involved and may never believe the results of later, more detailed and more realistic analyses if they indicate the risk is actually acceptable. Because of the cost and time required for more realistic analyses, risk management decisions may be based on worst-case results. This leads to bad decisions since the worst-case will overestimate actual results and thus lead to unnecessary expenditure on controls. Moreover, decisions often involve selection among different options. Worst case as a sole criterion is not a good selection method because the ratio of worst case to expected effects may not be constant among options. For example, an industry with a population some distance away and upwind but that has high emissions may yield a greater worst case risk, but a lower expected risk, than an industry with a population close by and downwind, but that has lower emissions.

The Council on Environmental Quality proposed that a worst-case scenario be examined in Environmental Impact Statements. Their goal was that incomplete or unavailable information be disclosed and reasonably foreseeable significant adverse impacts be considered even in the absence of all information. After considering many comments, CEQ decided that the concept of worst-case analysis was flawed, unproductive and inefficient, and that the goals could be better met in other ways (CEQ, 1986).

Probability of Causation

The possibility of after-the-fact liability claims can be an important influence on risk management. Determining cause and effect, however, can be a difficulty. Some cases are clear-cut; if an asbestos worker dies of mesotheleoma, there may be little question of the responsibility. If, on the other hand, a chemical worker dies of lung cancer, the question of whether it was related to his work exposure may be difficult to resolve. One approach to such a question is to work the usual risk assessment formula backward: instead of calculating the probability of cancer given an exposure, calculate the probability, given the cancer exists, of a known exposure being its cause. If a particular cancer has a background incidence (I_B) in people with a given set of characteristics (age, sex, time since exposure, etc.) but without the particular exposure, and a higher incidence (I_E) in people with the same characteristics except with the particular exposure, then the probability of causation (PC) that the appearance of that particular cancer in a person with those characteristics was due to the the particular exposure received is defined as (NIH, 1985):

$$PC = \frac{IE - I_B}{I_E} \tag{1}$$

The calculation is specific for a particular quantitative exposure or dose and to the set of personal characteristics. Lagakos and Mosteller (1986) illustrate this by an example of two similar groups in which there were 100 cases in the exposed group (I_E) and 80 cases in the unexposed group (I_B). The 20 extra cases in the exposed group might be interpreted as meaning that 20 cases in the 100 were caused by the exposure and the remaining 80 by other factors. The ratio ($20/100 = 0.2$) is the probability that any randomly selected case from the exposed group was caused by that exposure.

The assumption that the cancer is or is not caused by the exposure is an oversimplification. Interactive and synergistic effects are well known, but not sufficiently quantified or understood to include them in the calculation. If there is a synergistic effect, Eq. (1) assigns the full contribution of the interaction to the exposure of interest while assigning no share to the interacting agent, which remains part of the general background.

Thus, if the probability of causation of numerous factors, some interacting synergistically, could all be calculated, their sum would exceed 100% (Cox, 1987). Assuming sufficient data were available to examine the role of more than one toxic agent, the calculation becomes much more complex, especially if the error terms associated with each probability of causation are also determined (Seiler and Scott, 1987).

The most extensive application of probability of causation or assigned share, as some would rather call it, has been for cancers attributed to radiation exposure. The Orphan Drug Act of 1983 included a clause directing the Secretary of Health and Human Services to "devise and publish" tables estimating the likelihood that persons with cancers, who received specific doses of radiation prior to the onset of the cancer, developed their cancer as a result of the radiation exposure. It was hoped that this would lead to greater rationality and consistency in court cases awarding damages to cancer victims who had been exposed to radiation. The National Institutes of Health produced these tables (NIH, 1985), but difficulties remain in their application and interpretation.

Uncertainty in estimating cause and effect in a single individual is higher than for a population. Nygaard (1986) listed some of the uncertainties as:

1. Geographic, ethnic, and lifestyle variations affecting baseline cancer incidence
2. Uncertain estimates of the radiation dose received by the individual
3. Assumption of a linear quadratic dose–response model for all cancers without regard to the uncertainty in model choice
4. High-to low-dose extrapolation
5. Uncertainty in time-related factors such as minimal latent period, time-response variations, age at exposure
6. Host factors and competing etiological influences such as smoking that may affect the susceptibility to radiation-induced cancer and influence the baseline rate

For the radiological probability of causation (PC) values, Nygaard (1986) estimated:

A PC of 2% or less would have an upper bound of 7%
A PC of 5–10% might have limits of from 1–30%
A PC of 20% may have limits of 5–40%

The only possibilities are that an individual's cancer was due to his exposure, was not due to his exposure, or contributed to the exposure through some interaction with other factors such as smoking. Except in the latter sense (not generally used because of the inability to describe joint dose–response functions of multiple agents), a cancer either was or was not caused by the exposure. It makes no sense to say it was 5% caused by the exposure. The 5% simply means that in a group of 100 similar cancer victims with the same exposure, it is estimated that 5 cancers were due to the exposure and 95 were not. Since it is impossible to say which 5, we say they each had a 5% probability of being caused by the exposure.

Beyond the uncertainties, much of the argument over use of assigned shares focuses on how to use the results and their implications for the victim, the defendant (the person or organization responsible for the exposure) and for the management of risk. Three possible uses are (Lagakos and Mosteller, 1986):

1. The estimated PC could be used directly in a formula to calculate a claimant's award
2. The estimated PC could be "personalized" by using additional information on the individual's background that might affect cancer incidence
3. The PC could be considered as one piece of evidence along with other evidence presented

The first two uses lead to a radical change in the way compensation claims are awarded. Compensation in the current tort system is either all or none based on a decision of whether an exposure was or was not the cause of the cancer. Using the example above, awarding 5% of full compensation to 100 people in a given category is radically different than awarding 100% compensation to some percentage of the claimants based on the apparent strength of their claim (or the eloquence of their lawyer).

Reaction to the use of probability of causation varies. Resistance to its use even in principle has been reported as widespread in the insurance industry, the legal profession, and even the Justice Department (Nygaard, 1986). A Harvard law professor argues that the approach does not even purport that it can enable determinations of causation and compensation for individuals, but, at the same time, argues for the admission of probabilistic evidence (Rosenberg, 1986). Others note that political, scientific, and legal commentators have recommended use of the method for guiding compensation award decisions (Cox, 1987).

The use of probability of causation can be considered in light of three different functions of tort law (Rosenberg, 1986): First, distributional justice, which focuses on the victim's need. Since the evidence of the cancer is certain, this need is clear. Second, corrective justice, based on a finding that the defendant wrongfully injured the plaintiff. Rosenberg

(1986) argues that probability of causation cannot address this issue since it is based on population and population subgroup data and cannot be sufficiently individualized. Yet, the same limitations that apply to the probability of causation approach also apply to any other presentation of scientific data in a court. He ignores the possibility that probability of causation might be used alongside other evidence leading to a guilty or not guilty determination instead of a fractional rate of compensation. Third, the threat of liability for injuries is a deterrent to those who might otherwise wantonly expose people to carcinogens. It thus serves as one of society's tools for risk management.

Lave (1986) raises the issue that use of PC bases the decision on the scientific understanding of the time; he asks us to imagine being informed just after a case was concluded that new data have led to a significant revision in the probability of causation. The findings in any toxic tort case, however, can do no better than the current scientific understanding; PC does not change anything in this regard.

Quantitative Management Techniques

Formalized methods of decisionmaking, relying on quantitative analysis, have long been used in aiding public policy decisions. They have not always been well-received. Perhaps the first large-scale application was in The Flood Control Act of 1926 that required the Army Corps of Engineers to calculate costs and benefits of proposed water-resource projects and submit only those with benefits exceeding costs for Congressional action. In principal, this was an excellent example of the use of benefit/cost analysis; a consistent set of methods to be used were set forth ahead of time by Congress. Water resources was a traditional port-barrel area in Congress, however, and the Corps had a reputation for wanting to build a dam in every valley. Because of this, benefit/cost analysis was often seen as a means of justifying decisions already made for other reasons. It may have been this case that Quade (1975) had in mind when he said, in what is perhaps the best work on the application of analysis to public policy decisions, that it "... was often the wrong sort of analysis, by people who did not really understand its many limitations, in an environment beset with politics and special interests."

Yet, cost-benefit analysis is a good place to begin a discussion of quantitative decision methods. A proposal involves both costs and benefits; one would like the latter to exceed the former. Faced with a decision among competing proposals, one wants to choose the best. When these methods were applied to defense spending, people talked about "getting *the most bang for the buck.*" But how do we define best? Mathematics demands precision in definitions and one important contribution of quantitative decision analysis to public decisionmaking can be to enforce clear thinking about goals. For example, a businessman might wish to maximize net profits; this would be [benefits–costs]. The smarter businessman realizes he must consider the return on his investment, and wishes to maximize [(benefits – costs)/costs]. The latter is similar to the form usually used in cost-benefit analysis, [benefits/cost]. As benefits approach costs, the net return on investment approaches zero and the benefit/cost ratio approaches 1.

Incidentally, while most people would agree that clarifying goals and objectives in public decisionmaking is a good idea, decisionmakers themselves often try to avoid this. Public decisions are usually compromises among people with different goals. Clearly stated objectives may make compromise more difficult, especially when the decisionmakers must explain the results to their constituencies. It is only later, when the decisions begin to be implemented, that the effects of differences in interpretation become apparent and one or more parties to the agreement feel betrayed.

One can calculate the benefit/cost ratio of each option and select the one with the highest ratio or use the analysis as a screening tool, eliminating all options with a benefit/cost ratio below a given value (say 1.2). But, it is not so simple. Neither benefits nor costs can be measured entirely in monetary units; both are often composed of many kinds of things that have no common metric in which they can be measured. Of course, it is not necessary to have a common metric in order to compare different things or to decide among them. It is said that one cannot compare apples and oranges, but people routinely make decisions between apples and oranges; they do not become immobilized with indecision while standing before the fruit bins of the grocery store. People demonstrate daily that they can strike a balance between seemingly incommensurable things in the both large and small decisions affecting their lives. The need for a common metric is not because people cannot make decisions without it, but because people can only juggle a limited number of factors affecting a decision in their mind at the same time. Risk management decisions involve hundreds of different factors; some must be aggregated so as to reduce the detail that must be actively grappled with in a single decision. It is convenient to have a common metric for aggregation to avoid the need to make hundreds of individual decisions.

Introducing health risks in the benefit/cost calculation adds an additional complication. Although the basic approach remains the same, people feel differently about balancing health risks against monetary costs and benefits. Attempts have been made to keep the health risks separate from other risks in a decision. Terms such as "risk-benefit," "risk-cost-benefit," and "risk-risk" have emerged. Lave (1981) discusses eight such decision frameworks. But there are many social and environmental factors that have an emotional attachment equal to health. Indeed, in many cases, health may be a relatively minor part of a decision. There seems to be little justification for separating it out as something different.

The benefit/cost ratio is only one way to express the results of a quantitative, analytical approach. Cost-effectiveness is a different way of using the same data. Cost-effectiveness is the quotient of the annualized cost of a risk management option divided by a measure of its effectiveness, e.g., dollars per cancer averted. One advantage of this approach is that there is no need to even consider reducing the effects (e.g., cancers) to monetary terms to match the costs. Also unlike benefit/cost analysis, there is usually no attempt made to include all the benefits. Cost-effectiveness generally refers to effectiveness in terms of a particular benefit. It is a single-focus measure. One must, thus, keep in mind that an option that is not cost effective in terms of cancer risk may have a high overall benefit/cost ratio due to other benefits. One study comparing individual risk levels, cost-effectiveness of the proposed action, and after-the-fact information on whether the regulatory agency did impose regulations, found that substances with lifetime cancer risks above 4×10^{-3} were regulated regardless of cost; for cancer risks below that level, regulation was imposed if the cost-per-cancer-averted was less than about \$2 million (Travis et al., 1987). This is simply an observation from a limited data set, however. It implies no absolute rules for risk management decisions. Others cite much higher costs-per-cancer-averted for some actions. It is a useful measure for a decisionmaker to see. A high cost should make one wonder if the money might not be better spent elsewhere.

Another item that quantitative benefit/cost analyses have come to be known under in the 1980s is "benefits analysis." This stems from an Executive Order issued by President Reagan in 1981 requiring federal agencies to perform benefits assessments of proposed major regulations and prohibiting them from taking regulatory action unless potential benefits exceed potential costs to society. Much general background on benefit/cost analysis, its application to regulatory problems, and the evaluation of benefits is contained in a book produced with the support of the National Science Foundation (Bentkover et al., 1986).

Because of the differences in values involved and the difficulties of measuring many different kinds of costs and benefits in comparable units, benefit/cost analysis is too limited to be used blindly in making risk-management decisions. Another limitation of benefit/cost analysis is that it looks only at net efficiency. It compares the costs, whoever pays them, with the benefits, to whomsoever they accrue. It does not consider distributional effects, equity, or similar goals.

Decision analysis is a different approach to quantitative decisionmaking techniques. It draws on a wide range of disciplines, including statistical decision theory, psychology, systems engineering, systems science, operations research, management science, and economics. Different "schools" of decision analysis may slant their approach more toward one or another disciplinary base (Covello, 1987). Most applications have been in business (Schlaifer, 1959), but more recently decision analysis has been used widely to address public policy problems. Decision analysis begins with a clear definition of the objective sought in a decision. This is the most crucial part. For example, in the Nuclear Waste Management Act, the Department of Energy was required to select three potential nuclear repository sites for detailed investigation. Decision analysis techniques were used to select the three sites out of nine identified in a preliminary process. Which three were chosen depended on a subtle point in the definition of the objective. If the three sites chosen are the best, the second best, and the third best as determined by a given set of criteria, one set of sites is selected. If the objective were defined to choose the best portfolio of three sites so as to maximize the likelihood that at least one would be found acceptable in the second round of decisions, a different set of sites would be selected, perhaps three with different geologic characteristics (Merkoher and Keeney, 1987). The latter objective is similar to an investor trying to diversify his stock portfolio.

A characteristic feature of decision analysis is the use of probability. Uncertain parameters in the analysis and future events that may affect the results favorably or unfavorably are described as probability density functions. Decision analysts must work closely with experts in each area to define these probabilities. Often there are insufficient data to define these probability functions, so they must be developed using the expert's subjective judgment. A literature has developed on how to elicit this information from experts and the various biases and cognitive "traps" that experts can fall into when applying their judgment to predict probabilities of occurrences beyond their direct experimental knowledge (Tversky and Kaneman, 1981; Spetzler and Stael von Holstein, 1975; Morgan et al., 1979, 1985).

While the most straightforward approach to decision analysis is to maximize a single objective, in most real decisions not one, but many different aims are sought. Decision theory can accommodate multiobjective and multicriteria decisionmaking (Keeney and Raiffa, 1976; Bell et al., 1977; Steuer, 1986). Here, instead of (or in addition to) eliciting information from experts, the analyst must elicit from decision-makers quantitative value judgments on their preferences and willingness to make trade-offs among objectives or criteria. The strength of the formalized process is that it requires decisionmakers to make explicit judgments about their relative value of different aims apart from the complications and "overtones" imposed by the specific problem being addressed. A key complication, especially in public policy problems, is that there is never a single decisionmaker; many people, with different values, influence or are concerned in the decision. Sensitivity analysis, calculating, comparing, and discussing outcomes under different value sets are ways of dealing with this circumstance. They allow the effect of different values to be brought to the surface so the political decision can be based on the values as it should be. A newer approach to decision analysis explicitly recognizes the lack of a single, all powerful, decisionmaker. Rather than multiple criteria for a single decisionmaker, this approach deals with decisionmaking in a multidecision-maker environment, making use of research findings in behavioral science on how people understand, process, and communicate information, and how decisions are actually made in this interactive process (Von Winterfeld and Edwards, 1986).

Both the formal structure imposed by quantitative analysis and the comparative judgments that can be made from the results can be helpful to decisionmakers. Ways that quantitative analyses can be used in decisionmaking include:

Evaluating proposed regulations. Regulations developed through other means can be tested against quantitative benefit/cost analysis. If the results do not fit preconceived expectations, regulators might have second thoughts, at least sufficient to consider what led to the unexpected results.

Improve regulations. In one analysis, a level of control less stringent than that proposed yielded most of the benefits gained by the proposed standard at far lower cost (Haigh et al., 1984).

Organizing scientific and economic information into a consistent framework. Simply forcing the collection of a consistent set of information is an important contribution.

Making the criteria used in decisionmaking explicit. The formal structure can require decisionmakers to explicitly explain to themselves and others how the decision was made, on what specific information it was based, and how much weight was given to each type of evidence.

Best Available Technology

One practical approach to managing risks of emissions to the environment is to require that the best available technology (BAT) be applied to controlling the emissions. The use of BAT implicitly recognizes that demanding zero emissions is impracticable and would lead to shut-down of industries and home furnaces. EPA applied this approach instead of a strict interpretation of Section 112 of the Clean Air Act (dealing with hazardous air pollutants), which would require zero-discharge standards for carcinogens (Haigh et al., 1984).

While rejecting the application of a zero-risk, zero-discharge approach, BAT implicitly assumes a zero-risk goal, albeit unreachable. It implies that only the best technology can be acceptable, rejecting the possibility that less than the best control on emissions might be good enough, thus ignoring the rule of diminishing returns. It contrasts most sharply with a quantitative risk analysis approach when one considers that BAT for different situations may lead to vastly different risks. In comparing the implications of proposed BAT standards for benzene, coke ovens, and acrylonitrile emissions, Haigh et al. (1984) found that cost effectiveness, in terms of dollars per cancers averted, ranged from 2.3 to 144 millions. EPA later withdrew these proposals, presumably due, at least in part, to such quantitative risk arguments (Luken, 1985).

Discussions of BAT are abstract until one begins to come to grips with the question of how to define what is the best control technology available. Does "available" mean it can be bought off the shelf? No. Control technologies for industrial emissions are often complex, engineered systems, each uniquely designed for its specific application and costing tens, or hundreds of millions of dollars. They are never bought "off the shelf." The technology may not even have ever been used in a full-scale application. But, is it sufficient that EPA engineers decide the technology is technically feasible? To what extent does cost enter into a decision that a technology is available? The owner of a factory with a total value under $1 million cannot consider a control technology that would cost $100 million as "available." The purpose of BAT is to do the best that can be done to control emissions without closing down the factory (or at least not closing down a significant fraction of all the factories of a particular kind). Thus, "available" must be interpreted to mean "available at an affordable cost." It becomes clear that what at first seems a purely technical decision of selecting the "best" technology, is instead a complex socioeconomic–political decision that can include a great deal of consideration of questions such as how much the industry should be made to spend, and what will be the effect on competition between large and small firms within the industry.

MANAGEMENT FORMATS

Individual Risk Management

Individuals make risk management decisions for themselves in deciding what to eat, where to live, where to work, how to heat their homes, what hobbies to pursue, and many other decisions. Some of these are routine, taken with little thought; others are major decisions of one's life. Despite their seeming importance, cancer risks, or other risks to life and health, are generally only a minor consideration in these decisions, if considered at all. Quite apart from differences among individuals, decisions made on an individual level often do not reach the same results as decisions made on an organizational or societal level. Two effects come into play. In the first, preferences remain constant but relative costs change. A person with a strong preference for safety would like to buy a car with air bags, but, because few cars are so equipped, the cost is too high; there is, after all, a limit on how much one is willing to pay for the added safety. The same person, placed in a position to dictate national policy on highway safety, might find the expected cost of air bags under mass production conditions low enough to exercise a preference for safety, and impose this additional cost on all new cars sold. This is the "tragedy of the commons" reversed; costs, fixed by current societal conditions, can tend to force the cost of what we would like to be too great for us to opt for it. As in all such trade-offs, this is not a choice between safety and costs, but between a particular aspect of health or safety and all other things that could be had for the same money, including other kinds of health benefits.

The second kind of effect is that organizational values or "role values" substitute for individual values when one moves from individual to organizational decisionmaking. Individuals in a decisionmaking position, say in a government regulatory agency, can use their office to impose their personal values, but more frequently the office itself imposes organizational values on its occupant. Taking a different view of the air bag example, an individual might be personally willing, and financially able, to pay the high cost to equip his own car, but, faced with the need to consider the impact on the national economy, may find the cost to so equip all cars staggering and opt to see that money spent on more cost-effective ends.

Despite the limited scope of individual risk decisions, a distinct advantage of risk decisionmaking on the individual level is the ability to act directly on broadreaching trade-offs. If the highway safety administrator decides that funds could benefit population health much more effectively in antismoking campaigns than air bags, there is little that can be done to effect such a switch. One is caught in the compartmentalized budget boundaries of the bureaucracy. Individuals, on the other hand, can readily reallocate their money from an air-bag-equipped car to a stop-smoking clinic.

Owner Management

Owners of enterprises make risk management decisions within the scope of their own values and of societal attitudes expressed in many ways, including government regulation. It is said that when Dupont first established his explosives factory in America, he built his home on the factory grounds as a testament to his dedication to safety and, perhaps, to force himself to consider his workers' safety as much as his own. Electric utility officials, attacked in nuclear power controversies for endangering the community's safety sometimes counter with, "my family lives here, too." Regulatory agencies can make all kinds of rules on occupational exposure and environmental emission control, but it is the owners and managers who make the final risk management decisions. These may go far beyond legal requirements or they may be conscious decisions to ignore or evade the law. "Owners" in this sense does not mean solely an individual entrepreneur, but the person or group that has decisionmaking control over an enterprise. In a corporation, this might be the CEO or the Board of Directors, but the concept should not be limited to corporations.

Risk management in enterprise is not limited to industrial hygiene and environmental engineering at factory operations. It goes to the roots of enterprise in the development of new technologies and products. More and more, health risk considerations are part of this development process. Sometimes this is rigidly defined by government regulation as in the development of new pharmaceutical drugs, in other cases it is simply ingrained in management philosophy. Although the two must go hand in hand, there is a balancing act to be played between technological development and risk management. Society's risk adversity usually favors the old and familiar over the new. The nature of risk assessment and its frequent use of "upper bound" risk estimates works against the new, since scarcity of data leads to higher upper bound estimates. There is a "risk" that premature estimates of potential risks of a new technology will kill it before it has a chance to prove itself. The corollary to this is that the development-minded fear risk assessment and try to quash its application or at least the publication of results. This is a policy that can backfire and a tendency that should be fought. In the early days of nuclear energy, its benefits were loudly touted and its risks suppressed. The ultimate result was a complete lack of trust on the part of the public and an unwillingness to understand or believe any rational arguments about radiation risks. In contrast, the Department of Energy and private concerns involved in developing photovoltaic technologies have openly explored every conceivable hazard right from the beginning. Risk management must be built into new technologies, not welded on afterwards. The goal must be to involve the public in technological development, develop their trust, and facilitate their understanding and participation in risk management.

Government Regulation

The concept of risk management is closely tied to government regulation, probably too much so, because it draws attention away from other risk-management arenas. The variety of laws and regulations dealing with managing health risks exhibit a wide range of regulatory approaches. It is clear the United States is still seeking an appropriate risk-management philosophy of regulation. In a 1985 booklet, the Environmental Protection Agency states that despite an enormous apparatus for controlling pollution, EPA has always experienced difficulty in relating its actions to the actual reduction of risk (EPA, 1985).

Lester Lave, an economist who has contributed much to an understanding of health and environmental regulation in the 1980s (Lave, 1981, 1982; Crandall and Lave, 1981; Lave and Upton, 1987) strongly advocates that regulatory decisions be based on careful review of scientific evidence and quantitative risk assessment. "Regulation without these elements is uninformed, arbitrary, and unlikely to withstand litigation, induce co-operation from those being regulated, or produce the results desired" (Lave, 1982). He offers four steps to better regulation (Lave, 1981):

1. Decide what to regulate
2. Present information, prepare analyses, and provide decision frameworks that clarify the implications of regulatory alternatives
3. Ensure regulations are appropriate and not more stringent than necessary
4. Implement regulations efficiently and quickly, without endless litigation or unnecessary social costs.

Although Lave offers numerous examples, his steps remain much easier said than done. Deciding what to regulate seems obvious, but Congress too often states regulatory goals either in broad terms or defines them too narrowly. Likewise, agencies too often get side-tracked on second-or third-order priorities. OSHA and EPA have been criticized on the small number of carcinogens they have brought under regulation. While it has long been recognized by most participants in the process that it is hopeless to have separate regulations on every possible chemical, none of the alternatives that have been advanced have met with success.

Assuring regulations are "not more stringent than necessary" not only raises the question of how stringent is necessary, but also philosophical differences over whether to approach regulation this way or from the position of "at least as stringent as necessary."

The charge to implement regulations without endless litigation or unnecessary social costs seems impossible to meet in today's litigious climate in which virtually every regulation results in a lawsuit from one side or the other. The problem is not in the implementation itself, but in designing regulations in a form that will be accepted. This will require not simply better regulations, but a change in the regulatory climate that can only be brought about by a better and more widespread understanding of the nature of risk and of people's concerns about risk, the limitations of scientific understanding if it, and the technologic and economic limitations on our ability to eliminate it.

Toxic Torts

Courts have a role in the review of government regulatory decisions, but their unique role in cancer risk management is in litigation about responsibility for cancers (or other chronic diseases) caused by exposure to chemicals in the environment or on the job, and to pharmaceuticals and other products. These are sometimes called toxic tort cases. A tort is a legal term for a civil wrong calling for compensation. If a person trips on your sidewalk because of your negligence in failing to repair a crack, you are responsible for compensating their loss. Toxic torts can be much more complex because the link between cause and effect is more difficult to prove, especially at the individual level. Years may have passed between the exposure and the resulting cancer. Other exposures that may have caused or contributed to the cancer may have preceded or followed the exposure of interest. Unlike a criminal case, which must be proved "beyond the shadow of a doubt," in a civil case the plaintiff must only prove that the causal link between an exposure and the cancer is more likely true than not (Black, 1988). In some states, the burden of proof has been shifted to the defendant in toxic tort cases, biasing the result toward compensation of the plaintiff (Fiksel, 1986).

Toxic torts have two roles in risk management: fear and compensation. The fear of being taken to court and having large penalties assessed can restrain an industry or government agency from what otherwise might be a willingness to expose people to carcinogens. This restraint acts independently from regulation and even in the absence of regulation. Its effectiveness depends on the ability of people to bring tort cases to court and the manner in which the courts receive and decide them. The liability policy that has evolved over decades of court cases encourages quality and diligence in manufacturing and service industries. Because of the latency period in cancer development, there is a built-in delay in the process. Cases being tried now reflect exposures from over 20 years ago, and thus industries' past perception of the risks of court judgments. As with regulation, if the effect of fear is too great, it will overly stifle industrial development, rather than prudently control it. It also can inhibit innovation; industries may opt not to introduce a new product because of the fear of lawsuits.

Toxic tort cases are relatively new and, although few actual statistics are available, appear to be increasing rapidly. Moreover, jury awards also appear to be increasing (Harrington and Litan, 1988). One drawback of the tort system, especially in a new area such as toxic torts, is lack of consistency. Three plaintiffs presenting similar cases in different courts, with different juries, and different sets of lawyers may receive radically different results. The development of tabular data on probability of causation discussed above was an attempt to address this problem by providing a standard base for judgment.

Another undesirable characteristic is that large numbers of "undeserving" victims may be compensated, distorting economic markets. This is due to the uncertainty in judging causation in toxic tort cases. For example, one study concluded that radiation from atomic bomb testing led to an increase in leukemia in southern Utah (Lyon et al., 1979). Setting aside criticisms of the validity of these claims (Hamilton, 1983) for the purpose of illustration, obviously, not all leukemia cases in southern Utah were caused by radiation exposure, but it was impossible to differentiate those that were (assuming any were) and those that were not. When doubt exists in criminal law, it is better to let a criminal go free than to risk convicting an innocent person. In toxic torts, where a cancer victim is pitted against a large corporation or the government, the benefit of the doubt generally goes to the victim. If all the Utah leukemia cases receive compensation from the court, perhaps most of those compensated were not affected by the radiation. Yet, of their cousins in Colorado who received a lower radiation exposure, none are compensated because the probability of any one case being attributable to the radiation exposure was too small. Although, if some in Utah were affected then some smaller percentage in Colorado may have been affected also. The difficulty is that cancer is a common disease afflicting perhaps 30% of the population and small increments are impossible to distinguish from the background noise (see Chap. 11).

A further difficulty with the tort system is that the cases often extend over such extended time periods that, even if successful, the compensation comes too late to be of any help to the victim.

Much of the evidence presented in toxic tort cases relies on expert witnesses. Experts can make judgments and bring to bear evidence that would be ruled inadmissible as hearsay if given by a witness of fact. Often a case becomes a contest of who's expert witness is more convincing or easiest to understand (Budinger, 1987). Discussion of the use of epidemiologic data in toxic tort cases by expert witnesses is given by Hoffman (1984) and Lilienfeld and Black (1986). Sometimes juries may be swayed by the expert witness testimony of clinicians. Faust and Ziskin (1988) note that, "The clinician, who is limited by the state of his scientific field and likely disregards or undervalues actuarial data combinations, depends mainly on subjective methods of data interpretation. Without the safeguards of the scientific method, clinicians are highly vulnerable to the problematic judgment practices and cognitive limitations common to human beings."

A risk assessment document itself might become evidence in a court, or the document's author or other risk assessment experts might be called upon as expert witnesses to describe the risk assessment process and findings. Risk assessments conducted by government agencies are more likely to be acceptable by courts as evidence, but their authors, as government employees, may be barred by their agencies from testifying (Walker, 1988). A risk assessment document may still be challenged under rules of hearsay, on the basis that the inability to cross-examine would limit understanding of a highly technical document, or that the analysis might contain regulatory policy decisions as well as factual material. Even if inadmissible as evidence, however, a risk assessment may be discussed in court by an expert witness, and used as a basis of an expert opinion (Walker, 1988).

Insurance

Insurance is the way industries protect themselves from losses due to liability in toxic tort claims. With the increase in toxic tort liability, insurance companies have become more aggressive in demanding limits to routine and accidental exposures. New risk assessment consulting firms have been established to inspect industrial facilities and advise them on levels of environmental risks as a basis for setting rates. Companies then "internalize" the balancing of costs of environmental and occupational exposure control against mounting insurance costs, or even the possibility of not being able to find an insurer. Insurance becomes the practical mechanism whereby the risk management policies developed by the courts in tort law cases are translated from vague fears to practical business decisions.

Ideally, insurance premiums must equal the time-discounted value of expected future costs (Harrington and Litan, 1988). Rates are based on the size of expected future claims, when they will occur in the future, and the intervening interest rate. In an automobile accident, claims are often paid the same year the premium was paid. The insurance company pays out the money only shortly after it comes in. In a toxic tort case, the claim may be 20 years after the premium was paid. Since the insurance company earns interest on the premiums in the meanwhile, the premium can be lower for an equal size claim. The decades-long latent period for cancers, resulting in claims far in the future, affects rates in three ways. First, premiums will tend to be lower per dollar in claims, reflecting the time-discounting of money; second, premiums will be more dependent on interest rates, high interest rates tending to result in lower premiums; and third, premiums will tend to be higher reflecting the greater financial risks associated with possible changes in social policy, claim rates, claim amounts, and changes in interest rates. Resulting rates will depend on the insurers judgment as the relative importance of these factors.

SUMMARY

Risk management is the process by which society and the individuals in it manage or otherwise adjust themselves or their environment to the risks they face. Risk assessment provides the scientific and analytical basis for risk management decisions, while the management aspect itself is a political, economic, and social process built on a management philosophy. Risk management takes place within several different formats, of which government regulation is only one. There are many techniques used in risk management; the kind of information that must be provided by analysis and assessment may vary among the different techniques. Risk analysts must have some independence from risk managers to assure objectivity, but must not forget their role is to supply information on which risk management decisions are based.

REFERENCES

Abelson, P.H. 1987. California's proposition 65, *Science* 237:1553.
Bell, D.E., R.L. Keeney, and H. Raiffa. 1977. *Conflicting Objectives in Decisions*. John Wiley, Chichester, England.

Bentkover, J.D., V.T. Covello, and J. Mumpower. 1986. *Benefits Assessment: The State of the Art*. D. Reidel Publishing Co., Dordrecht, Holland.

Black, B. 1988. Evolving legal standards for the admissibility of scientific evidence. *Science* 239:1508–1512.

Budinger, F.C. 1987. Engineers in court. *Civil Eng*.   (8):52–54.

Butterfield, F. 1988. Nuclear arms industry eroded as science lost leading role. *New York Times* CXXXVII (47,731), December 26, p.1.

CEQ. 1986. Council on Environmental Quality, National Environmental Policy Act regulations: incomplete or unavailable information, Final Rule. *Fed. Reg*. 51:15618–15626.

Comar, C.L. 1979. Risk: a pragmatic *de minimus* approach. *Science* 203:319.

Covello, V.T. 1987. Decision analysis and risk management decision making: issues and methods. *Risk Analysis* 7:131–139.

Cox, L.A., Jr. 1987. Statistical issues in the estimation of assigned shares for carcinogenesis liability. *Risk Analysis* 7:71–80.

Crandall, R.W. and L.B. Lave (eds.). 1981. *The Scientific Basis of Health and Safety Regulation*. The Brookings Institution, Washington, DC.

Elkins, C.L. 1988. Toxic chemicals, the right response. *The New York Times* (November 13), p. F3.

Faust, D. and J. Ziskin. 1988. The expert witness in psychology and psychiatry. *Science* 241:31–35.

Fiksel, J. 1985. Toward a *de minimus* policy in risk regulation. *Risk Analysis* 5:257–259.

Fiksel, J. 1986. Victim compensation. *Environ. Sci. Technol*. 20:425–430.

Fisher, P.W., R.M. Currie, and R.J. Churchill. 1988. SARA Title III, Section 313—looking ahead. *J. Air Pollut. Control Assoc*. 38:1376–1379.

Freudenburg, W.R. 1988. Perceived risk, real risk: social science and the art of probabilistic risk assessment. *Science* 242:44–49.

Haigh, J.A., D. Harrison, Jr., and A.L. Nichols. 1984. Benefit-cost analysis of environmental regulation: case studies of hazardous air pollutants. *Harvard Environ. Law Rev*. 8:395–434.

Hamilton, L.D. 1983. Alternative interpretations of statistics on health effects of low-level radiation. *Am. Statist*. 37:442–451.

Harrington, S. and R. E. Litan. 1988. Causes of the liability insurance crisis. *Science* 239:737–741.

Hoffman, R.E. 1984. The use of epidemiologic data in the courts. *Am. J. Epidemiol*. 120:190–202.

Kasperson, R.E., O. Renn, P. Slovic, H.S. Brown, J. Emel, R. Goble, J.X. Kasperson, and S. Ratick. 1988. The social amplification of risk: a conceptual framework. *Risk Analysis* 8:177–191.

Keeney, R.L. and H. Raiffa. 1976. *Decisions with Multiple Objectives: Preferences and Value Tradeoffs*. John Wiley, New York.

Lagakos, S.W. and F. Mosteller. 1986. Assigned shares in compensation for radiation-related cancers. *Risk Analysis* 6:345–357.

Lave, L.B. 1981. The Strategy of Social Regulation:Decision Frameworks for Policy, The Brookings Institution, Washington, D.C.

Lave, L.B. (ed). 1982. *Quantitative Risk Assessment in Regulation*, The Brookings Institution. Washington, D.C.

Lave, L.B. and A.C. Upton. 1987. Regulating toxic chemicals in the environment, Chapter 10 in L.B. Lave and A.C. Upton (eds.). *Toxic Chemicals, Health, and the Environment*. The Johns Hopkins University Press, Baltimore, pp. 280–293.

Lave, L.B. 1986. Who needs causation probabilities. *Risk Analysis* 6:359–361.

Levin, M.H. 1988. State and Federal air toxics developments: disclosure strategies overtake regulations, *J. Air Pollut. Control Assoc.* 38:1371–1375.

Lilienfeld, D.E. and B. Black. 1986. the epidemiologist in court: some comments. *Am. J. Epidemiol.* 123:961–964.

Luken, R.A. 1985. The emerging rile of benefit-cost analysis in the regulatory process at EPA. *Environ. Health Perspect.* 62:373–379.

Lyon, J.L., M.R. Klauber, J.W. Gardner, and K.S. Udall. 1979. Childhood leukemias associated with fallout from nuclear testing. *N. Engl. J. Med.* 300:397–402.

Merkhofer, M. and R. Keeney. 1987. A multiattribute utility analysis of alternative sites for the disposal of nuclear waste. *Risk Analysis* 7:173–194.

Morgan, M.G., M. Henrion, and S.C. Morris. 1979. Expert judgments for policy analysis (BNL 51358), Brookhaven National Laboratory, Upton, NY.

Morgan, M.G., M. Henrion. S.C. Morris, and D.A.L. Amaral. 1985. Uncertainty in risk assessment. *Environ. Sci. Technol.* 19:662–667.

Mumpower, J. 1986. An analysis of the *de minimus* strategy for risk management. *Risk Analysis* 6:437–446.

NAS. 1978. *Saccharin: Technical Assessment of Risks and Benefits, Part I: Study of Saccharin and Food Safety Policy*. Committee for a Study on Saccharin and Food Safety Policy, National Academy of Sciences, Washington, DC.

NAS. 1979. *Saccharin: Technical Assessment of Risks and Benefits, Part II: Food Safety Regulation and Societal Impact*. Committee for a Study on Saccharin and Food Safety Policy, National Academy of Sciences, Washington, DC.

NAS. 1987. *Regulating Pesticides in Food: the Delaney Paradox*. Committee on Scientific and Regulatory Issues Underlying Pesticide Use Patterns and Agricultural Innovation, National Research Council. National Academy Press, Washington, DC.

NIH. 1985. Report of the National Institutes of Health ad hoc Working Group to Develop Radioepidemiological Tables (NIH Publ. No. 85-2748). National Institutes of Health, Washington, DC.

Nygaard, O.F. 1986. Probability of causation. In P. Oftedal and A. Brogger (eds.) *Risk and Reason: Risk Assessment in Relation to Environmental Mutagens and Carcinogens*, Alan R. Liss, Inc., New York, pp. 85–88.

Quade, E.S. 1975. *Analysis for Public Decisions*, American Elsevier Publishing Company, New York.

Rosenberg, D. 1986. The uncertainties of assigned shares tort compensation: what we don't know can hurt us. *Risk Analysis* 6:363–369.

Ruckelshous, W.D. 1984. Risk in a free society. *Risk Analysis* 4:157–162.

Schlaifer, R. 1959. *Probability and Statistics for Business Decisions*. McGraw-Hill, New York.

Seiler, F.A. and B.R. Scott. 1987. Mixtures of toxic agents and attributable risk calculations. *Risk Analysis* 7:81–90.

Slovik, P., B. Fischoff, and S. Lichtenstein. 1980. Facts and fears: understanding perceived risk. In R.C. Schwing and W.A. Albers, Jr. (eds.), *Societal Risk Assessment*. Plenum Press, New York, pp. 182–214.

Spetzler, C.S. and C-A. S. Stael von Holstein. 1975. Probability encoding in decision analysis, *Management Sci*. 22:340–358.

Steuer, R.E. 1986. *Multiple Criteria Optimization: Theory, Computation and Application*. John Wiley, New York.

Taylor, M.R. 1987. *De minimus* risk: progress and paradox. *Environ. Sci. Technol.* 11:1027.

Travis, C.C., S.R. Packer, and A. Fisher. 1987. Cost-effectiveness as a factor in cancer risk management. *Environ. Int.* 13:469–474.

Tversky, A. and D. Kaneman. 1981. The framing of decisions and the psychology of choice. *Science* 211:453–458.

Von Winterfeld, D. and W. Edwards, W. 1986. *Decision Analysis and Behavioral Research*. Cambridge University Press, New York.

Walker, V.R. 1988. Quantitative risk assessments as evidence in civil litigation. *Risk Analysis* 8:605–614.

Wildavsky, A. 1979. No risk is the highest risk of all. *Am. Sci.* 67:32–37.

17

Future Directions for Quantitative Health Risk Analysis

INTRODUCTION

Quantitative cancer risk assessment has become an integral part of regulatory decisionmaking. Although this might have led to stifling of development in the interest of consistent regulatory policy, such is not the case; quantitative risk assessment seems to be in a stage of rapid development. Three important factors helping to drive these advances are:

a. Improvements in biomedical research, such as micro dose measurements and better understanding of carcinogenic processes
b. Increasingly widespread use by state governments, leading to innovative approaches to new problems, especially in assessment of hazardous waste sites
c. Increasing recognition of the high cost of pollution control and remedial action, forcing quantitative assessments of cost-effectiveness

Some areas in which advances are especially striking are discussed below with the opportunities and implications of developments in these areas.

MORE COMPLETE PICTURE OF DOSE AND EFFECTS PROCESSES

Early high-to low-dose extrapolation models in cancer risk assessment were based on concepts of genotoxicity and cancer initiation such as the 1-hit model. The multistage model recognized that more than a single event was involved in the process, but did not allow much diversity in the kinds of processes included. It is now recognized that extrapolation models must include the full scope of events from exposure to ultimate expression of cancer in clinical form, including submodels addressing exposure-to-tissue (or cell) dose, initiation, promotion, immune control and

397

suppression, and progression. Many of these have the potential of introducing substantial nonlinearities into the calculation. Biomedical research has far outreached the mathematical models based on concepts of the 1950s that are still used in quantitative cancer risk assessment. Until recently, however, it has been difficult to apply new biological findings in risk assessment. That is changing; biomedical researchers now have a sufficient knowledge base to develop research models (e.g., Thompson and Brown, 1987) that are on the verge of being linked together as assessment models.

REALISTIC MODELS

Closely coupled with the recognition of the need to incorporate multiple processes into assessment models is the rapidly evolving transition from empirical models that are basically curve-fitting to physiologically based mechanistic models such as physiologically based pharmacokinetic models (NAS, 1987) and the Moogavkar-Venzon-Knudson cancer risk model (Moolgavkar et al., 1988). This, again, is supported by advancing biomedical research that provides the improved understanding of concepts needed to develop physiologically based models as well as the data needed to drive them. The result will be to replace much of the uncertainty and consequent conservatism in current models with knowledge, yielding more realistic estimates of risk.

UNCERTAINTY

The explicit treatment of uncertainty in quantitative assessment of health risk has been a concern for at least a decade. Nonetheless, most source term, environmental transport, and dose–response models still do not allow explicit estimation of uncertainty, and those that do often include only some aspects of the overall uncertainty. While many advances have been made in this area, much remains to be done and it is still an area of active development. There remains a need to move from upper-bound estimates and built-in conservatisms to a more complete consideration of uncertainty using best estimates and uncertainty parameters, with propagation of uncertainty through the different stages of analysis including exposure and dose–response components. Advancing scientific knowledge in both transport and effects and the development of realistic rather than empirical models provide the means to treat uncertainty better. Moreover, the ability to deal explicitly with uncertainty in mathematical models no longer requires large computers and sophisticated mathematical and programming expertise. Complete treatment of uncertainty can be included in simple microcomputer-based models using readily available tools that work with spreadsheet programs to allow explicit treatment of uncertainty. This puts sophisticated methods in the hands of all risk analysts.

LONG-RANGE POLLUTION TRANSPORT

In the past dozen years there has been increasing concern with effects of pollutants that travel great distances from their sources. Long-range transport models were commonly coupled with linear, no-threshold dose–response models. More recently, parallel analysis has applied the same principles to groundwater pollutants traveling over great time periods. Regulations under the Nuclear Waste Policy Act require consideration of ground water transport of contaminants for 10,000 years. Only recently has significant consideration been given to the interaction of uncertainty in long-range transport and low-dose extrapolation of effects information (Seiler, 1987). This is an area of key importance in risk management. Improvements in long-range transport models applicable to risk analysis, and their appropriate use with population-projection and dose–response information could yield significant changes in how many pollutants with the potential for long-range transport are treated. It needs much more attention then it is receiving.

HUMAN VARIABILITY

Quantitative health risk assessment has generally focused on "reference man" or other standardized notions of the exposed population. Greater consideration of human variability in susceptibility to environmentally induced disease is now being considered. This area is likely to have considerable impact on broadening the uncertainty bounds on health effect estimates.

NEW METHODS OF EXPRESSING RESULTS

Quantitative risk assessments have tended to present either abstract individual risk levels (e.g., lifetime increase in cancer risk) or "body counts" (increased number of cancers expected annually in the population). Although occasionally making for a good headline, these have never proved to be a satisfactory way to communicate meaningful information on risk to decisionmakers to the public. Benefit/cost analysis has always been viewed with suspicion because of the need to express health effects in monetary terms. Quantitative health risk assessment aims to aid decisionmaking. The ultimate decisionmaking instrument is the budget (Wildavsky, 1964). Cost-effectiveness has increasingly become recognized as a powerful way to express health risk in terms that make sense when developing a budget.

EXPERT SYSTEMS

Artificial intelligence, knowledge-based databases, and expert systems can be applied to quantitative health risk assessment in two ways. The first is to assist analysts to better incorporate biomedical research findings in their models. This has not yet shown any promise as a growth area, but may make substantial impacts as these tools begin to be applied in the research field that risk assessment draws upon. The second kind of application is growing rapidly. This is to give people in the field (e.g., those evaluating hazardous waste sites or the potential hazards of new chemicals) the benefit of "expert" advice and the ability to do more sophisticated health risk analyses. To cope with the number of expert systems being developed, the EPA Office of Solid Waste and Emergency Response developed a working paper to provide guidance on the design, development, and operational issues associated with expert systems.

RISK COMMUNICATION

The field of risk communication is growing rapidly. Many regulatory agencies already employ "risk communicators" to interface with the public. Risk communication is not simply public relations or public education; ideally it involves two-way communication. That means it will feedback public perceptions to agency management and risk analysts. Not only must risk analysts give more consideration to how their results are presented to make them more understandable to the public, but this feedback loop may affect what is addressed in analyses and how the analysis is done. The risk communications movement will clearly have an impact on risk analysis, although the nature of that impact may be difficult to predict. People doing quantitative health risk analysis may become much more involved in public communication as well as becoming an important link between the biomedical research scientist and the risk communicator.

CONCLUSIONS

Cancer risk analysis has grown rapidly over the past two decades and has established itself as a integral part of regulatory decisionmaking. It remains, however, a young field with much opportunity for growth and development. Indeed, substantial advances are taking place in the field. Equally as important, the experiences in cancer risk analysis are being increasingly applied to analysis of risks for other health endpoints such as reproductive and neurotoxic effects.

REFERENCES

Moolgavkar, S.H., A. Dewanji, and D.J. Venzon. 1988. A stochastic two-stage model for cancer risk assessment. I. The hazard function and the probability of tumor. *Risk Analysis* 8:383–392.

NAS. 1987. *Pharmacokinetics in Risk Assessment*. Subcommittee on Pharmacokinetics in risk Assessment, Safe Drinking Water Committee. National Research Council, National Academy Press, Washington, DC.

Seiler, F. 1987. A methodology for the selection of environmental dispersion models in health risk assessments. *Environ. Int.* 13:351–357.

Thompson, J.R. and B.W. Brown (eds.). 1987. *Cancer Modeling*. Marcel Dekker, New York.

Wildavsky, A. 1964. *The Politics of the Budgetary Process*. Little, Brown and Company, Boston.

Index

Absolute risk model, 282, 297
Acceptable risk, 374–375
Accountability, 9
Adversarial review, 354–355
Albert, R. E., 185, 194, 237, 297, 300
Allometry, 155–157
Ames, B. N., 28, 44, 97, 231
Ames test, 97, 100, 231–234, 298
Antagonisms, 191–193
Arsenic, 26, 75, 365
Asbestos, 22, 291
Ashby, J., 227, 231, 233, 235–236
Assigned share (*see* Probability of causation)
Atom bomb survivors, 245
Autopsy data, 247

Background cancer rate (*see* Cancer)
Benefit/cost analysis, 12, 381–382
Benefits analysis, 383
Benign tumors (*see* Tumors)
Benzene, 273–275
Benzene-soluble organics, 80
Benzo[a]pyrene, 80, 257, 278–282, 295, 352
Bioassay,
  blind, 181
  controls, 178
  design, 171–179, 217–218
  dose, 174–176

false positives, 189
interpretation, 180
positive controls, 178
test species, 172–175
use in relative potency method, 297–299
Biological monitoring, 94–99
Biologically effective dose, 155
Biomarkers, 268–269
Breathing rate, 142

Calibration, 360
Cancer
  atlas, 257–258, 273
  background rate, 186
  clusters, 273–274
  estimates of number, 399
  initiation, 23–24
  registries, 249
Cancers (*see also* Carcinoma; Tumors)
  bladder, 43
  breast, 43
  colon and rectum, 42
  lymphoma, 19
  liver, 292
  lung, 41, 292, 257
  myeloma, 43–44
  prostate, 43
Carcinogen
  ambiguous, 185

classification, 184
complete, 25
Carcinogenic activity indicator
(CAI), 194
Carcinoma, 19
Causation, inferring, 269–271
CERCLA (*see* Comprehensive
Environmental Response,
Compensation, and Liability
Act)
Chemical fractionation, 239–240
Chemotherapy drugs, 255
Chinese hamster ovary (CHO) assay,
234
Chloridane, 376
Chromosome aberrations, 97,
235–236
Cigarettes, 238, 262, 279–280, 298
Clayson, D. B., 184, 195, 220
Clean Air Act, 362
Clearance mechanisms, 159
Coal tar pitch volatiles (CPTV), 247,
281–284
Coke oven
bioassay of emissions, 298
emissions, 247
gas, 238
workers, 246, 281, 283–284
Compensation, 390
Complex mixtures, 79, 99–100,
122–123, 176, 191–193, 238–240,
337
Complex terrain, 121
Comprehensive Environmental
Response, Compensation, and
Liability Act (CERCLA), 63,
146
Computer-automated structure
evaluation program (CASE),
230–231
Confidence building, 356
Consensus, 333
Conservatisms, 10–11, 210, 306,
363–365, 398
Consistency, 361
Consumer Product Safety
Commission, 12, 210

Corps of Engineers, U.S. Army, 381
Cost effectiveness, 383, 400
Cost-benefit analysis (*see* Benefit/cost
analysis)
Costs, 45–47
Cothern, R., 313–314
Council on Environmental Quality,
377
Credible, 315, 375
Crump, K. S., 204, 206, 208–211,
213, 219, 293–294
Cuddihy, R. G., 282, 298–300, 308

De minimus, 371–375
Decision analysis, 295–296, 384–385
Decision making
multidecesionmaker, 385
multiobjective, 384
Delaney Amendment, 3, 7, 13, 185,
364–367
DES, 22
Diesel exhaust, 284, 297–300
DNA, 19–20, 22, 24, 26, 95
adducts, 98–99, 213, 237
strand breaks, 237
Doll, R., 7, 29, 34, 40–41, 44–45,
208, 213, 271, 279
Dose
in bioassay, 175–177
committed, 74
extrapolation, high to low, 203–220
maximum tolerated (MTD),
176–177
patterns in epidemiology, 246
route of administration, 175
Dose–response
additivity, 212
characteristics, 78
dose–rate effect, 188–189
effect of age, 188–189
from epidemiological studies,
274–285
extrapolation from animal to man,
155, 220–222
function, shape of, 202
index of exposure in, 247
interaction with background, 211

low-dose linearity, 207, 212
time-pattern dependency, 213

Ecological fallacy, 256, 258
Economic impacts, 45–47
Emergency Planning and Community
    Right-to-Know Act (SARA Title
    III), 370
Emission factors, 114
Emissions, 90, 113–116
Energy, U.S. Department of, 12,
    239, 360, 384
Environmental commitment, 74
Environmental contamination, 146
Environmental Protection Agency
    (EPA), 3, 12, 210, 239, 281,
    367, 389
  benzene standard, 275
  Carcinogen Assessment Group,
    276, 279
  Environmental Research
    Laboratory, Athens, GA, 129
  EXAMS model, 109, 127
  Guidelines, 58–61
  Kerr Environmental Research
    Laboratory, 131
  cancer potency methods, 194
  Valley model, 121
Enzyme-altered foci, 24
Epidemiology
  analytical, 255
  case-control, 258–261
  cohort studies, 261–265, 292
  cross-sectional, 255–258
  descriptive, 255
  design, 251–268
  ecological, 256–258
  nested case-control, 265
  occupational studies, 263–265
  proportional mortality studies,
    266–268
  prospective, 251
  retrospective, 251–252
  selection of controls, 260
  similarities with toxicology, 245
Error propagation (see Uncertainty)
Excess cancers, 334

Expert judgment, 316–320, 384
Expert systems, 400
Expert witnesses, 392
Exposure, 74
  air, 90, 116–125, 140–143
  background, 79
  food, (see also Food chains) 94,
    102, 132–135, 144–146
  groundwater, 130–132
  hand-to-mouth, 93
  occupational, 90–92, 265
  personal, 85
  skin contact, 91
  soil, 93–94
  water, 92–93, 101–102, 125–129,
    143–144

Fault trees, 325
Fence-post individual (see Individual)
Flamm, W. G., 4–5
Flexibility, 359
Flood Control Act of 1926, 381
Food and Drug Administration
    (FDA), 7, 12–13, 94, 366
Food chains, 132–135, 144
Food, Drug, and Cosmetic Act, 13

Gamma multihit model, 208
Gas retort workers, 280, 284
Gaussian plume model, 116–120
Gehring, P. J., 154, 158, 160–161
Gene mutation tests (see also Ames
    test), 232–235
Generalized k-hit dose–response
    model (see Gamma Multihit
    model)
Generic risk assessment, 308
Genes
  oncogene, 20–21
  protooncogenes, 24
  ras, 21
Guess, H. A., 206, 208–211

Hamilton, L. D., 267, 308, 391
Harris, J. E., 297–298, 300
Healthy worker effect 266, 284
Higginson, J., 6

High-risk groups, 138–139
Hoel, D., 210–212, 220

Immune system, 22, 25
Incidence rate, 250–251
Individual
  exposure, 73
  fence post, 77, 377
  risk, 335
  maximally exposed (MEI), 335
Initiation (see Cancer)
Insurance, 392–393
International Agency for Research
  on Cancer (IARC), 63
International Atomic Energy
  Agency, 12
International Ground Water
  Modeling Center, 131
International Program on Chemical
  Safety, 234

Krewski, D., 178, 204, 206, 213, 216

Latent period, 34, 157, 178, 262, 281
Latin hypercube, 316
Lave, L. B., 10, 84, 255–256, 389
Lawrence Livermore National
  Laboratory, 121
Leukemia, 19
Limit of detection, 89
Linear hypothesis, 145
Litigation, 390–392
Log-normal model, 204, 295
Long-range transport, 123–125, 399
Love Canal, 131
Lymphoma (see Cancers)

Mantel, N., 203–204, 293–294
Mantel-Bryan procedure, 294–295
Margin of safety, 207, 211, 376
Maximally exposed individual (MEI)
  (see Individual)
Maximum credible, 315
Maximum likelihood estimate
  (MLE), 210–212, 294

Maximum tolerated dose (see also
  Bioassay), 219
Mazumdar, S., 246, 280
McClellan, R. O., 298–300
Meta analysis 292–293
Michaelis-Menten equation, 158
Microenvironment, 86
Monitoring Trigger Levels (MTL),
  64, 66
Monte Carlo analysis, 316, 321–324
Moolgavkar, S. H., 213, 215–216
Moolgavkar-Venzon-Knudson
  (MVK) model, 214, 216–218,
  398
Morgan, M. G., 86, 140, 310,
  317–318, 322
Mortality
  data, 249
  rates, 248
  ratio, 266–267
Mouse lymphoma cells mutagenesis
  assay, 235
Mouse skin bioassay, 236, 298–299
Multicollinearity, 256–257
Multihit model, 207–208
Multimedia Environmental Goals
  (MEG), 64, 66
Multistage model, 208–213, 295
  confidence limits, 210
  theory, 27
  time-varying dose version, 214
Myeloma (see Cancers)

National Cancer Institute, 172, 250
National Cancer Survey, 29
National Center for Health Statistics,
  249
National Climatic Center, 119
National Council on Radiation
  Protection (NCRP), 262
National Environmental Policy Act,
  370
National Institute of Environmental
  Health Sciences, 172
National Institute of Occupational
  Safety and Health (OSHA), 172

National Institutes of Health, 379
National Science Foundation, 383
National Toxicology Program, 56–57,
   63, 172, 218
Noncarcinogenic substitute
   chemicals, 229
Nuclear Waste Management Act, 384

Oak Ridge National Laboratory, 162
Occupational Safety and Health
   Administration (OSHA), 12,
   246, 275
Odds ratio, 277
One-hit model, 206–207
Orphan Drug Act, 379

Peer review, 352–354
Perception of risk (*see* Risk)
Personal exposure monitoring, 85
Pharmacokinetic models, 159–163,
   220
   physiologically based, 160–163, 398
Pike, M., 257, 279, 284
Pittsburgh Steelworkers Study, 263,
   281
Poisson distribution, 316–319
Policy
   analysis, 308
   uncertainty, 307–309, 327
Polycyclic organic matter (POM),
   275, 279–285
Population
   activity patterns, 137
   exposure, 73
   migration, 137–138
   mobility, 137
   projection, 136–137
Portsmouth Naval Shipyard, 267
Potency, 64, 193–196, 296
Pott, P., 5–6.
Prevalence rates, 251
Probability analysis, 310
Probability of causation, 378–381
Probit model, 22, 204–205
Promotion, 25
   index, 25

Propagation of uncertainty (*see*
   Uncertainty)
Proportionate mortality ratio (PMR),
   267
Proposition 65, 370

Quality assurance, 348–349

Radiation, 35
Rat liver initiation–promotion
   bioassay, 25, 236
Reference location, 308
Reference man, 399
Regulation, 10, 389
Regulatory impact analysis, 12–13
Relative potency, 296–301
Relative risk, 263
Relative risk model, 283, 298
Replication, 351
Reversability, 25
Risk
   communication, 344–345, 400
   individual, 383
   management, 306
   models, 283, 298
   perceived, 368
   perception, 340–343
   unit, 194
Risk–benefit (*see* Benefit/cost
   analysis)
Risk–cost–benefit (*see* Benefit/cost
   analysis)
Roofing tar, 238, 298
Rowe, M. D., 124, 308
Ruckelshaus, W., 3

Saccharin, 7, 364
Safety factor, 205
SARA (*see* Superfund Amendments
   and Reauthorization Act)
Sarcoma, 19
Schneiderman, M., 41–42, 204
SEER (*see* Surveillance,
   Epidemiology, and End Results
   program)
Seiler, F., 123

Sensitivity analysis, 326, 385
Sielken, R. L., 11, 217
Simulation of Human Air Pollution
    Exposures (SHAPE), 141
Sister chromatid exchange, 235–236
S9 rat liver microsomal enzyme, 232
Social impacts, 45–47
Somatic mutation, 21
Standard man (*see also* Reference
    man), 143
Standard mortality ratio (SMR),
    266–267
Statistical power, 271–272
Stigma, 341
Structure–activity relationship,
    227–232
  substructural analysis, 229
Superfund Amendments and
    Reauthorization Act of 1986
    (ASRA), 370–371
Surveillance, Epidemiology, and End
    Results (SEER) program, 28–29,
    250
Survival, 34–35
Synergism, 191–193, 337
Synthesis, 330

TD_{50}, 195
Technology, best available, 386
Three Mile Island Nuclear Power
    Plant, 342, 368
Threshold Limit Values (TLV), 64,
    95
Tobacco, 44, 96
Total Exposure Assessment
    Methodology (TEAM) Study,
    87–89
Toxicology
  general principles, 170
  similarities with epidemiology, 245
TOXIWASP, 127
Travis, C. C., 94, 133, 140, 220
Tumors
  benign, 25

diagnosis, 181
fatal vs. incidental, 187–188
malignant vs. benign, 182–183
time to, 188

Uncertainty, 298
  in knowledge, 310–312
  in long-range transport, 123–124
  methods of characterizing, 313–321
  in multistage model, 209–213
  natural variability, 309–310
  policy, 305–307
  policy applications, 327
  propagation of, 316, 320–325, 398
  quantitative vs. qualitative
    expression, 312–313
  reasons for estimating, 306
  in water quality models, 129
Unit risk (*see also* Potency), 194
United National Environment
    Programme, 12
Upper-bound estimates, 10, 211, 398
Uranium mill tailings, 325
Urban gradient, 33

Validation, 112, 349–352
Value of life, 337
Van Ryzin, J., 204, 206–207
Variability, 309
Verification, 112, 350
Virtually safe dose, 204
Volatile organic compounds, 313

Weibull model, 205–206, 219
Weight of evidence, 60, 63, 333
Whittemore, A., 209
Wilson, R., 279
Worst-case analysis, 130, 307, 376

Xeroderma pigmentosa, 22

Years of life lost, 335–336

Zero risk, 366

Milton Keynes UK
Ingram Content Group UK Ltd.
UKHW021829071024
449327UK00021B/1468